Estrogens in the Environment II

Influences on Development

Estrogens in the Environment II
Influences on Development

Proceedings of the symposium, Estrogens in the Environment:
Influences on Development, Raleigh, North Carolina, United States,
April 10–12, 1985

Editor

John A. McLachlan, Ph.D.
Laboratory of Reproductive and Developmental Toxicology
National Institute of Environmental Health Sciences
Research Triangle Park, North Carolina, United States

Elsevier
New York • Amsterdam • Oxford

Elsevier Science Publishing Co., Inc.
52 Vanderbilt Avenue, New York, New York 10017

Sole distributors outside the United States and Canada:

Elsevier Science Publishers B.V.
P.O. Box 211, 1000 AE Amsterdam, The Netherlands

Library of Congress Cataloging in Publication Data

Main entry under title:
Estrogens in the environment II.

    Proceedings of the Second Symposium on Estrogens in the Environment, sponsored
by the National Institute of Environmental Health Sciences.
    Includes bibliographies and index.
    1. Estrogen — Congresses. 2. Estrogen — Physiological effect — Congresses.
3. Estrogen — Toxicology — Congresses. 4. Environmentally induced diseases —
Congresses. I. McLachlan, John A. II. Symposium on Estrogens in the Environ-
ment (2nd : 1985 : Raleigh, N.C.) III. National Institute of Environmental Health
Sciences. IV. Title: Estrogens in the environment. 2. [DNLM: 1. Environmental
Pollutants — congresses. 2. Estrogens — congresses. 3. Growth — drug effects —
congresses. WP 522 E817 1985]
QP572.E85E84 1985   599'.03   85-24567
ISBN 0-444-01029-7

Current printing (last digit)
10 9 8 7 6 5 4 3 2 1

Manufactured in the United States of America

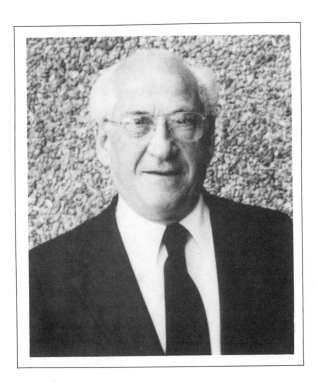

This book is dedicated to Roy Hertz
whose remarkable intellect and
uncompromising social concern
are a continuing inspiration.

Contents

Participants   xi

Foreword   xix

THE ESTROGEN PROBLEM--RETROSPECT AND PROSPECT   1
    R. Hertz

Structure-Activity Relationships of Estrogenic Chemicals

    STRUCTURE-ACTIVITY RELATIONSHIPS OF ESTROGENIC CHEMICALS   15
    W. L. Duax and J. F. Griffin

    STRUCTURE-ACTIVITY RELATIONSHIPS OF STEROID ESTROGENS   24
    J. P. Raynaud, T. Ojasoo, M. M. Bouton, E. Bignon, M. Pons,
    and A. Crastes de Paulet

    STEREOCHEMICAL ANALYSIS OF STILBENE ESTROGENS: RECEPTOR
    BINDING AND HORMONE RESPONSIVENESS   43
    K. S. Korach, L. A. Levy, and P. J. Sarver

    NATURALLY OCCURRING NON-STEROIDAL ESTROGENS OF DIETARY
    ORIGIN   69
    K. D. R. Setchell

    MORPHOLOGICAL ANALYSIS OF CHLORDECONE (KEPONE) ACTION IN
    DIFFERENT MOUSE ORGANS: CHOROID PLEXUS IN ADULT MALES
    AND VAGINAL EPITHELIUM IN SUCKLING NEONATES   86
    V. P. Eroschenko

Analysis and Characterization of Estrogenic Xenobiotics and
Natural Products

    ANALYSIS AND CHARACTERIZATION OF ESTROGENIC XENOBIOTICS AND
    NATURAL PRODUCTS   107
    A. K. Robison, V. R. Mukku, and G. M. Stancel

    CHEMICAL ANALYSIS AND CHARACTERIZATION OF ESTROGENS   116
    J. D. Henion, T. R. Covey, D. R. Silvestre, and K. K. Cuddy

    BIOCHEMICAL ANALYSIS OF ESTROGENS   139
    D. C. Collins and P. I. Musey

    DOES ESTROGEN-INDUCED GENOTOXICITY REQUIRE RECEPTOR-MEDIATED
    EVENTS?   146
    R. H. Purdy, N. J. Maclusky, and F. Naftolin

    SOME BIOLOGICAL AND TOXICOLOGICAL STUDIES OF VARIOUS ESTROGEN
    MYCOTOXINS AND PHYTOESTROGENS   168
    J. J. Li, S. A. Li, J. K. Klicka, and J. A. Heller

Role of Metabolism in Determination of Hormonal Activity
of Estrogens

ROLE OF METABOLISM IN DETERMINATION OF HORMONAL ACTIVITY
OF ESTROGENS: INTRODUCTORY REMARKS   187
   M. Metzler

IMPRINTING OF HEPATIC ESTROGEN ACTION   190
   G. W. Lucier, T. C. Sloop, and C. L. Thompson

ESTROGEN PRODUCTION AND METABOLISM IN RELATION TO CANCER   203
   P. K. Sitteri, J. Murai, and N. Simberg

PROLACTIN SYNTHESIS BY CULTURED RAT PITUITARY CELLS: AN ASSAY
TO STUDY ESTROGENS, ANTIESTROGENS AND THEIR METABOLITES
IN VITRO   221
   V. C. Jordan, R. Koch, and R. R. Bain

METABOLISM OF ZEARALENONE TO A MORE ESTROGENICALLY ACTIVE FORM   238
   M. E. Wilson and W. M. Hagler, Jr.

Developmental Biology of Estrogens

DEVELOPMENTAL BIOLOGY OF ESTROGENS: INTRODUCTORY COMMENTS   251
   J. A. McLachlan

BIOLOGICAL EFFECTS OF ESTROGENS AND ANTIESTROGENS IN THE FETUS
AND NEWBORNS   252
   J. R. Pasqualini, C. Sumida, and N. Giambiagi

STROMAL-EPITHELIAL INTERACTIONS IN THE DETERMINATION OF
HORMONAL RESPONSIVENESS   273
   G. R. Cunha, R. M. Bigsby, P. S. Cooke, and Y. Sugimura

DIETHYLSTILBESTROL-ASSOCIATED DEFECTS IN MURINE GENITAL
TRACT DEVELOPMENT   288
   R. R. Newbold and J. A. McLachlan

ESTROGEN-ASSOCIATED DEFECTS IN RODENT MAMMARY GLAND DEVELOPMENT 319
   H. A. Bern, K. T. Mills, and M. Edery

OVARIAN STRUCTURE AND FUNCTION IN NEONATALLY ESTROGEN-TREATED
FEMALE MICE   327
   J.-G. Forsberg, A. Tenenbaum, C. Rydberg, and C. Sernvi

Critical Evaluation of the Role of Environmental Estrogens
in Premature Sexual Development

PREMATURE THELARCHE AND ESTROGEN INTOXICATION   349
   M. I. New

PREMATURE SEXUAL DEVELOPMENT IN PUERTO RICO: BACKGROUND
AND CURRENT STATUS   358
   L. Haddock, G. Lebrón, R. Martinez, J. F. Cordero, L. W.
   Freni-Titulaer, F. Carrión, C. Cintron, and L. González

PREMATURE THELARCHE IN PUERTO RICO: DESIGN OF A CASE-CONTROL STUDY 380
J. F. Cordero, L. Haddock, G. Lebrón, R. Martinez, L. W. Freni-Titulaer, and J. L. Mills

ESTROGENS IN FOOD PRODUCTS AS DETERMINED BY CYTOSOL RECEPTOR ASSAY 398
A. M. Bongiovanni

EFFECTS OF ENVIRONMENT HORMONAL CONTAMINATION IN PUERTO RICO 404
C. Sáenz de Rodriguez, A. M. Bongiovanni, and L. Conde de Borrego

ENDOCRINOLOGY OF PREMATURE THELARCHE 412
J. L. Mills

Index 429

Participants

Dr. Yusuf Abul-Hajj
University of Minnesota
College of Pharmacy
Health Sciences, Unit F
308 Harvard Street, S.E.
Minneapolis, MN 55455

Mr. Stephen P. Adams
Toxicology Training Program
University of Rochester School
  of Medicine and Dentistry
Box RBB/TOX
Rochester, NY 14642

Dr. Herman Adlercreutz
Department of Clinical Chemistry
University of Helsinki
SF-00290 Helsinki
FINLAND

Dr. Miriam N. Alicea
Pediatric Endocrinology
  Section
San Juan City Hospital
San Juan, P. R. 00920

Dr. Calvin E. Anthony
1809 Haney Street
El Dorado, AR 71730

Dr. Martha Arcos
Food and Drug Adminsitration
HFV-156
5600 Fishers Lane
Rockville, MD 20857

Dr. Raymond B. Baggs
University of Rochester
601 Elmwood Avenue
P.O. Box 674
Rochester, NY 14642

Ms. Donna Baird
National Institute of
  Environmental Health Sciences
National Institutes of Health
Research Triangle Park, NC 27709

Dr. Howard A. Bern
Professor of Zoology and
  Member, Cancer Research
  Laboratory
University of California, Berkeley
Berkeley, Ca 94720

Dr. Robert M. Bigsby
Department of Anatomy, 51334
University of California
San Francisco, CA 94143

Dr. Alfred Bongiovanni
Professor of Pediatrics,
  Obstetrics and Gynecology
  and Medicine
Pennsylvania Hospital
Department for Sick and Injured
University of Pennsylvania
Eighth and Spruce Streets
Philadelphia, PA 19107
(In Absentia)

Dr. Bent G. Boving
Department of Anatomy
  and OB-GYN
C. S. Mott Center for
  Human Growth and Development
Wayne State University
275 East Hancock
Detroit, MI 48201

Dr. Renee L. Boving
Department of Anatomy
  and Ob-Gyn
C. S. Mott Center for Human
  Growth and Development
Wayne State University
275 East Hancock
Detroit, MI 48201

Dr. Elizabeth S. Boylan
Department of Biology
Queens College of City
  University of New York
Flushing, NY 11367

Dr. Carlos Bourdony
Member of the Commission of the
  Secretary of Health to Study
  the Problem of Thelarche and
  Precocious Sexual Development
  in Puerto Rico
Director, Pediatric
  Endocrinology
San Juan City Hospital
San Juan, Puerto Rico

Dr. Algie C. Brown
Director, Dermatopathology
  Laboratory
Atlanta Skin and Cancer Clinic
817 Douglas Road
Atlanta, GA 30342

Dr. Robert W. Brueggemeier
College of Pharmacy
The Ohio State University
500 West 12th Avenue
Columbus, OH 43210

Dr. William H. Bulger
The Worcester Foundation for
  Experimental Biology
222 Maple Avenue
Shrewsbury, MA 01545

Dr. Chaiyod Bunyagidj
Laboratory of Reproductive and
  Developmental Toxicology
National Institute of
  Environmental Health Sciences
National Institutes of Health
Research Triangle Park, NC 27709

Ms. Diane Campen
National Institute of
  Environmental Health Sciences
National Institutes of Health
Research Triangle Park, NC 27709

Dr. Delwood C. Collins
Professor, Department of
  Biochemistry
Emory University
Atlanta, GA 30033

Dr. Jose F. Cordero
Epidemiologist, Birth Defects Branch
Chronic Disease Division
Center for Environmental Health
Centers for Disease Control
1600 Clifton Road
Chamblee, Building 5
Atlanta, GA 30333

Dr. Thomas R. Covey
Equine Drug Testing and Toxicology
New York State College
  of Veterinary Medicine
Cornell University
925 Warren Drive
Ithaca, NY 14850

Dr. Gerald R. Cunha
Associate Professor
Department of Anatomy
School of Medicine
University of California, SF
San Francisco, CA 94143

Dr. Margaret Davis
National Institute of
  Environmental Health Sciences
National Institutes of Health
Research Triangle Park, NC 27709

Dr. Gisela H. Degen
Institute of Toxicology of the
  University of Wurzburg
Versbacher Strasse 9
D-8700 WURZBURG
Federal Republic of Germany
WEST GERMANY

Dr. William L. Duax
Head, Molecular Biophysics Department
Medical Foundation of Buffalo
73 High Street
Buffalo, NY 14203

Dr. Richard L. Ellis
Director, Chemistry Division
USDA/FSIS/SCI
300 12th Street
Room 404, Annex Bldg.
Washington, DC 20250

Mr. Bruce Wells Ennis
Department of Anatomy
University of North Carolina
111 Swing Building
Chapel Hill, NC 27514

Dr. Victor P. Eroschenko
Associate Professor
Department of Biological Sciences
University of Idaho
Moscow, ID 83843

Dr. Charles R. Fish
Mayo Clinic
200 1st Street, S.W.
Rochester, MN 55905

Dr. John-Gunnar Forsberg
Chairman, Department of Anatomy
University of Lund
Biskopsgaten 7
S-223 62 Lund, SWEDEN

Dr. John E. Fortunato
Squibb Institute for
  Medical Research
P.O. Box 4000, Room A4201
Princeton, NJ 08540

Dr. Theodore Fotsis
Department of Clinical Chemistry
University of Helsinki
SF-00290 Helsinki
FINLAND

Dr. Lambertina W. Freni-Titulaer
Cancer Branch
Chronic Disease Division
Centers for Disease Control
1600 Clifton Road
Chamblee, Building 5
Atlanta, GA 30333

Dr. Michael Galvin
Extramural Program
National Institute of
  Environmental Health Sciences
National Institutes of Health
Research Triangle Park, NC 27709

Dr. Simon J. Gaskell
Laboratory of Molecular Biophysics
National Institute of
  Environmental Health Sciences
National Institutes of Health
Research Triangle Park, NC 27709

Dr. Beth Gladen
National Institute of
  Environmental Health Sciences
National Institutes of Health
Research Triangle Park, NC 27709

Dr. Joseph W. Goldzieher
Baylor College of Medicine
6720 Bertner, 23rd Floor
Houston, TX 77030

Ms. Tamra Goodrow
National Institute of
  Environmental Health Sciences
National Institutes of Health
Research Triangle Park, NC 27709

Mr. Thomas Golding
Laboratory of Reproductive
  and Developmental Toxicology
National Institute of
  Environmental Health Sciences
National Institutes of Health
Research Triangle Park, NC 27709

Dr. Earl Gray
U.S. Environmental Protection
  Agency, MD-72
Research Triangle Park, NC 27711

Dr. Lillian Haddock
Professor of Pediatrics
School of Medicine
University of Puerto Rico
Medical Sciences Campus
G.P.O. Box 5067
San Juan, Puerto Rico 00936

Dr. Winston M. Hagler
Associate Professor
Mycotoxin Laboratory
Department of Poultry Science
North Carolina State University
Raleigh, NC 27695

Dr. A. F. Haney
Professor and Director, Division
  of Endocrinology and Fertility
Department of Obstetrics and
  Gynecology
Duke University Medical Center
Box 2971
Durham, NC 27710

Dr. Jack D. Henion
Professor, Equine Drug Testing
  and Toxicology
New York State College of
  Veterinary Medicine
Cornell University
925 Warren Drive
Ithaca, NY 14850

Dr. Roy Hertz
Professor Emeritus
Departments of Pharmacology
  and Obstetrics and Gynecology
George Washington University
  Medical Center
2100 Eye Street, N.W.
Washington, D.C. 20037

Dr. Rex Hess
U.S. Environmental Protection
  Agency, MD-72
Research Triangle Park, NC 27711

Dr. Robert Hill
Centers for Disease Control
1600 Clifton Road
Cham 17/2113
Atlanta, GA 30333

Dr. Tsuneyoshi Horigome
Laboratory of Reproductive
  and Developmental Toxicology
National Institute of
  Environmental Health Sciences
National Institutes of Health
Research Triangle Park, NC 27709

Ms. Susan Hughes
Duke University Medical Center
Box 2971
Durham, NC 27710

Dr. Alvin M. Janski
International Minerals and
  Chemical Corporation
Box 207
Terre Haute, IN 47808

Dr. John A. Jefferies
Mayo Clinic
200 S.W. 1st Street
Rochester, MN 55905

Dr. Lovell Jones
Department of Gynecology
M.D. Anderson Hospital
  & Tumor Institute
6723 Bertner Avenue, Box 67
Houston, TX 77030

Dr. Craig Jordan
Associate Professor
Department of Human Oncology
Wisconsin Clinical Cancer Center
University of Wisconsin
600 Highland Avenue
Madison, WI 53729

Dr. Paul Juniewicz
Department of Population Dynamics
Johns Hopkins University
Baltimore, MD 21205

Dr. Rajan Kapur
V.A. Medical Center
Lyons, NJ 08801

Mr. George M. Kingman
Office of Program Planning
  and Evaluation
National Institute of
  Environmental Health Sciences
National Institutes of Health
Research Triangle Park, NC 27709

Dr. John Kirkland
Department of Pediatrics
Baylor College of Medicine
Texas Medical Center
Houston, TX 77030

Dr. Rick Koch
Human Oncology Department
K4/653 Clinical Science Center
600 Highland Avenue
Madison, WI 53792

Dr. Vera Kolb-Meyers
Department of Chemistry
  and Biochemisty
Southern Illinois University
Carbondale, IL 62901

Dr. Kenneth S. Korach
Research Endocrinologist
Laboratory of Reproductive
  and Developmental Toxicology
National Institute of
  Environmental Health Sciences
National Institutes of Health
Research Triangle Park, NC 27709

Dr. Donald R. Koritnik
Department of Comparative
  Medicine
Bowman-Gray Medical School
Wake Forest University
300 South Hawthorne Road
Winston-Salem, NC 27103

Dr. David Kupfer
Worcester Foundation for
  Experimental Biology
222 Maple Avenue
Shrewsbury, MA 01545

Mr. Hugh J. Lee
Information Officer
National Institute of
  Environmental Health Sciences
National Institutes of Health
Research Triangle Park, NC 27709

Dr. Jonathan J. Li
Senior Scientist
Medical Research Laboratories
Veterans Administration Medical
  Center
54th Street and 48th Avenue, South
Minneapolis, MN 55417

Dr. George W. Lucier
Chief, Biochemical Applications
Biometry and Risk Assessment
   Program
National Institute of
   Environmental Health Sciences
National Institutes of Health
Research Triangle Park, NC 27709

Dr. Bruce W. Martin
International Minerals
   & Chemical Corp.
1401 South Third Street
P.O. Box 207
Terre Haute, IN 47808

Dr. David Maxwell
U.S. Environmental Protection
   Agency, MD-72
Research Triangle Park, NC 27711

Mr. Zadock McCoy
National Institute of
   Environmental Health Sciences
National Institutes of Health
Research Triangle Park, NC 27709

Dr. John A. McLachlan
Chief, Laboratory of Reproductive
   and Developmental Toxicology
National Institute of
   Environmental Health Sciences
National Institutes of Health
Research Triangle Park, NC 27709

Dr. Manfred Metzler
Professor, Institute of
   Pharmacology and Toxicology
University of Würzburg
8700 Würzburg
FEDERAL REPUBLIC OF GERMANY

Dr. Cal Y. Meyers
Department of Chemistry
   and Biochemistry
Southern Illinois University
Carbondale, IL 62901

Dr. James L. Mills
Senior Epidemiologist
Epidemiology and Biometry Branch
National Institute of Child
   Health and Human Development
National Institutes of Health
Bethesda, MD 20205

Dr. Kathleen S. Morgan
National Institute of
   Environmental Health Sciences
National Institutes of Health
Research Triangle Park, NC 27709

Dr. Paul Munson
University of North Carolina
   at Chapel Hill
Chapel Hill, NC 27514

Dr. Cathy S. Murphy
Human Oncology Department
K4/613 Clinical Science Center
600 Highland Avenue
Madison, WI 53792

Dr. Paul I. Musey
Veterans Administration
   Medical Center
1670 Clairmont Road
Decatur, GA 20033

Dr. Frederick Naftolin
Chairman, Department of
   Obstetrics and Gynecology
Yale School of Medicine
333 Cedar Street
P.O. Box 3333
New Haven, CN 06510

Dr. Rehan H. Naqvi
EG&G Mason Research Institute
57 Union Street
Worcester, MA 01608

Dr. Mike Naslund
Johns Hopkins Hospital
Marburg 105
600 North Wolfe Street
Baltimore, MD 21205

Dr. Bruce Naumann
Ciba-Geigy Corporation
556 Morrts Avenue
Summitt, NJ 07901

Dr. Karen Nelson
Biometry and Risk Assessment
   Program
National Institute of
   Environmental Health Sciences
Nationl Institutes of Health
Research Triangle Park, NC 27709

Dr. Maria I. New
Professor and Chairman
Department of Pediatrics
New York Hospital
Cornell Medical Center
525 East 68th Street
New York, NY 10021

Ms. Retha R. Newbold
Biologist, Laboratory of
  Reproductive and Developmental
  Toxicology
National Institute of
  Environmental Health Sciences
National Institutes of Health
Research Triangle Park, NC 27709

Dr. Godfrey P. Oakley, Jr.
Centers for Disease Control
Chamblee, Building 5
1600 Clifton Road, N.E.
Atlanta GA 30333

Dr. Edward O'Neill
Director, Department of
  Obstetrics and Gynecology
San Juan City Hospital
281 TTE. Cesar Gonzalez
Hato Rey, P.R. 00918

Dr. James Overpeck
Food and Drug Administration
200 C Street
Washington, DC 20204

Dr. Arthur J. Pallotta
Biomedical Consultants, Inc.
1515 Wilson Boulevard
P.O. Box 12021
Arlington, VA 22209

Dr. Samuel W. Page
Food and Drug Administration
HFF-454, 200 C Street, N.W.
Washington, DC 20204

Dr. Chandra K. Parekh
International Minerals and
  Chemical Corporation
1810 Frontage Road
Northbrook, IL 60062

Dr. Carol Parker
Laboratory of Molecular
  Biophysics
National Institute of
  Environmental Health Sciences
National Institutes of Health
Research Triangle Park, NC 27709

Dr. Jorge R. Pasqualini
Director of Research
C.N.R.S. Steroid Hormone
  Research Unit
Foundation for Hormone Research
26 Boulevard Brune
F-75014 Paris, France

Dr. Herbert S. Posner
National Institute of
  Environmental Health Sciences
National Institutes of Health
Research Triangle Park, NC 27709

Dr. Robert M. Pratt
Laboratory of Reproductive
  and Developmental Toxicology
National Institute of
  Environmental Health Sciences
National Institutes of Health
Research Triangle Park, NC 27709

Dr. Thomas E. Pratt
Squibb Institute for
  Medical Research
P.O. Box 4000, Room A4203
Princeton, NJ 08540

Dr. Anna Prieto
Ciba-Geigy Corporation
Old Mill Road
Suffern, NY 10901

Dr. Robert H. Purdy
Senior Scientist
Department of Organic Chemistry
Southwest Foundation for
  Biomedical Research
P. O. Box 28147
West Loop 410 at Military Drive
San Antonio, TX 78284

Dr. Valerie Quarmby
Labs for Reproductive Biology
University of North Carolina
Box 4, Macnider Building, 202H
Chapel Hill, NC 27514

Dr. James Rabinowitz
U.S. Environmental Protection
  Agency, HERL - MD-68
Research Triangle Park, NC 27711

Dr. David P. Rall
Director, National Institute of
  Environmental Health Sciences
National Institutes of Health
Research Triangle Park, NC 27709

Dr. Jean-Pierre-Raynaud
Director, Roussel-UCLAF Group
35 Boulevard Des Invalides
75007 Paris, FRANCE

Dr. Ann Richard
U.S. Environmental Protection
Agency, MD-68
Research Triangle Park, NC 27709

Dr. Simon Robinson
Human Oncology Department
K4/613 Clinical Science Center
600 Highland Avenue
Madison, WI 53792

Dr. Jorge Rodriguez
De Diego Hospital
Box 46397
Santurce, Puerto Rico 00940

Dr. Leslie Rubin
U.S. Department of Agriculture
Food Safety and Inspection
Service
300 12th Street, S.W.
Washington, DC 20250

Dr. Carmen A. Saenz
Pediatric Endocrinologist
De Diego Hospital
Box 46397
Santurce, Puerto Rico 00940

Dr. Risto Santti
Department of Anatomy
Institute of Biomedicine
University of Turku
Kiinamyllynk. 10
Turku 20 520
FINLAND

Ms. Pamela J. Sarver
Laboratory of Reproductive and
Developmental Toxicology
National Institute of
Environmental Health Sciences
National Institutes of Health
Research Triangle Park, NC 27709

Dr. K. D. R. Setchell
Head, Clinical Mass Spectrometry
Laboratory
Department of Pediatric
Gastroenterology and Nutrition
Children's Hospital Medical Center
Elland and Bethesda Avenue
Cincinnati, OH 45229

Dr. Helen Shu
Syntex Corporation
3401 Hillview Avenue
Palo Alto, CA 94304

Dr. Pentti K. Siiteri
Professor, Department of
Obstetrics and Gynecology
University of California, SF
San Francisco, Ca 94143

Ms. Tracy Sloop
National Institute of
Environmental Health Sciences
National Institutes of Health
Research Triangle Park, NC 27709

Dr. Carlos Sonnenschein
Tufts University School
of Medicine
136 Harrison Avenue
Boston, MA 02111

Dr. George M. Stancel
Professor, Department of
Pharmacology
University of Texas Medical
School at Houston
P. O. Box 20708
Houston, TX 77025

Dr. Walter E. Stumpf
Department of Anatomy
University of North Carolina
111 Swing Building
Chapel Hill, NC 27514

Dr. Geoffrey Sunahara
National Institute of
Environmental Health Sciences
National Institutes of Health
Research Triangle Park, NC 27709

Dr. Martin K. Terry
International Minerals
and Chemical Corporation
1401 South 3rd Street
Terre Haute, IN 47808

Dr. John A. Thomas
Travenol Labs., Inc.
6301 Lincoln Avenue
MGO2M
Morton Grove, IL 60035

Dr. Claudia Thompson
National Institute of
Environmental Health Sciences
National Institutes of Health
Research Triangle Park, NC 27709

Dr. Yasuhiro Tomooka
Laboratory of Reproductive
  and Developmental Toxicology
National Institute of
  Environmental Health Sciences
National Institutes of Health
Research Triangle Park, NC 27709

Dr. Tuchmann-Duplessis
Faculte of Medecine
45, rue de St-Peres
Paris, FRANCE

Dr. Alison Vickers
National Institute of
  Environmental Health Sciences
National Institutes of Health
Research Triangle Park, NC 27709

Dr. Morgan M. W. Weber
Schering-Plough Corporation
Galloping Hill Road
Kenilworth, NJ 07033

Dr. Patricia L. Whitten
Associate Research Scientist
Department of Obstetrics and Gynecology
Yale School of Medicine
P.O. Box 3333
333 Cedar Street
New Haven, CT 06510

Dr. Thomas Wong
National Institute of Environmental
  Health Sciences
National Institutes of Health
Research Triangle Park, NC 27709

Foreword

This book represents the proceedings of the Second Symposium on Estrogens in the Environment sponsored by the National Institute of Environmental Health Sciences and held in Raleigh, North Carolina, on April 10-12, 1985. As in an earlier Symposium held in 1979 (Estrogens in the Environment, J.A. McLachlan, ed., Elsevier, NY, 1980), the present meeting continued to address the chemical and biological bases for estrogenic activity among various chemicals. However, in this current meeting, the influence of estrogenic compounds on development in animals and humans was a new and important focus.

Estrogens are a class of chemical defined more by their biological function than their structure. The expression of hormonal activity by chemicals other than those having a steroid nucleus is apparently unique to estrogens. Exposures to environmental estrogens may take a variety of routes. There are many naturally occurring estrogenic substances in plants, and some fungi produce estrogenic mycotoxins. Another source of estrogens in the environment arise from synthetic processes. In some cases, an environmental estrogen is made and used as a hormone (e.g., DES), while in others, the products are synthesized for nonhormonal purposes but have estrogenic activity (e.g., DDT). In the latter case, metabolism of these compounds from hormonally inactive (prohormone) to more active forms may become an important factor. The special sensitivity of the developing mammary gland or genital tract to estrogens and the subsequent long term modifications of these organs pose a unique problem for the immature individual exposed to these compounds. Recent reports concerning precocious breast development in young girls in Puerto Rico underline the pertinence of this area of investigation. The question raised many years ago concerning the structural diversity of estrogenic chemicals remains unanswered. However, the current environmental implications of the question compel us to seek its solution.

I want to thank several people who helped in the successful completion of the book: Ms. Jacqueline Russell, for administrative support before and during the meeting; Ms. Vickie Englebright, for superb secretarial help and advice before, during, and after the meeting, including great help in preparation of this volume; Ms. Christopher Allen Baley McLachlan, for, among many other things, the calligraphy on the dedication page; and the energetic speakers and participants who discussed difficult subjects with wit and grace. I also need to mention the sad absence of Dr. Alfred M. Bongiovanni, who was, and is, recovering from major surgery. Although he could not attend the meeting, his intellectual presence was strongly felt. Several times the statement was heard, "If Bongi were here, he would say. . . ." I only hope these statements did justice to Dr. Bongiovanni's clarity of thought in the area of estrogens and human development. They certainly added spice to the meeting.

John A. McLachlan, Ph.D.
July 1985

THE ESTROGEN PROBLEM--RETROSPECT AND PROSPECT

Roy Hertz, M.D., Ph.D., Professor Emeritus--Pharmacology, and Obstetrics
and Gynecology, The George Washington University, Washington, D. C.

The estrogen problem may be defined as those concerns arising from
the exposure of man and animals to estrogens. An estrogen is a substance
which reproduces or simulates the morphological, physiological, biochemical and behavioral effects of the naturally occurring hormones secreted
by the granulosa cells of the Graafian follicle, the interstitial cells of
the testis, and the cells of the adrenal cortex. The primary effect of
an estrogen is the stimulation of mitotic activity in the tissues of the
female genital tract both in early ontogeny, in pubescence, and in the
adult organism. This primary effect may be accompanied by numerous
other responses such as: increased vascularity of the affected tissue,
alteration of motility of affected muscular elements, alteration of fluid
balance and of lipid and calcium metabolism. In addition, such distal
responses as profound effects on the mammary glands and other secondary
sex organs, a positive or a negative feed-back effect upon pituitary
gonadotropic function, the promotion of epiphyseal closure in the long
bones, and effects on the differentiation of the central nervous system
and associated behavioral patterns also prove to be characteristic of
estrogens. Notwithstanding this complex array of variably associated
effects of estrogens, the sine qua non of estrogenic activity remains the
mitotic stimulation of the tissues of the female genital tract. A
substance which can directly elicit this response is an estrogen; one that
cannot do this is not an estrogen.

This characterization stems from the historical development of our
knowledge of "the female sex hormone." An initial step in this development was the trail-blazing description by Dr. George Papanicolaou in the
guinea pig and Dr. Herbert Evans in the rat of the chronological

association of cyclic pre-ovulatory swelling of the follicle with uterine engorgement and vaginal cornification [1,2] (Fig. 1).

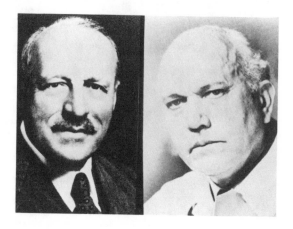

FIG. 1.   Dr. G. Papanicolaou (left) and Dr. H. M. Evans (right).

These observations signaled the probable existence of a humoral ovarian effect on these processes.   It then remained for Dr. Edgar Allen and Dr. Edward Doisy to exploit the biological end-point of vaginal cornification for the purification of the active agent and to first show this effect to be due to a steroid named "estrone" [3] (Fig. 2).

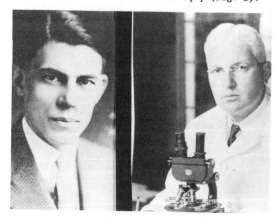

FIG. 2.   Dr. Edward Doisy (left) and Dr. Edgar Allen (right).

In a classic study Drs. Allen and Gardner then used the mitotic-
blocking agent, colchicine, to bring out the profound mitotic effect of
estrone on the uterus and on the vagina of the mouse [4] (Fig. 3).

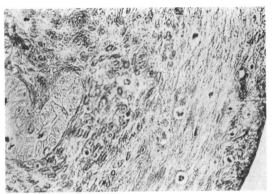

FIG. 3.   Colchicine arrested mitoses in estrogen treated mouse uterus
(reference 4).

Hence, for the first time the experimentalist had in hand a naturally
occurring substance which could augment the mitotic activity of a given
tissue to an extreme degree.

Some decades earlier the clinical pathologists had emphasized that
excessive mitotic activity was an essential feature of malignant tissue.
This similarity between estrogen-induced tissue growth and malignant
tissue in such sites as the endometrium and the cervical mucosa naturally
led to a persistent concern regarding the ultimate effect of estrogenic
stimulation on these tissues. The basis for this concern was early emphasized by the demonstration by Hisaw and Lendrum of a striking epidermiza-
tion of the cervical glandular epithelium in the rhesus monkey [5]
(Fig. 4). However, such estrogen-induced lesions showed no invasiveness
and were, therefore, considered to represent metaplasia rather than
neoplasia. For the next several decades, several workers tried by continuous estrogen administration combined with chronic trauma to induce
cancers in the cervix of the rhesus monkey [6]. Such efforts proved

fruitless and helped support the idea that women could be expected to be
resistant to potential carcinogenic effects of estrogens even on prolonged exposure.

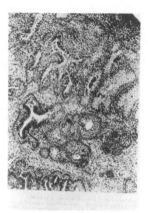

FIG. 4.   Squamous metaplasia of cervical epithelium in estrogen treated
monkey (reference 5).

Meanwhile, however, extensive experimentation in literally hundreds
of laboratories proved over the next decades that estrogens can induce
neoplastic growth in numerous species of animals, including the squirrel
monkey, and in numerous tissue sites [7].

Moreover, the occurrence of estrogenic substances in the diet and in
the environment came to be appreciated from some early studies which are
of historic interest.   For it was Dr. Bernard Zondek (Fig. 5) who
demonstrated in the early 1920's that the flowers of the female willow
tree contain a biologically active estrogen.   He also showed that the
mud at the bottom of the Dead Sea, which he reasoned was made up largely
of decaying plant materials, also contained an estrogenic substance.

Another early experience with environmental estrogen of plant origin
was the occurrence in New Zealand of frequent abortions and of male
infertility in sheep exposed to a variant form of clover in which
excessive estrogenic activity had developed.   The active compound was

identified as a genistein [8]. There has, of course, since been extensive study of the biological and economic impact of a variety of plant estrogens [9].

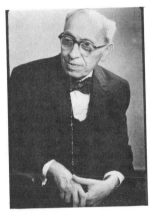

FIG. 5. Dr. Bernard Zondek.

It is also instructive to recall several of our early laboratory and clinical experiences with the problem of accidental estrogen exposure. About 1950, the Director of our Rocky Mountain Laboratory complained that their previously fertile mouse breeding colony had virtually stopped producing any litters. Also many of the male mice had developed large inguinal hernias which caused them to drag their intestines behind them. This latter effect suggested that an estrogen may be involved since Gardner had previously observed such an effect in male mice [10]. Accordingly, we tested the chow fed this colony by bioassay of ether-extracts and found this diet to contain a potent estrogenic substance which subsequent isolation proved to be diethylstilbestrol. Further investigation at the milling plant revealed that several batches of this mouse chow had been processed on equipment just previously used to incorporate potent stilbestrol concentrates into cattle feed. These findings resulted in the requirement that each bag of chow exhibit a label indicating that the feed was free of estrogenic activity. However, with improved milling procedures that requirement was later dropped.

Shortly after this experience, there were referred to our clinic a girl about 4 years old and her brother about 6 years old, both of whom exhibited recent nodular breast enlargement. The occurrence of two cases in a single household suggested a dietary or environmental cause. Intensive study of the habits of this family revealed that the mother was most conscientious in providing each child with a daily vitamin capsule. For budgetary reasons the parents were spared this daily medication. For the same reason, the vitamins used were of an off-brand and had been purchased in the corner grocery store. Bioassay of an ether-extract of these vitamin capsules and chemical analysis proved the presence of substantial amounts of diethylstilbestrol. The FDA found that in the garage in which these capsules had been prepared, stilbestrol was also being processed without proper cleaning of the equipment between runs.

A similar phenomenon was observed shortly after this in two young brothers, but in their case stilbestrol was found in capsules of "isoniazide" which had been contaminated during careless manufacturing [11].

These experiences were extended by several reports from various sources. For example, Dr. Sox, then the Health Officer of San Francisco, reported that an outbreak of gynecomastia had occurred among some boys in a tuberculosis sanitarium due to their use of estrogen-contaminated isoniazide. Also, an earlier report from a kibbutz in Israel attributed an outbreak of gynecomastia to the ingestion of chicken necks in which estrogen pellets had been implanted.

Meanwhile, clinical observation had drawn attention to the relationship of gynecomastia to impairment of hepatic function especially from cirhossis in adult males. This effect was presumed to have been mediated through liver damage. Of course, inactivation of estrogen by rat liver slices _in_ _vitro_ was soon demonstrated. Later on, we were able to show in man that the estrogen content of hepatic vein blood was much lower than simultaneously obtained peripheral vein blood when both samples were drawn during the course of a sustained intravenous infusion of estrone sulfate [12].

This involvement of the liver in estrogen metabolism opened up the consideration of the potential role of hepato-toxins in effecting accidentally induced estrogen responses. It was this consideration which led to the extensive studies on the estrogenic effects of a wide variety of hydrocarbons.

One of our experiences in this connection merits recounting. We noted a spotty occurrence of an apparently spontaneous uterotrophic effect in our totally untreated weanling rats coming from the breeding colony at NIH. We sought high and low for a cause of this disturbing complication. Detailed review of the practices in this facility revealed that a dusting powder to combat ectoparasite infestation had been recently introduced into daily usage. We could observe the rats licking this material from each others coats. Bioassay of the dusting powder and of each of its constituents demonstrated the estrogenic potency of the ingredient, methoxychlor. Upon elimination of the use of this dusting powder the problem was solved [13].

It was this background that had sensitized some of us to the potential harm that could result from prolonged exposure of women to exogenous estrogen either through accident or by clinical usage. For decades it had become common clinical practice to give most middle-aged women estrogens in various forms and in varied dosages. The low cost of stilbestrol and the increasing ease of the synthesis of steroid estrogens made this practice more feasible. However, it was interesting that far and away the most popular estrogen preparation used was Premarin, a trade name derived from the contraction of the first letters of the natural source of the hormonal preparation, namely, pregnant mares urine. For it had been Dr. Zondek who had demonstrated the very high level of estrogenic activity in the urine of the pregnant mare [14].

There were attributed to this universal estrogen usage many benefits both to the psyche and the body. One commercial proponent used the term: "Forever feminine" to describe these effects. The possible pertinence of the vast body of pre-existing animal data was denied as representing bizarre effects of massive dosages peculiar to susceptible rodents and not then reproducible in primates.

It was not until the 1960's when the estrogen-progestin contraceptive pill was proposed to be used by millions of completely normal young women that anything approaching a statistically valid epidemiological approach to the problem of long-term hormone usage was proposed [15]. However, it remained for the workers whose data are summarized in Table 1 to show that chronic estrogen administration to menopausal women is indeed associated with an increased incidence of endometrial cancer [19]. Moreover, these studies parallel the earlier animal observations that dosage and duration of exposure are determining factors for the extent of endometrial cancer in an estrogen-treated population.

However, the question arises as to why some animal studies showed an almost uniform incidence of cancer in estrogen-treated animals whereas the clinical experience indicates that susceptible women constitute only a very small fraction of those treated. This discrepancy may be considered to stem from the genetic heterogeneity of the human population as contrasted with the genetic uniformity of many strains of test rats and mice. We can, in this respect, be grateful that in effect we are such mongrels.

It is interesting to recall that as early as 1951 an observer of the problem of chronic estrogen usage made the following recommendation: "From a practical point of view, it would seem appropriate (a) to restrict the clinical use of estrogen to only those patients who present a clear

indication for its use, (b) to take all available steps to eliminate the

possible pre-existence of carcinoma in the breasts or pelvis of any patient

to be given estrogens, and (c) to follow carefully all estrogenized

patients by frequent physical examination and cytological study of the

vaginal smear. Under these conditions available evidence would indicate

that prolonged estrogenization is a reasonably safe form of therapy [16].

TABLE I. Salient features of six epidemiological studies regarding
menopausal estrogen use and endometrial cancer.

Senior Author*	Source of Patient Recruitment	No. of Cases	No. of Controls	Risk Ratio	Risk Ratio by Duration of Use	Method of Assessment of Drug Use
Zeil	Prepaid medical service	94	188	7.6	5.6(5+ yrs) 13.9(7+ yrs)	Medical records
Mack	Affluent retirement community	55	191	8.0 8.8	2.8(1 yr) 8.8(8+ yrs)	Clinical records Local pharm- acy interviews
Smith	Local hospital admissions	317	317	4.5	Not sought	Hospital records
Dunn	University hospital admissions	55	78	1.0	Not sought	Hospital records
Gray	Private practice	205	205	3.1	11.5(10+ yrs)	Private files
McDonald	Olmsted county	145	580	1.0	7.9(3+ yrs)	Clinic records

*See reference (19) for documentation of each study.

The resemblance of this counsel to that adopted by the FDA just a few

years ago provides a lesson for the future introduction of potent drugs

by large segments of the human population. For it took the introduction

of sound epidemiologic principles into the process of initial drug
evaluation and follow-up to bring us to our current level of
sophistication in such matters.

It is noteworthy that our initial point of departure for an
epidemiological approach to the estrogen problem was the phenomenon of
thromboembolism and related thrombotic disorders first noted in the early
days of the high dosage steroid contraceptives used by young women.
Thus, an early recommendation for an epidemiologic study of this problem
came from an advisory group chaired in 1963 by Dr. Irving S. Wright of
Cornell Medical School when he wrote: "This Committee recommends that a
carefully planned controlled prospective study be initiated with the
objective of obtaining more conclusive data regarding the incidence of
thromboembolism and death from such conditions in both untreated females
and those under treatment of this type among the pertinent age groups"
[17].

In contrast it should be recalled that the initial approval of the
first steroid contraceptive was actually based on prior experience with
only 400 case reports submitted by the manufacturer [18].

It is difficult for a current reader to visualize the resistance with
which the now accepted statistical criteria for drug evaluation and
surveillance were first met. In retrospect, one must ask what such
resistance may have cost in cummulative morbidity and mortality over the
years. Conversely, looking to the future, it is fair to ask whether we
have learned our lesson sufficiently well to feel secure that history
will not repeat itself.

For example, we are now confronted with the non-biological,
legalistic thinking which permits the zearalenone type of estrogen to
continue to be used after it has taken 20 years or more to have stilbestrol
removed from use in the poultry and beef industry. The justification for

this is that although both stilbestrol and zearanol now being used for the same purposes for which stilbestrol was used are both estrogens, zearanol merits a completely new approach for its evaluation.

It is this purely legalistic approach coupled with an ever more widely indiscriminate attitude against all "regulation" which can in time vitiate many of the hard-earned gains in keeping estrogens in their environmental place. We are just beginning to get a firm hold on some of these problems through the good offices of our newly developed epidemiologically oriented agencies. It would be unfortunate to have these fine efforts arrested or even slowed down.

REFERENCES

1. J.A. Long and H.M. Evans, The Oestrous Cycle in the Rat and its Associated Phenomena. Mem. Univ. Calif. 6, 1 (1922).
2. C.R. Stockard and G.N. Papanicolaou, Am. J. Anat. 22, 225 (1917).
3. E. Allen and E.A. Doisy, JAMA 81, 819 (1923).
4. E. Allen, G.M. Smith and W.V. Gardner, Am. J. Anat. 61, 321 (1937).
5. F.L. Hisaw and F.C. Lendrum, Endocrinology 20, 228, (1936).
6. M.D. Overholser and E. Allen, Surg. Gyn. and Obst. 60, 129, (1935).
7. R. Hertz, Pediatrics 62, 1138, (1978).
8. H.W. Bennetts, Australian Veterinary Journal 17, 85, (1946).
9. J.D. Biggers, in: The Pharmacology of Plant Phenols, J.W. Fairbairn, ed. (Academic Press, London 1959) p. 51.
10. W.V. Gardner, C.A. Pfeiffer and J.J. Trentin in: Pathophysiology of Cancer, F Homburger and W.H. Fisherman, eds. (Harper and Row, New York 1959) p. 152.
11. R. Hertz, Pediatrics, 21, 203, (1958).
12. J.M. Evans, Young, J.P., W.W. Tullner, R. Hertz, G. Wilmer and O. Wood, J. Clin. Endoc. and Met. 12, 495 (1952).
13. W.W. Tullner, Science 133, 647 (1961).
14. B. Zondek, Klin. Wchnschr. 9, 2285 (1928).
15. R. Hertz and J.C. Bailar, III, JAMA 28, 1000 (1966).
16. R. Hertz, Cancer Res. 11, 393 (1951).
17. I.S. Wright, J. New Drugs, 3, 201 (1963).
18. A. Ruskin, Acting Director, Division of New Drugs, FDA, official correspondence, Feb. 4, 1964.
19. R. Hertz, J. Steroid Biochem. 11, 435 (1979).

Structure-Activity Relationships of Estrogenic Chemicals

STRUCTURE-ACTIVITY RELATIONSHIPS OF ESTROGENIC CHEMICALS

William L. Duax and J. F. Griffin
Medical Foundation of Buffalo, Inc., 73 High Street, Buffalo, NY 14203,
U.S.A.

In 1962, Huggins speculated that the molecular basis for steroid
hormone action was the intercalation of steroids in DNA. He also
proposed that carcinogens by virtue of their structural resemblance to
both steroids and base pairs might be acting by intercalation at the
growth sensitive sites in the DNA that are the natural target of
steroids [1]. Subsequently Jensen discovered that steroid action was
contingent upon binding to cytosolic receptors [2], and specific protein
receptors for most of the known hormonal steroids have been isolated
and identified.   The natural hormones exhibit a fair degree of
selectivity for their respective receptors [3] and many investigators
have concluded that the steroid must be completely buried in the
receptor in order to account for the high binding affinity [4]. It has
been demonstrated that most steroid receptors undergo a temperature
dependent conformational change that appears to be crucial to hormone
function. This conformational change is contingent upon steroid binding
and was long considered essential to facilitate entry of the steroid
receptor complex into the nucleus of the target cell where specific
interaction with DNA is presumed to take place. The steroid was assumed
to promote receptor transport into the nucleus. Recent studies using
radio immunoassay techiques have demonstrated the presence of the
receptor in the cell nucleus [5,6] independent of the presence of
steroid. This observation suggests that the function of the steroid is
to induce or stabilize the conformational change in the receptor that is
required for appropriate interaction with DNA.

X-Ray crystallographic data provide reliable information on the
overall conformation of estrogen agonists and antagonists that may be
used to gain insight into the conformational flexibility of these
molecules, the structural similarities that might account for their
binding to a common site and the structural differences that might
account for varying degrees of hormonal response. In general X-ray
determinations provide information on the most stable conformation of a

molecule. Since the receptor bound and/or active form of an estrogen agonist or antagonist may not be the most stable form, empirical energy calculations can be useful for the exploration of conformational space and the determination of metastable states that may account for binding and activity. The X-ray results on ground state conformation provide a useful basis for evaluating the accuracy and utility of theoretical energy calculations [7].

Estrogens

Compounds having remarkably different structures have been found to compete for the traditional estrogen binding site on the estrogen receptor and elicit varying degrees of response (FIG. 1). A phenolic ring is the structural feature that appears to promote high affinity for the estrogen receptor and most investigators have suggested that when binding to the receptor site the phenolic ring mimics the steroid A ring [8,9]. The potent nonsteroidal estrogen diethylstilbestrol (DES) has two phenolic rings capable of mimicing the A ring of estradiol. Recognizing the similarity in overall structures between estradiol and DES, Keasling and Schueler [10] suggested that the precise spacing of two hydroxyl groups at either end of an essentially planar and primarily hydrophobic molecule is the structural basis for estrogen function.

When the phenol rings of a sample of the compounds that compete for binding to the estrogen receptor are superimposed significant differences in the D ring region of the molecules are observed (FIG. 2). If there is a close association between estrogens and the receptor it would appear to be limited to the A and B rings. The receptor is either flexible in the D ring region or insensitive to it [11,12].

Metabolites of DES are of interest due to uncertainty concerning the form responsible for the carginogenic properties of DES and as additional probes of the structure-activity relationships of estrogens. The low affinity of indanesterol (FIG. 1e) for the estrogen receptor despite the presence of two phenolic rings indicates that the bent overall shape of the molecule (FIG. 3) is incompatible with receptor binding. It is evident that the precise location of steric bulk and functional groups relative to the phenolic ring will govern binding and activity. The subtlty of the details of molecular control is

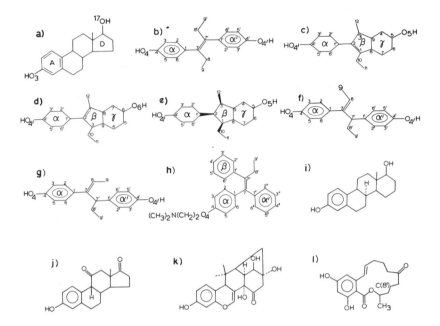

FIG. 1. Chemical diagrams, atomic numbering and ring identification for
(a) estradiol, E, (b) diethylstilbestrol, DES, (c) indenestrol A, IA,
(d) indenestrol B, IB, (e) indanestrol, I, (f) Z-pseudo
diethylstilbestrol, ZPD, (g) E-pseudo diethylstilbestrol, EPD, (h) trans
(Z) tamoxifen, (i) 8α-D-homoestradiol, (j) 11-keto-9β-estrone, (k)
mirestrol, and (l) trans-zearalenone.

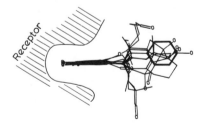

FIG. 2. Superposition of the phenol rings of six compounds (a,b,i,j,k,l
in FIG. 1.) that bind to the estrogen receptor, suggests that
variability in D-ring orientation is compatible with receptor binding
and some degree of activity.

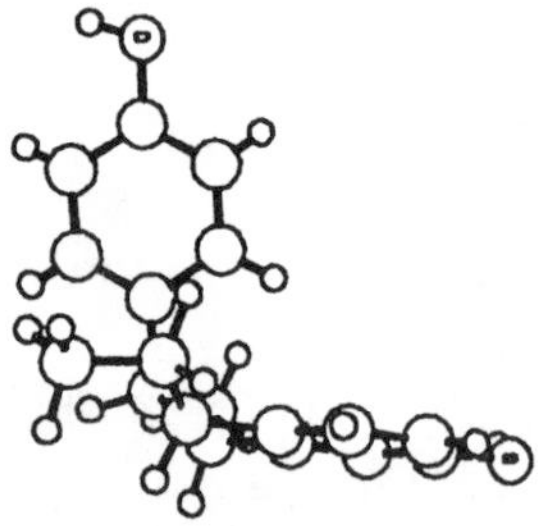

18

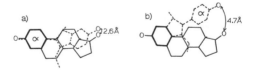

FIG. 3. Bent conformation of indanestrol observed in the solid state

exemplified by the case of the racemates of the dienestrol isomers (FIG.
1c and d). Korach finds that only one enantiomer of indenestrol A (IA)
has high affinity for the estrogen receptor and that both enantiomers of
indenestrol B (IB) have moderate affinity. Model studies using X-ray
crystallographically observed structures of IA and IB suggest that it is
the α-ring that mimics the estrogen A-ring [13] (FIG. 4) but it is
difficult to identify the structural basis for the enantiomeric effect
in IA and the weaker affinity of IB. It must be related to the topology
of the molecule in the region of the double bond. In this regard IA has
a high degree of similarity to the crystallographically observed
asymmetric form of DES in which the two methyl groups are on the same
side of the plane of the double bond. A comparison of the
crystallographically observed structures of estradiol, DES and IA, (FIG.
5), suggests that the C3-(R) enantiomer of IA, which has structural
features most closely resembling DES and estradiol, may be the active
enantiomer.

Crystallographic analysis of another DES analogue, pseudo DES (FIG.
1) together with empirical energy calculations provides additional

FIG. 4. Comparison of the conformations of IA with estradiol reveal
that the best fit is achieved when the α ring of IA is superimposed on
the A ring of estradiol with the double bond in the β ring overlapping
the C(8)–C(9) bond in estradiol.

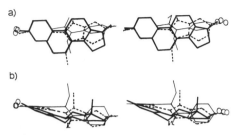

a)

b)

FIG 5. Stereo views illustrating the best fit of the hydroxyl groups
and the hydrophobic bulk of the structure of E (dark solid lines), DES
(light solid lines), and IA (dashed lines).

information on the importance of overall conformation to estrogenic
activity [14,15]. Pseudo DES exists as the Z and E isomers. While both
forms bind to the estrogen receptor only the Z form has appreciable
activity. X-Ray structure determinations revealed that both EPD and ZPD
have bent conformations completely unlike the conformation of
estradiol, DES and the indenestrol isomers. When the
crystallographically observed conformations of EPD and ZPD were
subjected to energy minimization the structures retained their overall
conformation with only minor changes in individual torsion angles that
average less than 4°.

The consistency between the crystallographic results and the energy
calculations suggests that the bent form is the energy minimum
conformation of ZPD and EPD. However, previous studies indicate that
this conformation is unlikely to be compatible with any significant
degree of estrogenic biological activity. For this reason it became
important to determine whether an extended DES-like conformation might
constitute a metastable state capable of accounting for the estrogenic
activity of ZPD. The crystallographically observed structures of ZPD
and EPD were transformed to the DES-like extended conformation and
subjected to energy minimization. As a result of extremely close
contacts between the hydrogens on C(9) and the α-ring in EPD (FIG. 6)
the extended conformation is energetically unfavorable and the molecule
refined to a bent conformation resembling in overall shape the
crystallographically observed structure. In contrast to this, the
extended conformation of the more active Z-isomer does not incorporate
intolerable non-bonding interactions and refinement indicates that a
metastable state exists which resembles the DES conformation (FIG. 6),
satisfactorily accounting for the observed activity.

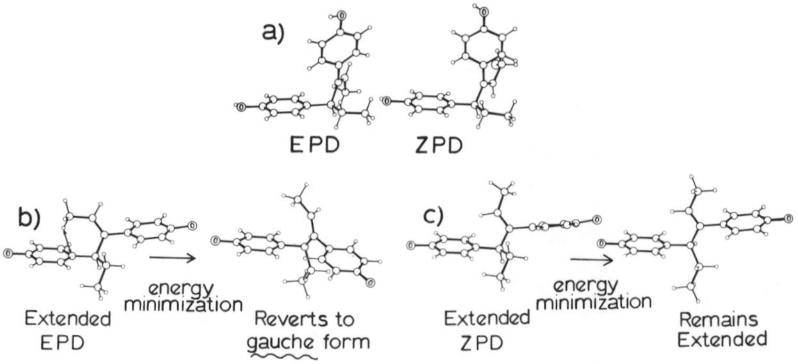

20

FIG. 6. (a) Crystallographically observed conformations of ZPD and EPD (b and c). Results of energy minimization of extended models of the inactive (EPD) and active (ZPD) isomers.

Estrogen Antagonists

Estrogen antagonists such as trans tamoxifen (FIG. 1h) compete for binding to estrogen receptors and elicit little or none of the characteristic hormonal response. Although at least two types of binding sites are present on the estrogen receptor [16] and it is possible that there is a specific antiestrogen binding site [17] it is clear that the clinical utility of the estrogen antagonists is a result of their competition for the traditional Type I estrogen binding site [18]. Consequently, estrogen and antiestrogen must share structural features that account for their ability to compete for binding to a common site and have structural differences that account for the degree of agonist or antagonist response elicited.

The 4-hydroxy metabolite of trans tamoxifen has been shown to be the potent competitor for the estrogen receptor responsible for the antagonist properties useful in breast cancer therapy [19]. This observation has led most investigators [20-23] to conclude that, at least in the case of the 4-hydroxy derivative of tamoxifen, it is the α ring that mimics the estradiol A ring in receptor interaction (FIG. 7). Pons, et al. [22] have explored the influence of hydroxyl substitution on all three of the rings in the triphenyl ethylene structures. They found that p-hydroxyl substitution on the α ring is most important for high affinity binding to the estrogen receptor. They also demonstrate

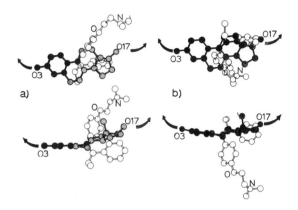

FIG. 7. Comparison of the crystallographically observed conformation
and hydrogen bonding of estradiol with that of tamoxifen. For purposes
of the comparison, the A ring of estradiol is superimposed on the phenyl
ring of tamoxifen that is hydroxylated in animal metabolism. The two
possible superpositions of these rings are illustrated in (a) and (b).
Common structural features are dark, agonist's structure is shaded and
antagonist's is light.

that mono-hydroxy substitution in the p-position on the α' ring results
in moderate competition for the estrogen binding site and optimum
binding occurs when both the α and α' rings are p-hydroxy substituted.
When only the β-ring is hydroxylated competition for receptor binding is
weak. However, p-hydroxy substitution on both the β and α' rings
permits near optimum receptor interaction [22]. These observations
suggest that tamoxifen will not bind with the β-ring substituting for
the A-ring of estradiol and that a p-hydroxylated α' ring may be able to
mimic the estradiol A ring but with somewhat impeded interaction. The
p-hydroxy group on either or both of the β and α' rings further enhances
receptor binding once the α-ring has taken up the position analogous to
the estradiol A ring relative to the receptor.

SUMMARY

These and related studies of the molecular structures of compounds
that compete for the estrogen binding site suggest that when estradiol
is bound to its receptor, there is a close fit only at the A-ring end of
the steroid (12). If a specific A-ring composition and conformation are
the primary requirement for binding to the estrogen receptor, the D-ring
region would be free to (a) influence the stability of the receptor

"dimer", [24] (b) induce a conformational change in the receptor, or (c) participate in a direct interaction with chromatin. The most potent antagonists have phenolic rings capable of mimicking the estradiol A ring in promoting high affinity binding to the receptor. They fail to stabilize the conformational change or molecular interaction needed to achieve hormonal response because they either lack an essential functional group (hydrogen bond donor) or they present a steric block or topological feature incompatible with transformation or interaction subsequent to the initiation of binding by the A ring or A ring analogues.

The similarity in shape between steroid structures, carcinogens, and base pairs [1,25], the binding of some carcinogens and their derivatives to estrogen receptors [26] and the possibility that direct contact between the receptor-bound steroid and DNA may occur, raises a further interesting possibility. One end of some carcinogens might mimic the steroid A ring, and thus bind to receptors; the receptor, activated by this binding could bring the carcinogen to the specific site(s) on DNA involved in the steroid-regulated growth response. In this way Huggins original hypothesis that carcinogens induce neoplastic growth by mimicking steroids in their molecular level interactions could prove to be correct.

ACKNOWLEDGEMENTS

Research supported in part by NIAMDD Grant No. AM-26546 and DDR Grant No. RR-05716. The organization and analysis of the data base associated with this investigation and several of the illustrations were carried out using the PROPHET system, a unique national computer resource sponsored by the NIH.

REFERENCES

1. C. Huggins and N. C. Yang, Science 137, 257–262 (1962).
2. E. V. Jensen and H. I. Jacobson in: Recent Progress in Hormone Research R. O. Greep, ed. (Academic Press, New York 1962) pp. 387–414.
3. J. P. Raynaud, T. Ojasov, M. M. Bouton and D. Philibert in: Drug Design E. J. Ariens, ed. (Academic Press, New York 1979) Vol. 8 pp. 169–214.

4. M. E. Wolff, J. D. Baxter, P. A. Kallman, D. L. Lee, I. D. Kuntz, E. Bloom, D. T. Matulich, and J. Morris, Biochemistry 78, 3201–3208 (1978).
5. W. J. King and G. L. Green, Nature (Lond.) 307, 745–747 (1984).
6. W. V. Welshons, M. E. Lieberman, and J. Gorski, Nature (Lond.) 307, 747–749 (1984).
7. W. L. Duax, J. F. Griffin, and D. C. Rohrer, J. Am. Chem. Soc. 103, 6705–6712 (1981).
8. C. Busetta, C. Courseille, F. Leroy, and M. Hospital, Acta Crystallogr. B28, 3293–3299 (1972).
9. W. L. Duax, C. M. Weeks, D. C. Rohrer, and J. F. Griffin Exerpta Medica International Congress V. H. T. James, ed. (1976) Series No. 403, pp. 565–569.
10. H. H. Keasling and F. W. Schueler, J. Am. Pharm. Assoc. 39, 87–90 (1950).
11. W. L. Duax, V. Cody, J. Griffin, J. Hazel, and C. M. Weeks, J. Steroid Biochem. 9, 901–907 (1978).
12. W. L. Duax and C. M. Weeks in: Estrogens in the Environment J. A. McLachlan, ed. (Elsevier, New York 1980) pp. 11–31.
13. W. L. Duax, D. C. Swenson, P. D. Strong, K. S. Korach, J. McLachlan, and M. Metzler, Molecular Pharmacology 26, 520–525 (1984).
14. K. S. Korach and W. L. Duax, Abstract No. 1047, 65 Annual Meeting of the Endocrine Society, San Antonio, Texas (1983).
15. W. L. Duax, J. F. Griffin, C. M. Weeks, and K. S. Korach, Environmental Health Perspective, in press (1985).
16. J. H. Clark, B. Markaverich, S. Upchurch, H. Eriksson, J. W. Hardin, and E. J. Peck, Recent Prog. Horm. Res. 36, 89–134 (1980).
17. R. L. Sutherland, L. C. Murphy, M. S. Foo, M. D. Green, A. M. Why-Bourne, and Z. S. Krozowski, Nature (Lond.) 288, 273–275 (1980).
18. J. H. Clark, J. Anderson, and E. J. Peck, Steroids 22, 707–718 (1973).
19. J. L. Borgna, E. Coezy, and H. Rocheport, Biochem. Pharmacol. 31, 3187–3191 (1982).
20. S. Durani, A. K. Agarwal, R. Saxena, B. S. Setty, R. C. Gupta, P. L. Kole, S. Ray, and N. Anand, J. Steroid Biochem. 11, 67–77 (1979).
21. W. L. Duax, J. F. Griffin, D. C. Rohrer, D. C. Swenson, and C. M. Weeks, J. Steroid Biochem. 15, 41–47 (1981).
22. M. Pons, F. Michel, A. Crastes De Paulet, J. Gilbert, J-F. Miquel, G. Precigoux, M. Hospital, T. Ojasso, J. P. Raynaud, J. Steroid Biochem. 20 137–145 (1984).
23. V. C. Jordan, Pharmacological Reviews 36, 245–276 (1984).
24. W. V. Vedeckis, W. T. Schrader, B. W. O'Malley, Biochemistry 2, 343–349 (1980).
25. L. B. Hendry, F. H. Witham, and O. L. Chapman in: Perspectives in Biology and Medicine R. L. Landau, ed. (Univ. of Chicago Press, Chicago 1977) Vol. 21, pp. 120–130.
26. S. L. Schneider, V. Alks, C. E. Morreal, D. K. Sinka, and T. L. Dao, J. Natl. Cancer Inst. 57, 1351–1354 (1976).

STRUCTURE-ACTIVITY RELATIONSHIPS OF STEROID ESTROGENS

J.P. RAYNAUD, T. OJASOO, M.M. BOUTON, E. BIGNON*, M. PONS* and A. CRASTES
de PAULET*
Roussel-Uclaf, 75007 Paris, France
*Inserm Unité 58, 34100 Montpellier, France.

INTRODUCTION

Over the years estrogens have rather unjustly earned a bad name : although crucial to female physiology, much emphasis has been laid on their possible carcinogenic properties. On the other hand, anti-estrogens have gained increasing favor, particularly as potential treatments of hormone-dependent neoplasms. Consequently, much recent work has been devoted to the study of anti-estrogenic compounds of, for instance, the triphenylethylene series whereas, apart from a few exceptions [6,14,20], steroid estrogens have been sadly neglected. It may be by comparing the results obtained with both these types of structure that new insight can be gained into the significance of binding to various proteins (estrogen receptor, alpha-fetoprotein, anti-estrogen binding site...) in the different manifestations of estrogen action. Interaction with an estrogen receptor may not necessarily be an absolute, or sole, requirement for the expression of estrogenic activity [34,54] ; it is an increasingly widely held opinion that multiple mechanisms of estrogen action exist [18,55].

BINDING TO THE ESTROGEN RECEPTOR : THE RECOGNITION STEP

The need for hydroxy groups at C-3 and C-17 of the estradiol molecule for effective binding to the estrogen receptor has often been stressed. The hydroxy group in C-3 is considered to be involved in the first recognition step [11,13,24,49] and acts as a H-bond donor. It is this donor H-bond rather than the conformation of the molecule that governs the interaction with the estrogen receptor as illustrated by the following examples :

a) Although prenortestosterone has a conformation, as determined by X-ray crystallography,closer to that of estradiol than of nortestosterone, it has no affinity for the estrogen receptor (Fig. 1) [12].

b) The 3-keto-Δ4,9,11-trienes, norgestrienone and gestrinone, have conformations close to those of ethynyl estradiol and 18-methyl estradiol respectively but, although they are highly flexible molecules and can bind to the progestin, androgen, mineralocorticoid and glucocorticoid receptors [49], they do not bind to the estrogen receptor (Fig. 2) [12].

c) The oxygen at C-3 of β-androstane is closer to that of estradiol than that of an A-nortestosterone derivative that binds to the estrogen receptor (Fig. 3). Nevertheless, it has no affinity for this receptor [43].

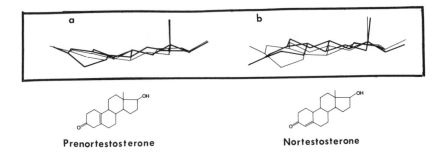

Prenortestosterone   **Nortestosterone**

FIG. 1. Best-fit superpositions of the crystalline conformations of prenortestosterone (bold line) and (a) estradiol, (b) nortestosterone (fine lines) [12].

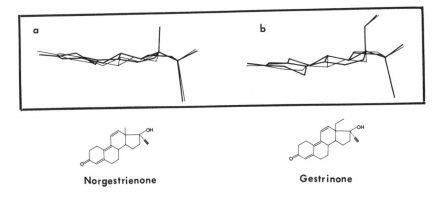

Norgestrienone   **Gestrinone**

FIG. 2. Best-fit superpositions of the crystalline conformations of (a) norgestrienone (bold line) and ethynyl estradiol (fine line), (b) gestrinone (bold line) and 18-methyl estradiol (fine line) [12].

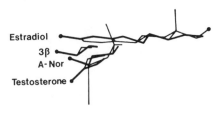

FIG. 3. Projection of the O(3) oxygen of 3β-androstane and of an A-nor derivative onto the C(13)–C(17)–C(18) plane [43].

d) In a study on a homologous series of A-nor derivatives, a hydroxy group in position 2β favored binding to the estrogen receptor and, in 2α, androgen binding. When the hydroxy group was replaced by a ketone, no binding to the estrogen receptor occurred, but there was noticeable affinity for the androgen receptor (Table I) [10].

TABLE I. Relative binding affinities for the estrogen receptor (ER) and androgen receptor (AR) [10].

			ER	AR
2αOH	2β C≡CH		0.1	<0.1
2βOH	2α C≡CH		12	14
2 = O			<0.1	46
2α OH	2β C≡CH } 17α C≡CH		0.2	–
2β OH	2α C≡CH		20	0.8
2α OH	} 17α C≡CH		0.6	0.3
2β OH			12	0.2
2 = O			<0.1	10
2α OH	2β C≡CH } 17α CH_3		0.1	17
2β OH	2α C≡CH		11	18
2α OH	} 17α CH_3		0.3	7.8
2β OH			2.6	3.5
2 = O			<0.1	54

ER = mouse uterus cytosol incubated for 2 h at 0°C
AR = rat prostate cytosol incubated for 30 min at 0°C

e) The rank order in relative binding affinities for the estrogen receptor of a series of 7α-methyl-lynestrenol derivatives is as follows : 3β-OH > 3α-OH ≫ 3-deoxy > 3-keto [6]. Bergink et al. thus also conclude that since the keto group at site C-3 is inhibitory, unlike a C-17 keto group (estrone), "the hydroxyl group at site C-3 of 17β estradiol maintains a hydrogen bond with a hydrogen acceptor site in the binding groove of the receptor. The hydroxyl group at site C-17 may interact with a hydrogen bond donor or acceptor site".

Segaloff et al. have used a different approach to demonstrate the tolerance of the estrogen receptor to flexibility in overall molecular shape. They observed a remarkably high estrogenic activity for 3-hydroxy-9β -estra-1,3,5(10)-triene-11,17-dione despite its unusual bent conformation. The 9α -epimer, which has an overall shape nearly identical to that of estrone, is, on the other hand, much less active [52].

STRUCTURE-AFFINITY STUDIES OF STEROIDS

To correlate ligand structure with protein binding capacity and, ultimately, with an estrogenic response, a simple routine system is needed to evaluate the relative binding affinities (RBAs) of a series of test-compounds for the cytosol estrogen receptor under set conditions. This type of screening system is routine in our laboratories [37,48,49]. Cytosol is prepared from immature mouse uterus since uterotrophic response in this species is one of our basic biological tests for estrogenic activity. Incubation times and temperatures have been chosen as a function of the interaction kinetics of estradiol with the estrogen receptor. The first set of incubation conditions (2 h at 0°C) reflects differences in association rates and indicates whether an interaction between the ligand and receptor is feasible ; the second set (5 h at 25°C) reflects differences in dissociation rates and, by comparison with the first set of values, gives an idea of the stability of the receptor complex [1,7]. An increase in RBA on increasing time and temperature indicates that the complex formed by the test-compound is more stable than the estradiol-receptor complex ; a decrease in RBA that it is less stable.

1/ Substitution at C-17

For many years, interest has been focussed on C-17 esters of estradiol, from two carbon chains to the long chain fatty acids, all of which are potent long-acting estrogens. These compounds exert their estrogenic effects only after hydrolysis to the free parent steroid [26].

It is generally acknowledged that the presence of a C-17α ethynyl substituent enhances binding to the estrogen receptor as illustrated by the data in Table II. Its influence seems to be crucial. Several years ago we attempted to deduce the relative binding increment associated with a particular substituent in the total binding of a ligand to a receptor [30]. The increment was deduced by comparing pairs of ligands differing by a single substitution and then used to calculate the expected binding of another ligand. This calculated value was compared to the experimental value. The overall concordance between theoretical and experimental values was extremely good, but the principle of additivity did not seem to apply in the case of certain combinations of substituents, in particular when a 17α-ethynyl was present. The data in Table II clearly show that the combination of an 11β-methoxy or 11β-ethoxy substituent with a 17α-ethynyl is particularly effective in forming a highly stable estrogen receptor complex

(10-fold increase in RBA from 11 to 125 % compared to a 2-fold increase from 100 to 220 %), more effective than a combination with a 17α-methyl (6 to 31 %), 17α-but-2-yn-1-yl (12 to 19 %) or 17α-2-methylallyl (11 to 2.5 %).

2/ Lengthening the chain at C-13

Lengthening the C-13 chain of estradiol (methyl → ethyl → propyl → butyl) decreases binding affinity probably because of steric hindrance and also decreases complex stability (Table II). This decrease in stability is also noted for 16α-hydroxy estradiol derivatives but is less apparent for 11β-methoxy derivatives which retain little binding affinity.

TABLE II. Relative binding affinities for the mouse uterus estrogen receptor

Substituent at C-17α	Estradiol		11β-methoxy estradiol		11β-ethoxy estradiol	
	2h 0°	5h 25°	2h 0°	5h 25°	2h 0°	5h 25°
– H	100	100	7	28	10	11
– CH_3	67	35	6	31	7	11
– C≡CH	100	220	11	125	10	118
– C – C≡C – CH_3			12	19	14	28
– C – C = CH_2 　　CH_3			11	2.5		

Substituent at C-13	Estradiol		11β-methoxy estradiol		16α-hydroxy estradiol	
	2h 0°	5h 25°	2h 0°	5h 25°	2h 0°	5h 25°
– CH_3	100	100	11	125	26	20
– C_2H_5	53	33	7	6	22	5
– C_3H_7	30		1.5	0.5	19	16
– C_4H_9	14	4				

3/ Substitution at various points of the steroid skeleton

Before reviewing some of the literature on structure-affinity relationships of steroid estrogens, a word of caution is called for. Comparing published data can be misleading since it is unlikely that the experiments have been performed under comparable conditions. The choice of species, organ, radioactive ligand, buffer, etc... may vary and, most important of all, the choice of incubation time and temperature [53]. In our opinion, it is essential to determine RBA values under two sets of incubation conditions. This is neatly illustrated by some of the data in Table II. For instance, whereas the four diversely substituted 17α-derivatives of 11β-methoxy estradiol have RBAs at 2 h 0°C ranging from 6 to 12 that are not very different from that of the parent compound (i.e. 7), the RBAs after 5 h incubation at 25°C can be very high (e.g. 125) or very low (e.g. 2.5). It is thus possible to conclude that whereas recognition between ligand and receptor occurs at comparable rates in each case, the complexes formed have very different kinetic stabilities. The data from the literature given below should be considered with this in mind.

In a study to determine suitable positions in the estradiol molecule for substitution with cytotoxic groups, Zeelen and Bergink [56] used a methyl group as a hydrophobic probe. They found that positions where the introduction of a methyl group led to low or moderate affinity were the 1 (15 %), 2 (36 %), 6α (31 %), 15α (rac. 29 %), 15β (26 %) and 18 (31 %) positions. We had previously reported similar results for the mouse uterine receptor for the 2 (41 %), 9 (39 %) and 18 (31 %) methyl derivatives (see Fig. 5) [49] and here report a decreased RBA for 4-methylestradiol (27 %). Gabbard and Segaloff [20] also found a decreased affinity for 9α-methylestradiol (35 %) and Gonzalez et al. [23] for 2-methylestradiol and 16β-methylestradiol in rat uterus. However, Kirchhoff et al. [28] have recently published that 2-methylestradiol and 4-methylestradiol exhibit estrogen receptor affinities that are not significantly different from that of estradiol.

Positions where the introduction of a methyl group leads to a relatively high affinity are, according to Zeelen and Bergink [56], the 7 (104 %), 11β (65 %) and 17 (83 %) positions in confirmation of our results in the mouse with 7 (101 %) and 12β(111 %) methyl derivatives [49] (see Fig. 5). These observations have been substantiated by Gabbard and Segaloff [20] who have published an RBA of 124 % for 11β-methylestradiol and 104 % for 7α-methylestradiol.

When using a hydroxyl group as a probe, Bergink et al. [6] found RBAs of only 1 % for positions 6α, 7α, 11α and 15α, of 3 % for position 2, 7 % for position 11β and 17 % for position 16α. Some of our results are shown in Table VI (see later).

ANALOGIES WITH ESTROGENIC NON-STEROIDS

It is in the case of steroids substituted at C7 and/or C-11 that the greatest analogies can be made with non-steroid derivatives of the di and triphenylethylene type. This particular area of research has been extremely well analyzed by scientists at the Lucknow All-India Central Drug Research Institute who have drawn analogies among several classes of estrogen : seco-estradiols, chromans and chromenes, cyclofenil, distilbenes [16,17, 21]. Our interest has been focussed in two directions which we hope, on further analysis, will converge into a unifying whole : (1) substituting steroids in positions C-7 and C-11 (or neighbouring positions) with various side-chains to approach the conformation and nature of certain anti-estrogenic triphenylethylenes [5], (2) synthesizing analogs of triphenylethylenes in an attempt to delineate the relative importance of each phenyl ring and of the nature and position of diverse substituents [35,40,41,48].

1/ Substitution at positions C-7 and/or C-11 of steroids

The importance of the presence and orientation of a C-11 substituent can be exemplified by two compounds : moxestrol [2] and RU 16117 [3]. Moxestrol is the 11β-methoxy derivative of ethynyl estradiol and forms a slowly-dissociating complex with the estrogen receptor (Table III). It is a highly potent estrogen [8,46]. Its 11α-methoxy isomer, on the other hand, interacts fleetingly with the estrogen receptor and is a partial agonist/antagonist similar in activity to estriol on several biological parameters [8,45].

The data in Table II have already shown that, whatever the substituent in position 17α, an 11β-methoxy or ethoxy group tends to increase the stability of the estrogen receptor complex.

TABLE III. Relative binding affinities for the mouse uterus estrogen receptor

Substituent	Estradiol		17α-ethynyl estradiol	
	2h 0°	5h 25°	2h 0°	5h 25°
None	100	100	100	220
11β-methoxy	7	28	11	125
11α-methoxy	4	0.3	10	2.5
11β-hydroxy	5	1.5		
11β-hydroxy 13-ethyl			2	0.6
7α-methyl	116	330		
7α-methyl 11β-methoxy	0.4	3	< 0.1	< 0.1

7α-Methyl estradiol also binds with high affinity to the estrogen receptor to form a stable complex (the introduction of this substituent also induces some androgen binding [49] (see Fig. 5)). However, the combined effect of the simultaneous introduction of both 7α-methyl and 11β-hydroxy substituents leads to a compound that has lost virtually all affinity for the estrogen receptor. In the ethynyl estradiol series, such a disubstituted compound is effectively inert (Table III). An explanation for this could be steric hindrance impeding hydrogen bond formation between the C-3 hydroxyl and the receptor recognition site located at the deep end of a hydrophobic pocket and also impeding access to a second site that can bind either the C-11 or C-7 substituent. The two substituents projecting above and below the plane of the steroid skeleton would seem to bar entry into the pocket.

Several authors have noted the importance of substitution at the C-11 position in the 17α-ethynyl-4-estren-17β-ol series [4,9], later extended to a number of 11β-substituted 4,9-estradienes and 1,3,5(10)-estratrienes by the development of new synthetic pathways [5]. Relative binding affinities for the estrogen receptor, although systematically below that of estradiol after two hours incubation, increased to very high values at 5 hours in the case of the C-11 vinyl, allyl, i and n propyl substituents [5] (Table IV). All these compounds exert uterotrophic activity in the immature mouse.

TABLE IV. Relative binding affinities for the mouse uterus estrogen receptor of C-11 substituted ethynyl estradiol derivatives

Substituent at C-11	2h 0°C	5h 25°C	Substituent at C-11	2h 0°C	5h 25°C
H	112	245	p-methoxyphenyl	61	66
n-Pr	95	730	o-methoxyphenyl	15	8.5
i-Pr	84	710	2-thienyl	76	91
vinyl	91	415	benzyl	77	53
allyl	93	555			

2/ Triphenylacrylonitrile derivatives

Certain di and triphenylethylene (TPE) derivatives bind to the estrogen receptor and much fun and games have been had superposing these types of structure with estradiol [15,25,27]. X-ray crystallography studies have established that TPEs adopt a preferential conformation where the orientation of the α, α' and β-phenyl rings are fixed but each ring has a certain degree of freedom of rotation. According to our binding data in Table V, the most likely, but probably not unique, superposition is one where the α-phenyl ring of the TPEs adopts the position of the estradiol A-ring [40,41,48].

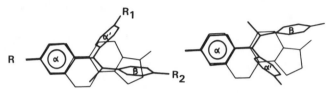

FIG. 4. Superposition of the α-phenyl ring of a TPE structure onto the A-ring of estradiol.

The reasons for this are as follows :

- the monohydroxy derivative with an OH-group on ring β (in R_2) has very low affinity for ER (5-3 %) thus suggesting that superposition of ring β of the TPE and ring A of estradiol is unlikely. The introduction of an OH-group in R of this molecule markedly enhances binding (75-200 %).

- the monohydroxy derivative with an OH-group on ring α' (in R_1) also has very low affinity for ER (7-14 %) ; the superposition of ring α' and ring A gives a very poor fit between ring D and a second phenyl ring of the TPE. The introduction of an OH-group in R of this molecule also markedly enhances binding (100-470 %).

- the monohydroxy derivative with an OH-group on ring α (in R) was the only compound with an RBA equivalent to that of estradiol. However, the complex formed was not as stable as the estradiol-receptor complex since the RBAs decreased with incubation time and temperature. A second OH-group, preferably in position R_1, is required for stabilisation of the binding.

These results suggest that the OH-group in R is the more important but that the presence of two hydroxyl groups is needed to maintain the stability of the complex. The need for a second hydroxyl group is confirmed by the negligible RBA recorded for 3-(hydroxyphenyl)-2-phenyl-acrylonitrile which has an OH group in R, a H in R_2 but no α'-phenyl ring. This α'-phenyl ring must consequently contribute in no small way to the interaction with the estrogen receptor, the interaction being even more effective when this ring is hydroxylated. The superposition in Fig. 4 indicates that this phenyl ring is located in the region of the C-11 or C-7,8 atoms of estradiol [40,41,48]. The presence of a methyl group is not conducive to binding.

TABLE V. Relative binding affinities for the estrogen receptor in mouse uterus cytosol and inhibition of prostaglandin synthase (PGS) in bovine seminal vesicle microsomes.

R	R_1	R_2	RBA 2h 0°C	RBA 5h 25°C	Inhibition of PGS $IC_{50}(\mu M)$
H	H	H	< 0.1	<0.1	3.5
CH	H	H	100	65	1.6
H	CH	H	7	14	0.2
H	H	CH	5	3	6.6
CH	CH	H	100	470	1.8
CH	H	CH	75	200	4.0
H	CH	OH	21	37	
CH	CH	CH	57	200	5.6
CH	CH_3	H	2	6.5	0.8
CH_3	CH	H	1	7	0.08
CH	CH	CH_3	24	147	4.0
CH_3	CH	CH	14	19	1.8
CH	CH_3	CH	24	195	3.2

INTERACTION WITH PROTEINS OTHER THAN THE ESTROGEN RECEPTOR

1/ Other steroid receptors

In our laboratories, the binding to five steroid hormone receptors is systematically measured [37,48,49]. Well-known steroid estrogen derivatives are highly specific to the estrogen receptor [49], but subtle modifications, particularly in C-11, can induce some, albeit weak, binding to the receptors of other hormone classes (Fig. 5).

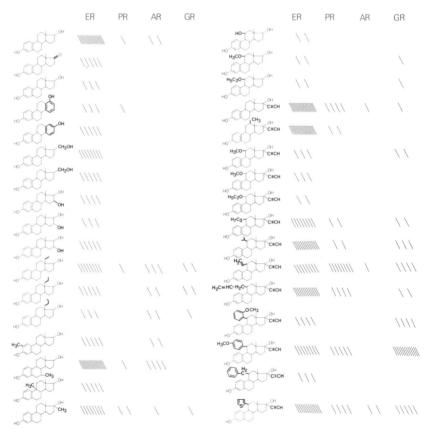

FIG. 5. RBAs for the estrogen receptor (ER) in mouse uterus, progestin receptor (PR) in rabbit uterus, androgen receptor (AR) in rat prostate and glucocorticoid receptor (GR) in rat liver after short incubation times. None of the compounds bound to the mineralocorticoid receptor.

\	< 1	\\\	10 - 15	\\\\\\ 50 - 75
\	1 - 3	\\\\	15 - 25	\\\\\\\ 75 - 100
\\	3 - 10	\\\\\	25 - 50	▨ 100 - 125

Ethynyl estradiol interacts quite noticeably with the progestin receptor, much less so with the androgen and glucocorticoid receptors. The introduction of an allyl or 2-thienyl substituent in position C-11 does not affect this progestin binding, a vinyl or p-methoxymethyl substituent enhances it [5]. In most cases, and in particular in the case of a p-methoxymethyl substituent, there is noticeable glucocorticoid binding. That for most of these compounds both progestin and glucocorticoid binding are simultaneously affected is not surprising in view of the close relationships that have been observed between these two types of binding for a whole series of progestins [38,47]. None of these C-11 substituted compounds manifested any progestational activity but several induced abortion in the rat at relatively high doses. Whether this abortive effect is due to an antiprogesterone effect or to their estrogenic activity is not yet known.

2/ Plasma and other proteins

As mentioned in the introduction, estrogens and anti-estrogens can also bind to proteins other than steroid hormone receptors. Estradiol binds to plasma sex-steroid binding protein (SBP), alphafetoprotein (AFP), and a more recently detected "unusual hepatic estrogen-binding protein" [39] whose functions remain unclear. A large majority of synthetic compounds have diminished affinity for these proteins [32,46]. Compounds with non-steroidal structures that mimic certain aspects of estrogenic activity tend not to bind to SBP and AFP but, on the other hand, interact with yet other proteins. For instance, certain triphenylethylene derivatives can inhibit prostaglandin synthase to the same extent as some well-known anti-inflammatory agents. The concentration of indomethacin inhibiting PGS in bovine vesicle microsomes to 50 % is 5.6 μM compared to less than 1 μM for two methylated TPE derivatives tested in Table V [22,40]. Inhibition of glutamate dehydrogenase has also been reported for estrogens and estrogen analogs [42]. None of these TPEs, however, interacted with the recently detected "anti-estrogen binding site" which would seem to necessitate the presence of an alkylamino-ether side-chain [27,29]. The contribution of these interactions to estrogenic activity (other than influencing the pharmacokinetics of access of the ligands to the estrogen receptor site) is not known.

3/ Metabolising enzymes

The study of the affinity and activity of hydroxylated derivatives of estradiol and of its analogs is of particular interest since hydroxylation is the main pathway of estrogen metabolism. There is much controversy on the formation and action of these compounds for instance in the liver and brain. According to certain authors, catecholestrogen formation would be a form of estrogen inactivation whereas others have advanced important anti-estrogenic and neuroendocrine properties for these molecules. The relevance of estrogen receptor interaction has been disputed in these effects even when account is taken for possible metabolism [33].

The RBAs of a few hydroxylated estradiol derivatives are given in Table VI. Hydroxylation of estradiol whether in C-2 or C-16 (estriol) results in compounds with decreasing RBAs and therefore with potential anti-estrogenic properties as a result of their rapid interaction kinetics with the estrogen receptor [8]. However, in view of the in situ formation of C-2 derivatives within the target tissues even a low but sustained concentration might produce estrogenic effects. According to data in the literature [31], C-4 hydroxylated estradiol surprisingly has an opposite effect ; it dissociates from the receptor at a significantly slower rate than estradiol. Whatever the position of hydroxylation of 11β-methoxy ethynyl estradiol (C2,C4 or C16) slowly-dissociating receptor complexes are formed.

TABLE VI. Relative binding affinities for the mouse uterus estrogen receptor

Substituent	Estradiol		Ethynyl estradiol		11β-methoxy ethynyl estradiol	
	2h 0°	5h 25°	2h 0°	5h 25°	2h 0°	5h 25°
None	100	100	100	220	11	125
2-hydroxy	28	2.5			2.6	27
4-hydroxy					2	9
16α-hydroxy	15	3	26	20	0.7	14
11β,16α-dihydroxy	0	0				

Correlations cannot be drawn with activity unless the degree of metabolic conversion is known in the target tissue and species under study. In general, the presence of a 17α-ethynyl group which protects the 17β-hydroxyl favors enzyme attack of the A-ring, whereas the presence of an 11β-methoxy group, even in the presence of a 17α-ethynyl, favors C-16 hydroxylation [50]. This observation is of particular relevance to the hypothesis that catechols are activated metabolites of estrogens and consequently could be involved in estrogen provoked mutagenicity [44]. The synthetic estrogen moxestrol gives rise to small amounts of catechols in the human, compared to considerably larger amounts in the monkey. In the dog, on the other hand, the vast majority of the compound is excreted intact in the urine (Table VII).

Enzyme systems that are present in some tissues are absent in others. The larger amounts of radioactivity found in the rat pituitary compared to the hypothalamus after injection of ethynyl estradiol compared to moxestrol could be explained by the formation of catechols of ethynyl estradiol by a hydroxylase present in the pituitary but not detected in the hypothalamus [51].

TABLE VII. Metabolites identified after oral administration of moxestrol

| | Metabolites (% excreted radioactivity) | | | | | Bile |
| | | Urine | | | | |
	Human	Dog	Rhesus	Baboon	Rat	Rat
Intact moxestrol	13.0	80	16.3	16.6	5.2	17.9
16β-OH	13.0	ND	ND	ND	11.1	13.5
16α-OH	18.5	ND	ND	ND	ND	ND
15α-OH	24.5	ND	1.9	1.0	ND	0.5
2 or 4-OH	1.5	ND	32.0	24.7	ND	5.4
2-OCH₃	1.0	ND	3.9	8.5	ND	11.9
D-homo	10.0	ND	5.1	4.1	6.3	4.5

ND = Not detected

STRUCTURE-ACTIVITY RELATIONSHIPS

In view of the above comments, it is obvious that the relative estrogenic activities of, for instance, compounds such as moxestrol and ethynyl estradiol may differ appreciably according to the specific end-point and species under consideration. The increasing use of in vitro tests, in particular of cell culture systems, will further the understanding of the relative potency of these compounds. We have already screened series of TPE derivatives on progesterone receptor induction and cell proliferation using MCF₇ cells (manuscript in preparation) and are doing similar studies with analogous steroid derivatives. Increasing recent evidence supports the hypothesis that there is a dichotomy between estrogens' effect on growth and progesterone receptor synthesis [18], i.e. on proliferation and protein synthesis [19]. It is yet too early to be able to distinguish which are the crucial positions and substituents, in series other than tamoxifen analogs [36], which are crucial to these activities.

CONCLUSIONS

Our studies in the field of estrogen protein binding support the hypothesis that the first interaction with the estrogen receptor is the formation of a H-bond between the C-3 hydroxy group of estradiol (or of its analogs) and a receptor subsite located at the deep end of a pocket. This hydroxy group is a H-bond donor. A second interaction occurs between a substituent at C-17 and another subsite, thus increasing the stability of the complex. However, somewhere between these two anchorage points, there is a third subsite to which certain substituents at other positions of the steroid skeleton, in particular at C-7 or C-11, can bind. This substituent may slow down the rate of association between the steroid and receptor but may also lead to extremely stable complexes.

The phenol rings of hydroxylated triphenylethylenes (TPE) can also interact with these subsites, the position of the TPE within the binding site depending upon the availability and position of the one or more hydroxy groups. In our opinion, therefore, by modifying the substituents at the strategic C-7 or C-11 positions noted by several authors (or maybe at neighbouring positions), it should be possible to design, at will, steroids with activity profiles more or less similar to those of TPEs.

ACKNOWLEDGEMENTS

1/ Chemical syntheses

The close collaboration of the following chemists is most gratefully acknowledged :
A-nor derivatives : J. Jacques, J. Canceill (Collège de France) [10].
Triphenylethylene derivatives : J. Gilbert, J.F. Miquel (CERCOA-CNRS) [22,35].
C-11 substituted steroids : A. Bélanger (Univ. Laval), G. Teutsch (Roussel-Uclaf) [5].

2/ X-ray crystallography

We are extremely privileged to be able to draw upon the expertise of :
- J. Delettré, J.P. Mornon (Univ. Paris VI) [12].
- G. Précigoux, M. Hospital (Bordeaux Univ.) [25,43].

3/ Metabolism

The metabolism studies have been performed by D. Coussedière and J. Salmon of the Roussel-Uclaf Research Centre.

REFERENCES

1. Aranyi, P. : Biochim. Biophys. Acta, 628 (1980) 220-227.

2. Azadian-Boulanger G. and Bertin D. : Chim. Ther., 78 (1973) 451-454.

3. Azadian-Boulanger G., Bouton M.M., Bucourt R., Nédélec L., Pierdet A., Torelli V. and Raynaud J.P. : Eur. J. Med. Chem., 13, n° 4 (1978) 313-319.

4. Baran J.S., Lennon H.D., Mares S.E. and Nutting E.F. : Experentia, 26 (1970) 762-

5. Bélanger A., Philibert D. and Teutsch G. : Steroids, 37 (1981) 361-382.

6. Bergink E.W., Kloosterboer H.J., van der Velden W.H.M., van der Vies J. and de Winter S. : In : Steroids and Endometrial Cancer, Jasonni V.M. et al. eds (Raven Press, New York 1983) pp. 77-84.

7. Bouton M.M. and Raynaud J.P. : J. steroid Biochem., 9 (1978) 9-15.

8. Bouton M.M. and Raynaud J.P. : Endocrinology, 105 (1979) 509-515.

9. Broek A.J. v.d., Broess A.I.A., Heuvel M.J. v.d., Jongh H.P. de, Leembuis J., Schönemann K.H., Smits J., de Visser J., van Vliet N.P. and Zeelen F.J. : Steroids, 30 (1977) 481-450.

10. Canceill J., Jacques J., Bouton M.M., Fortin M. and Tournemine C. : J. steroid Biochem., 18 (1983) 643-647.

11. Chernayaev G.A., Barkova T.I., Egorova V.V., Sorokiria I.B., Ananchenko S.N., Mataradze G.D., Sokolova N.A. and Rozen V.B. : J.steroid Biochem.,6 (1975) 1483-1488.

12. Delettré J., Mornon J.P., Ojasoo T. and Raynaud J.P. : In : Perspectives in Steroid Receptor Research, Bresciani F. ed (Raven Press, New York 1980) pp 1-21.

13. Duax W.L., Griffin J.F., Rohrer D.C. and Weeks C.M. : In : Hormone Antagonists, Agarwal M.K. ed (Walter de Gruyter and Co., Berlin 1982) pp. 3-24.

14. Duax W.L., Smith G.D., Swenson D.C., Strong P.D., Weeks C.M., Ananchenko S.N. and Egorova V.V. : J. steroid Biochem., 14 (1981) 1-7.

15. Duax W.L., Swenson D.C., Strong P.D., Korach K.S., McLachlan J. and Metzler M. : Mol. Pharmacol., 26 (1984) 520-525.

16. Durani S., Agarwal A.K., Saxena R., Setty B.S., Gupta R.C., Kole F.L., Ray S. and Anand N. : J. steroid Biochem., 11 (1979) 67-77.

17. Durani S. and Anand N. : Intl. J. Quantum Chem., XX (1981) 71-83.

18. Ederi M., Imagawa W., Larson L. and Nandi S. : Endocrinology, 116 (1984) 105-112.

19. Ederi M., McGrath M., Larson L. and Nandi S. : Endocrinology, 115, (1984) 1691-1697.

20. Gabbard R.B. and Segaloff A. : Steroids, 41 (1983) 791-805.

21. Garg S., Bindal R.D., Durani S. and Kapil R.S. : J. steroid Biochem., 18 (1983) 89-95.

22. Gilbert J., Miquel J.F., Précigoux G., Hospital M., Raynaud J.P., Michel F. and Crastes de Paulet A. : J. Med. Chem., 26 (1983) 693-699.

23. Gonzalez F.B., Neef G., Eder U., Wiechert R., Schillinger E. and Nishino Y. : Steroids, 40 (1982) 171-187.

24. Hähnel R., Twaddle E. and Ratajczak T. : J. steroid Biochem., 4 (1973) 21-31.

25. Hospital M., Busetta B., Courseille C. and Précigoux G. : J. steroid Biochem., 6 (1975) 221-225.

26. Janocko L., Larner J.M. and Hochberg R.B. : Endocrinology, 114 (1984) 1180-

27. Jordan V.C., Haldemann B. and Allen K.E. : Endocrinology, 108 (1981) 1353-1361.

28. Kirchhoff J., Wang X, Ghraf R., Ball P. and Knupper R. : Brain Res., 294 (1984) 354-358.

29. Kon O.L. : J. Biol. Chem., 258 (1983) 3173-3177.

30. Lepicard G., Mornon J.P., Delettré J., Ojasoo T. and Raynaud J.P. : J. steroid Biochem, 9 (1978) 830.

31. MacLusky N.J., Barnea E.R., Clark C.R. and Naftolin F. : In : Catechol Estrogens, Merriam G.R. and Lipsett M.B. eds (Raven Press, New York 1983) pp. 151-165.

32. McElvany K.D., Carlson K.E., Katzenellenbogen J.A. and Welch M.J. : J. steroid Biochem., 18 (1983) 635-641.

33. Merriam G.R. and Lipsett M.B. (eds) : Catechol Estrogens (Raven Press, New York 1983).

34. Meyers C.Y., Kolb V.M. and Dandliker W.B. : Res. Comm. Chem. Path. Pharmacol., 35 (1982) 165-168.

35. Miquel J.F., Sekera A. and Chaudron T. : Cr. hebd. Séanc. Acad. Sci. Paris, 286 (1978) 151-154.

36. Murphy L.C. and Sutherland R.L. : Endocrinology, 116 (1985) 1071-1078.

37. Ojasoo T. and Raynaud J.P. : Cancer Res., 38 (1978) 4186-4198.

38. Ojasoo T. and Raynaud J.P. : In : Steroids and Endometrial Cancer, Jasonni V.M. et al. eds (Raven Press, New York 1983) pp. 11-28.

39. Peetz A. : Acta Endocr., 102 (1983) 58.

40. Pons M., Michel M., Crastes de Paulet A., Gilbert J., Miquel J.F., Précigoux G., Hospital M., Ojasoo T. and Raynaud J.P. : J. steroid Biochem., 20 (1984) 137-145.

41. Pons M., Michel F., Bignon E., Crastes de Paulet A., Gilbert J., Miquel J.F., Précigoux G., Hospital M., Ojasoo T. and Raynaud J.P. : In : Hormones and Cancer 2, Bresciani F. et al. eds (Raven Press, New York 1984) pp. 27-36.

42. Pons M., Michel F., Descomps B. and Crastes de Paulet A. : Eur. J. Biochem., 84 (1978) 257-266.

43. Précigoux G. In : "Analyse radiocristallographique de molécules oestrogènes et androgènes et étude de leur affinité et de leur spécificité" (Ph.D. Thesis, Université de Bordeaux I, France) - (1978).

44. Purdy R.H. : In : Hormones and Cancer 2, Bresciani F. et al. eds (Raven Press, New York 1984) pp. 401-415.

45. Raynaud J.P., Azadian-Boulanger G., Bouton M.M., Faure N., Ferland L., Gautray J.P., Husson J.M., Kelly P., Labrie F., Ojasoo T. and Précigoux G. : J. steroid Biochem., 20 (1984) 981-993.

46. Raynaud J.P., Bouton M.M., Gallet-Bourquin D., Philibert D., Tournemine C. and Azadian-Boulanger G. : Mol. Pharmacol., 9 (1973) 520-533.

47. Raynaud J.P., Bouton M.M. and Ojasoo T. : Tips, 1 (1980) 324-327.

48. Raynaud J.P. and Ojasoo T. : In : Steroid Hormone Receptors : Structure and Function, Gustafsson J.A. and Eriksson H. eds (Elsevier, Amsterdam 1983) pp. 141-170.

49. Raynaud J.P., Ojasoo T., Bouton M.M. and Philibert D. : In : Drug Design, Vol. 8, Ariëns E.J. ed (Academic Press, New York 1979) pp. 169-214.

50. Salmon J., Coussedière D., Cousty C. and Raynaud J.P. : J. steroid Biochem., 18 (1983) 565-573.

51. Salmon J., Coussedière D., Cousty C. and Raynaud J.P. : J. steroid Biochem., 19 (1983) 1223-1234.

52. Segaloff A., Gabbard B., Flores A., Borne R.F., Baker J.K., Duax W.L., Strong P.D. and Rohrer D.C. : Steroids, 35 (1980) 335-349.

53. Shutt D.A. and Cox R.I. : J. Endocr., 52 (1972) 299-310.

54. Sonnenschein C. and Soto A.M. : JNCI, 64 (1980) 211-215.

55. Tchernitchin A.N. : J. steroid Biochem., 19 (1983) 95-100.

56. Zeelen F.J. and Bergink E.W. : In : Cytotoxic Estrogens in Hormone Receptive Tumors, Raus J., Martens H. and Leclercq G. eds (Academic Press, New York 1980) pp. 39-48.

DISCUSSION

MCLACHLAN: Are the differences seen in binding between C-3 hydroxyl or keto compounds the result of chemical bonding (generally) to the receptor, or a change in electron distribution as suggested by Dr. Duax?

RAYNAUD: It seems that hydrogen binding is achieved with both a hydrogen donor or acceptor at the C_3 position of the steroid molecule.

PURDY: Would you kindly provide information on the in vivo hormonal activity of the unusual A-nor derivative (2α-ethinyl, 2β-hydroxy) where the relative binding activity is 20% of that of estradiol?

RAYNAUD: They possess weak antagonist activity.

JORDAN: Do you observe antiestrogenic activity if you extend the 11-substitution in estradiol?

RAYNAUD: Yes, depending on the nature of the substitution. We can also obtain agonist activity with fairly bulky substitutions.

JORDAN: Do 11-substituted compounds exhibit the species differences in estrogenic/antiestrogenic activity similar to that observed with tamoxifen?

RAYNAUD: We have not tested these compounds in different species to a sufficient extent to deduce a definite answer.

SIITERI: How do you account for variations in nonspecific binding at equilibrium of various analogues? These interactions confound the interpretations of relative receptor binding potency. For example, we have not been able to demonstrate binding of tamoxifen (or 4-hydroxy tamoxifen) to receptor in rat uterine cytosol by equilibrium methods.

RAYNAUD: This is a very important question. For some compounds which have been tritium-labeled, we have measured the rate of association and dissociation and were able to deduce affinity constants at equilibrium. The values are generally higher than those measured by the DCC adsorption method. We cannot generalize to all the compounds we have studied because it will be unrealistic to label all but the most interesting compounds. The reason why we have developed multifraction/multitime incubation binding conditions is to evaluate to what extent the ligand-receptor complex is stable vis a vis the actual hormone receptor complex.

ABUL-HAJJ: Have you looked at the estrogen receptor binding activity of 4,9,11-estratriene-3β,17β-diol?

RAYNAUD: No.

Published by Elsevier Science Publishing Co., Inc.
Estrogens in the Environment, John A. McLachlan, Editor

STEREOCHEMICAL ANALYSIS OF STILBENE ESTROGENS: RECEPTOR BINDING AND
HORMONE RESPONSIVENESS

KENNETH S. KORACH[1], LOUIS A. LEVY[2] AND PAMELA J. SARVER[1]
[1]Laboratory of Reproductive and Developmental Toxicology, and
[2]Laboratory of Molecular Biology, National Institute of Environmental
Health Sciences, NIH, P.O. Box 12233, Research Triangle Park, North
Carolina 27709, U.S.A.

In earlier studies we reported the receptor binding and uterotropic

activity of a number of DES metabolites [1]. In those and later studies

we described that oxidative metabolism of DES [2] resulted in products

which retained some hormonal and receptor binding activity. Figure 1

lists some of these compounds and their respective activities.

BINDING AFFINITIES AND UTEROTROPIC ACTIVITIES OF DES METABOLITES

COMPOUND	c_{50}	K_d	UTEROTROPIC STIMULATION	COMPOUND	c_{50}	K_d	UTEROTROPIC STIMULATION
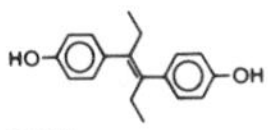 E-DES	0.5	0.5	5±1	INDANESTROL	60	0.006	1120±40
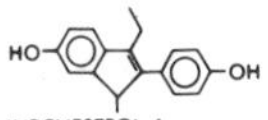 INDENESTROL A	0.7	0.45	107±14	Z-DES	130	0.003	–
INDENESTROL B	0.7	0.45	111±6	3,4 DIHYDROXY DES	334	0.001	3374±700
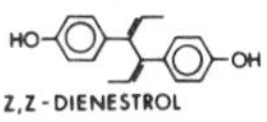 Z-PSEUDO DES	1.1	0.7	500±20	Z,Z-DIENESTROL	367	0.001	15000
17β-ESTRADIOL	1.2	0.8	5±2	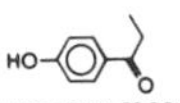 4-HYDROXY PROPIOPHENONE	<1000	–	–
E-DES 3,4 OXIDE	17	0.02	14±2				

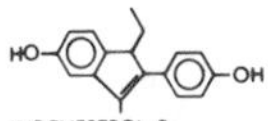

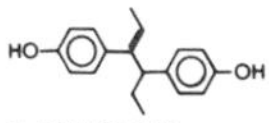

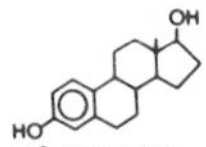

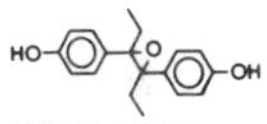

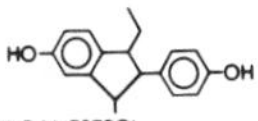

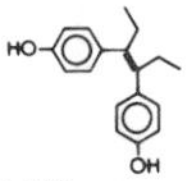

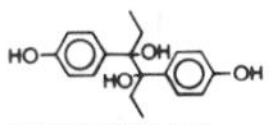

FIG. 1. Binding affinities (K_d), half maximal binding values (c_{50}) and
activities (µg/kg dose) of some DES metabolites and analogs in the mouse
uterus. K_d values expressed as nM^{-1} units.

One of the chemical features of DES which was thought to explain its

possible carcinogenicity is the stilbene double bond. Three of the compounds which are products of that metabolic pathway involving metabolism of the stilbene double bond are shown in the figure. Metabolic conversion of this bond to a 3,4 epoxide; 3,4 dihydroxy DES and finally 4-hydroxypropiophenone results in a progressive decrease in both receptor affinity and uterotropic activity. Several of the DES compounds were found to be more active at receptor binding than the endogenous ligand estradiol. Two groups of compounds, pseudo-DES and indanyl-DES, were of particular interest because they possessed these strong binding affinities but weak uterotropic activity [3]. These compounds exist in various isomeric forms which might explain their differences in biological activity. However, the structural variations are very subtle, and it was suspected that these differences would not be significant enough to be an explanation. In order to examine this poor biological activity, we have attempted to investigate the receptor mediated mechanism of estrogen action in the uterus (Fig. 2) and evaluate if certain steps or responses are compromised or altered due to treatment with these various compounds.

The DES derivative compounds indenestrol A (IA), indenestrol B (IB) and indanestrol (I) are structurally more rigid than DES because one of the side chains is bonded back onto the ring. Pseudo-DES (PD) is partly structurally restricted since the double bond is now shifted to one of the side chains. Moreover, PD can exist in E or Z isomeric forms. Preliminary studies with these isomers indicate that the uterine estrogen receptor binds the two isomers with different affinity. This suggests that the orientation of the terminal methyl group is influential in the receptor ligand interaction [4]. The strongest affinity is for the Z isomer shown in Fig. 1. The E-PD isomer is approximately 15 times weaker. The unsaturated indanyl compounds IA and IB differ in the position of the double bond but have equivalent binding affinities, which are themselves better than estradiol and in the same range as DES. Receptor interaction of the saturated isomer (indanestrol) is 100 times less.

Poor binding activity of indanestrol may be an explanation for the weak biological activity, since significant quantities of ligand receptor complexes would not be formed. This relationship of binding affinity, receptor occupancy and the ability of a compound to induce biological responses has been a long-standing concept in describing the mechanism of estrogen hormone action [5].

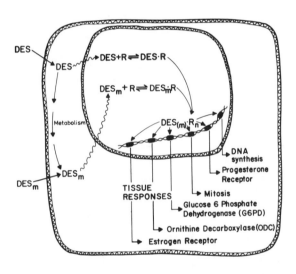

FIG. 2. Diagram of uterine estrogen target cell taken from the refined model of estrogen receptor localization [7]. Abbreviations used: (DES) diethylstilbestrol, (R) estrogen receptor, (R_n) activated form of estrogen receptor.

X-ray crystallographic analysis of the indanyl compounds illustrates that the unsaturated isomers exhibit a planar structure, while the saturated isomer (indanestrol), which has the weaker binding affinity, has a conformation in which the two phenyl rings are oriented at right angles to each other [6]. Considering the differences seen in binding affinity of these compounds, the molecular structure of indanestrol could explain its apparent activity. However, pseudo-DES also shows an angular molecular structure similar to indanestrol [4]. PD is a much higher affinity ligand than indanestrol, suggesting that a planar structure is not a requisite for high affinity and that the weak binding of indanestrol is not simply due to its angular molecular structure. We are presently involved in testing molecular mechanics programs and energy calculations in an attempt to explain these observations.

As shown in the model in Fig. 2 which is taken as a refinement [7] of the earlier two step model of estrogen hormone action [5], binding activity of the ligand is correlated to nuclear receptor levels resulting in the expression of various tissue responses. Nuclear estrogen receptor levels and their degree of retention in the nucleus have been suggested as a correlative to hormone responsiveness [8]. Therefore, it was possible that these compounds would not produce similar nuclear receptor levels or retention as the potent synthetic estrogen DES. Such an approach was used with steroidal compounds such as estriol, illustrating poor nuclear receptor retention resulting in weak and incomplete uterine stimulation [9]. Results of these types of studies are shown in Figures 3 and 4. Figure 3 illustrates the receptor distribution pattern after a 20 μg/kg dose of DES. Figure 4 shows the pattern after treatment with the three DES compounds having the highest binding affinity. Comparison of the nuclear receptor levels shows that the pattern of IA, IB, and PD are essentially the same as those with DES (Fig. 3). These compounds retain as much receptor in the nucleus as DES but are not active biologically (e.g., Fig. 1), suggesting that the presence of the receptor protein itself within the nucleus is not all that is needed for stimulation. These results would question the earlier ideas that long-term retention of estrogen receptor complex is all that is needed for uterine growth stimulation. The results also illustrate the bimodal pattern of nuclear receptor reported earlier with steroidal compounds [10].

In the past we have suggested the second increase in nuclear estrogen receptor may be linked to uterine growth and DNA synthesis [11]. On the

other hand, the presence of the peak occurred with both steroidal as well
as stilbene estrogens. These types of compounds share a phenolic ring
structure and have been reported to undergo enterohepatic recirculation
[12,13]. It was possible that the second peak was generated by enterohepatic recirculation producing a bolus of the compound which could
interact with receptor to cause a peak. We tested this possibility by
determining the receptor distribution pattern in germ free (axemic) CD-1
mice which are void of intestinal bacterial flora and demonstrate no
apparent enterohepatic recirculation metabolism [14]. The profile is
shown in Fig. 3. Levels of nuclear estrogen receptor are slightly lower
than those seen in the regular CD-1 animal but qualitatively similar.
The fact that the axemic animals exhibit a second peak and respond com-
parably with a uterotropic stimulation (data not presented) would suggest
this metabolic route is not an influence on the hormonal activity or
nuclear receptor pattern produced with DES.

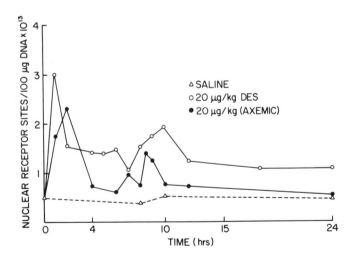

FIG. 3. Nuclear occupancy pattern after single IP injection of DES at
zero time into either normal (0) or axemic (●) mice. Receptor measurements quantified by the exchange assay as previously described.

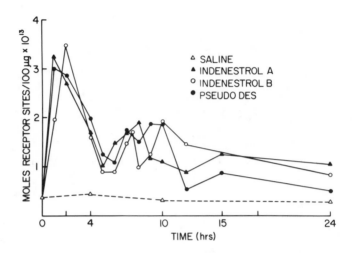

FIG. 4. Nuclear occupancy pattern after single IP injections at zero time of DES compounds. Nuclear receptor measured as described in Figure 3 legend.

Several years ago it had been demonstrated that total nuclear estrogen receptor levels were composed of salt extractable and salt resistant receptor sites. The non-extractable form was considered to be tightly associated with nuclear genomic structures [15]. It was also thought that the level of these salt resistant sites might be a better indication of tissue responsiveness. Preliminary results with the different DES compounds shown in Fig. 5 indicate that the level of salt resistant sites is comparable to DES. These levels are slightly lower than those detected with estradiol but are greater than 5X control. IA showed the lowest levels but was not significantly different than DES or the other DES compounds. We are continuing these studies and investigating the level of salt resistant sites at later times after stimulation to determine if this may show a better relationship to uterotropic activity.

Besides the nuclear estrogen receptor, new studies have suggested a
second nuclear binding site may be present and that binding of compounds
to this site is related to the mechanism of uterine growth stimulation
[16]. The possibility that the DES compounds were not active estrogens
because they did not bind to this type II site was tested. An argument
to support this relationship had been described earlier [17] for the
antiestrogenic activity of Nafoxidine in the rat uterus. Results of the
nuclear binding assay are shown in Fig. 6.

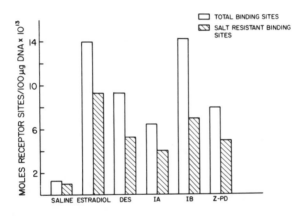

FIG. 5. Levels of total and 0.6 M KCl non-extractable nuclear receptor
sites 1h after IP injection of 20 μg/kg dose of compounds.

These assays measure the effectiveness of these unlabeled compounds to
act as competitors for the nuclear binding sites. Indanestrol and
Nafoxidine are both weak binders to the estrogen receptor type I site as
shown in the region of the binding curve below 10 nM estradiol. This is
consistent with the indanestrol data in Fig. 1 indicating a low affinity.
We have also determined that Nafoxidine binds approximately 60 times
poorer than estradiol to the mouse uterine estrogen receptor (unpublished
observations). When binding occurs in the type II region (10-40 nM), the
Nafoxidine is weakly active as reported [18], but indanestrol binds as
effectively as DES. The other DES compounds are effective binders in

both the type I and type II region. Interaction with the type II site
appears not to be an explanation for their poor biological activity,
since all the stilbene type compounds bind to the type II site but have
weak biological activity. Nafoxidine, on the other hand, is a potent
estrogen in the mouse uterus and does not bind to the type II sites.
Further work with additional compounds will be needed to more clearly
ascertain the possible function and role for this type II binding site.

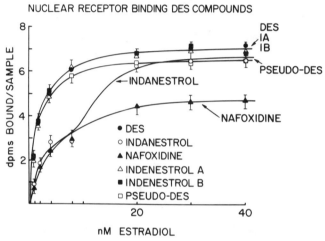

FIG. 6. Competitive binding of DES, DES compounds and Nafoxidine to
nuclear binding sites. Results are expressed as specific binding (dpms
bound) per common unit of sample DNA.

Figure 2 illustrates several uterine responses linked to estrogen
stimulation involving nuclear receptor genomic interactions. As mentioned
earlier, we have investigated the activity of several of these responses
as they relate to stimulation with these DES compounds. It was reported
earlier [19] that weak estrogens stimulate uterine biochemical responses
to a diminished degree. Therefore, it was expected that these DES compounds would demonstrate the same activity. Experiments were performed
at 20 μg/kg dose, which we have already demonstrated will result in the
same quantitative and qualitative pattern of nuclear estrogen receptor in
the uterus. Stimulation of glucose 6-phosphate dehydrogenase (G6PD) has

been used by many laboratories as a marker for estrogen action [20].

Results are shown in Fig. 7. Estradiol was the most active while IA

was similar to DES and slightly lower than estradiol. None of the other

compounds produced activity above the control group. Expanded dose

response studies confirmed this difference between IA and IB isomers.

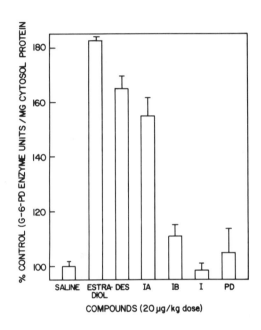

FIG. 7. Uterine glucose 6-phosphate dehydrogenase activity measured
24h after single treatment. Enzyme analysis performed as previously
described [20] and results taken from reference [33].

Indanestrol was not surprising since it gave very low nuclear receptor

levels at this dose, but PD was as low as IB, and both of these gave

significant nuclear receptor occupancy. Estradiol has been shown by

Barker and associates to stimulate G6PD at both a transcriptional and

translational level [21]. Similar studies with stilbene estrogens have

not been performed, so the various sites of stimulation may or may not be

the same as with estradiol. It is possible that there is a genomic site

for the receptor complex which results in transcriptional activity produced by estradiol, DES, or IA. On the other hand, estradiol could also have an affect on translational activity for G6PD thereby producing a slightly higher activity.

Ornithine decarboxylase (ODC) has been shown to correlate with estrogen stimulation in target tissues. The enzyme controls the rate limiting step in polyamine biosynthesis [22]. Activity is stimulated maximally by 16h in the rat uterus [23] and mouse uterus (data not presented) after a single treatment. Results of such experiments using the DES compounds are shown in Fig. 8, where activity with DES is increased 600 times control at both doses. Enzymatic activity is not significantly stimulated by PD at either dose, yet it is slightly above control at 20 μg/kg IA. The higher IA dose and both IB doses were approximately twice control. The pattern of activity is not the same as seen with G6PD stimulation (Fig. 7).

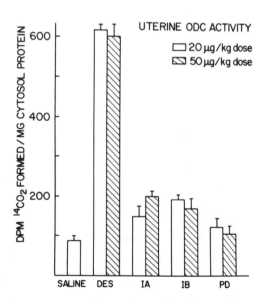

FIG. 8. Ornithine decarboxylase activity measured 16h after single treatment. Enzyme analysis performed as previously described [23].

Another estrogen protein synthetic response is stimulation of soluble
progesterone receptor levels. This induction has been shown to be relatively estrogen specific in target tissues such as the uterus or mammary
gland [19]. Results are taken from Scatchard plot analysis and are shown
in Fig. 9 as moles receptor per mg cytosol protein.

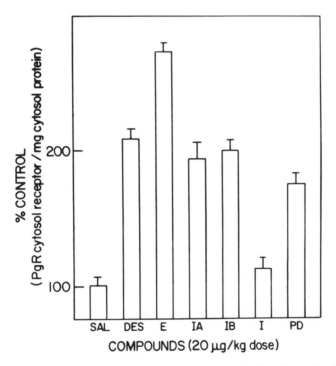

FIG. 9. Uterine soluble progesterone receptor levels after single
stimulation with compounds. Results taken from reference [33].

Estradiol was the most effective ligand, similarly to what was seen for
the G6PD response. However, all the DES compounds except indanestrol
produced comparable progesterone receptor levels. This was significantly
different from the G6PD response (Fig. 7) where IB and PD were not active
in stimulating that response. Such observations are particularly
interesting since past reports of poor stimulation of a variety of tissue

responses being related to weak receptor interactions of particular compounds such as estriol or dimethylstilbestrol [24].

A number of studies with mammary tumor cells (MCF-7) have correlated
progesterone stimulation with estrogen responsive cell growth. It was
interesting to evaluate the DNA synthesis and mitotic activity of these
DES compounds to determine if it correlated with the progesterone receptor
levels (Fig. 9). In the adult mouse uterus estrogen stimulation of DNA
synthesis is maximal at 16h after a single injection of hormone and specific for epithelial cells [25]. The dose response stimulation of uterine
DNA synthesis is shown in Fig. 10. Experiments investigating the time
course of DNA synthesis illustrated that the poor activity of the DES
compounds was not due to a shift in the response time. DES was the most
active while IB produced comparable stimulation at a 5X higher dose.

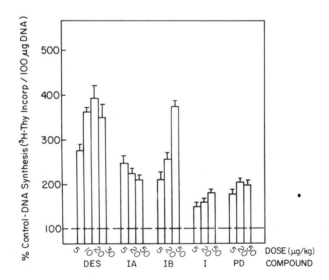

FIG. 10. Uterine DNA synthesis activity measured at 16h after single
treatment with varying doses of DES compounds. DNA synthesis assay performed as previously described [25].

Interestingly, IA did not show a dose increase but, in fact, gave a
slight dose-related decrease. Most importantly, the two unsaturated

isomers (IA and IB) gave very different results. PD and I gave low activity which was expected for indanestrol but unexpected for PD, particularly because PD produced similar stimulation of progesterone receptor levels as DES. IA also showed this same relationship of dissociating stimulation of progesterone receptor from DNA synthesis. Recently, this same concept has been suggested with estrogen responsive cells in culture [26]. This is the first indication of this varied responsiveness in an in vivo model system.

In the past, we have suggested that for uterine DNA synthesis there may be a requirement for a second nuclear receptor stimulation [11]. This event is correlated to a discontinuous requirement for estrogen stimulation which has been demonstrated with estriol in both the mouse [27] and rat [28] uterus. We attempted to evaluate whether this same phenomenon could be demonstrated with a stilbene estrogen. Indanestrol was selected since it was relatively inactive as far as DNA synthesis and had short receptor occupancy. Multiple injections of indanestrol were given at two different doses in a combination of different times. Results are shown in Fig. 11. Multiple injections of 25 µg/kg were unsuccessful in stimulating activity to the same extent as the DES treatment. Multiple treatments of 50 µg/kg dose of indanestrol given at 0 and 6h was the only treatment which stimulated DNA synthesis to the same extent as a single injection of DES. Combination doses at earlier or later times were not as effective, supporting the idea that a secondary stimulation at a particular time is necessary. The 6h stimulation time is consistent with the need to produce nuclear receptor around 7-8h [11]. Studies are underway to determine the uterotropic stimulation and receptor levels during this type of experimental protocol.

Uterine hyperplasia and hypertrophy are some of the primary physiological actions of estrogenic agents. There have been reports that certain types of triphenylethylene compounds may produce the hypertrophy

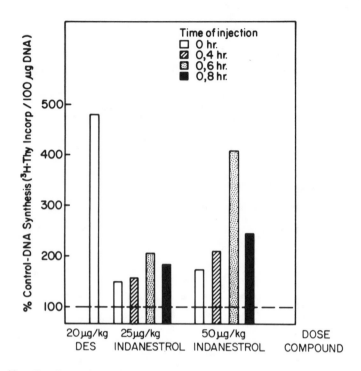

FIG. 11. Uterine DNA synthesis activity after multiple injections of varying doses of indanestrol.

response with no subsequent hyperplasia [29]. In an earlier study we had suggested a similar possibility for PD [3] after histological evaluation of uterine specimens. In order to further test this observation, we have quantified uterine mitotic activity by counting the number of colchicine arrested mitotic figures and the tissue hypertrophy by measuring the cell height after stimulation with different DES compounds. Results of those studies are listed in Fig. 12. The number of mitotic cells increase dramatically after treatment with DES as well as the cell hypertrophy in both the luminal and glandular epithelium. Stromal cells were not stimulated, thereby, indicating the activity of the DES compounds to be in the same tissue cell type as DES or estradiol. Levels of mitotic activity increase with the two indenestrol isomers but not to the same degree as with DES. Cell height stimulation is comparable to DES. Indanestrol

effects were indistinguishable from saline controls. Results obtained

with PD were very different with no apparent increase in mitotis but a

significant hypertrophy response. The responses in glandular epithelium

to PD were not the same as luminal since there were no increases in

either mitotic activity or tissue hypertrophy, although treatment with

DES or the other compounds showed consistent results in both tissue

types. It is unclear at the present time whether this difference in

responsiveness of the two types of epithelium to PD is of physiological

importance. It has been shown, however, that there is a clear compartmen-

talization of tissue response to triphenylethylenes in the rat uterus

[30]. Most importantly, the results with PD in luminal epithelium suggest

a dissociation of hypertrophy from hyperplasia because the cells were

stimulated to increase in size but not in division. A similar observation

was made earlier concerning Nafoxidine stimulation of uterine tissue cell

types [17].

MITOTIC ACTIVITY OF UTERINE EPITHELIAL COMPARTMENTS
AFTER STIMULATION WITH DES ANALOGS

TREATMENT	LUMINAL EPITHELIUM		GLANDULAR EPITHELIUM	
	MITOSIS/SECTION	CELL HEIGHT	MITOSIS/SECTION	
SALINE	2	13 ± 1	0	7 ± 1
DES	48	21 ± 1	11	14 ± 2
IA	23	23 ± 2	13	11 ± 2
IB	20	18 ± 2	6	10 ± 1
I	3	13 ± 1	2	7 ± 0
PD	3	18 ± 1	0	9 ± 1

ANIMALS WERE SACRIFICED 24 HRS. AFTER IP INJECTION OF 20μg/KGDOSE
OF THE COMPOUNDS. COLCHICINE 5μgWAS GIVEN IP 2 HRS. PRIOR TO
SACRIFICE.

FIG. 12. Uterine epithelial cell mitotic activity and hypertrophy
response.

As originally mentioned, our interest in these DES compounds arises from their differential biological activity and chemical structures. In the course of our studies with these compounds we had observed that at doses of 10 μg/kg or less, nuclear receptor levels were lower in the IA group than with DES, PD, or IB, even though the binding affinities were comparable to each. This was particularly surprising in comparing the indenestrol isomers which differed only in the position of the double bond and had the same apparent binding affinity (Fig. 1). An illustration of this difference is shown in Fig. 13.

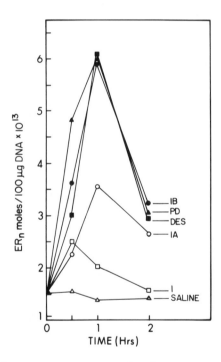

FIG. 13. Nuclear estrogen receptor levels at varying times after single treatment of 10 μg/kg DES compounds. Receptor levels measured as described in Fig. 3 legend.

The IA levels at 1h are approximately 55% of the DES or IB levels. An in vivo pharmacokinetic difference of these isomers where IA was either metabolized or excreted more readily than IB or the other compounds could be an explanation. At the present time, information on further metabolism of these metabolites is not known and will await synthesis of radiolabeled ligand for such studies to be performed. Another point which was considered was the fact that the indenestrol compounds possessed a single chiral carbon atom and exist as a mixture of enantiomers (Fig. 14). Our studies described above and in previous work [2,3] had utilized a racemic mixture of the enantiomers of IA or IB. Therefore, it was possible that the lower nuclear receptor levels observed with IA at low doses could be because the receptor had a binding preference for one of the enantiomers. The IA enantiomers were separated by HPLC utilizing a chiral stationary phase and the separated enantiomers shown to have identical mass spectra and nuclear magnetic resonance spectra but opposite optical rotation spectrum. Enantiomer peak 1 has $[\alpha]^D$ +205 and peak 2 has $[\alpha]^D$ −211. Results of the competitive estrogen receptor binding assays are shown in Fig. 15. There is a 20-fold difference in the binding activity of the two enantiomers. The racemic mixture binds with a value between that found with the separate enantiomers.

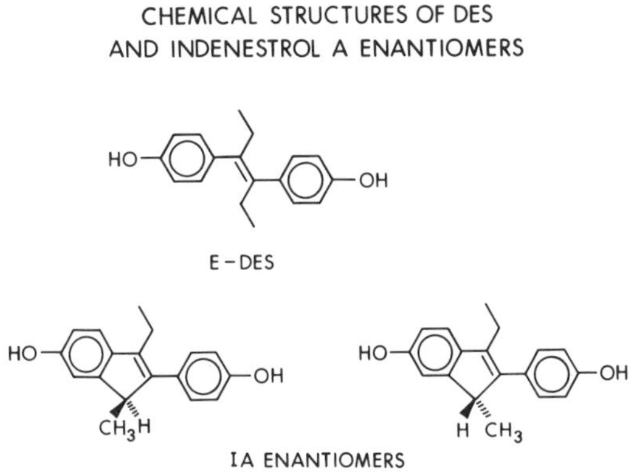

CHEMICAL STRUCTURES OF DES
AND INDENESTROL A ENANTIOMERS

E – DES

IA ENANTIOMERS

FIG. 14. Diethylstilbestrol and indenestrol A structures.

It was interesting to see that enantiomer peak 2 bound as well as DES, which is one of the highest affinity ligands for the estrogen receptor binding site. Studies have been reported by Katzenellenbogen and associates [30] analyzing the stereochemistry of hexestrol in attempts to describe its binding mode to the estrogen receptor in relation to estradiol. Those studies did not demonstrate significant differences in the binding of hexestrol enantiomers but showed some differences using norhexestrol derivatives. Our studies are consistent with the idea that the estrogen receptor binding site demonstrates stereochemical recognition.

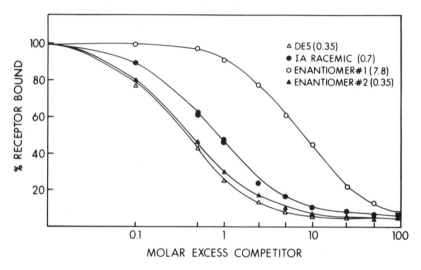

FIG. 15. Competitive binding activity of DES and indenestrol A mixture and enantiomers. Values in parentheses are the C_{50} values and represent the molar excess of competitor required to occupy 50% of the receptor binding sites.

In an attempt to determine if this binding difference was an explanation for the nuclear receptor levels seen in earlier investigations (Fig. 13), individual enantiomers were tested for their ability to increase nuclear receptor levels. Results shown in Fig. 16 are based on a 10 µg/kg dose of DES as a positive control. The difference between the two enantiomers were dramatic. The IA racemic mixture gave results similar

to those seen earlier (Fig. 13) where an identical dose gave about half
the nuclear receptor levels while the levels were the same with the 20
μg/kg dose. Enantiomer peak 1 which had the lowest binding activity
showed very weak in vivo activity to occupy nuclear receptors; only at a
dose of 200-300 μg/kg did the levels approach those of either DES or the
IA racemic mixture. On the other hand, enantiomer peak 2 was quite active
and was equal to the DES effect at a similar 10 μg/kg dose. Higher doses
of IA-2 did not increase the receptor level, illustrating the saturation
of the receptor system at the 10 μg/kg dose.

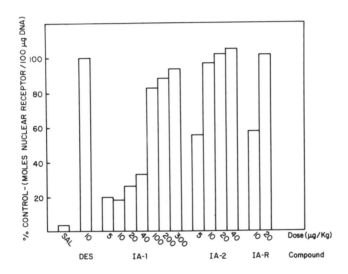

FIG. 16. Uterine nuclear estrogen receptor levels 1h after single
treatment with varying dose of compounds. Levels quantified as described
in Fig. 3 legend.

Comparison of the doses of enantiomer required to saturate the nuclear
receptor levels would indicate a similar 20X activity difference as seen
in the different binding affinities. Therefore, it is clear that the
nuclear receptor values produced by the IA racemate are due to the
activity of only one enantiomer (e.g. peak 2). Enantiomer peak 1 is not
appreciably active at the doses used with the IA racemate. Moreover, the

biological response data described earlier is apparently due to the activity of the one enantiomer. Interestingly, the structure of that enantiomer allows it to bind and interact as well as DES, but comparable biological activity does not result suggesting that the ligand structure may play a more significant role in hormone stimulation than simply to occupy or activate the estrogen receptor.

Our earlier work had analyzed the molecular structure of these indanyl compounds and compared them to DES and estradiol. Those analyses suggested the possibility that the indenestrol compounds (i.e. IA and IB) could have different binding modes. Figure 17 illustrates a molecular comparison of the conformation of the two IA enantiomers taken from the x-ray crystallography studies [6].

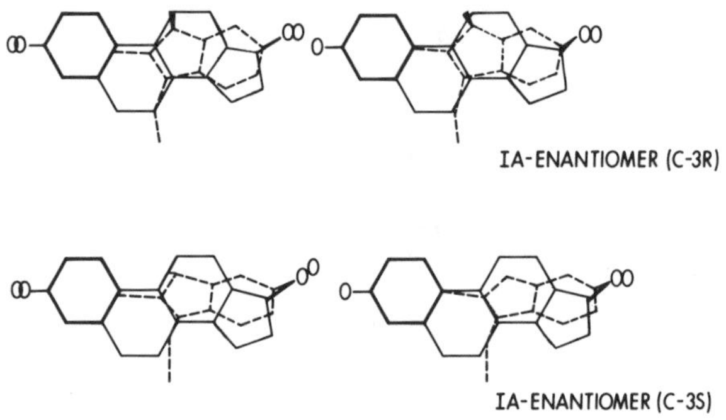

IA-ENANTIOMER (C-3R)

IA-ENANTIOMER (C-3S)

FIG. 17. Diagrammatic representation of molecular structures of estradiol (solid line) and indenestrol enantiomers (dotted line). Figures are compiled from results in reference [6].

When the α-ring of IA is aligned with the A-ring of estradiol, the chiral center of IA most closely aligns with carbon 11 of the steroid structure. In the case of the C-3R enantiomer conformation, the methyl group is in a β-orientation while in the C-3S enantiomer there is an α-orientation. We

are presently synthesizing bromoacetoxy derivatives of the indanyl compounds in order to separate the enantiomers in a form that can be analyzed
by x-ray crystallographic analysis to deduce the absolute molecular configuration of the enantiomer peaks 1 and 2. It is probable that the C-3R
enantiomer is the active form since studies from Bouton and Raynaud using
estradiol derivatives have indicated that the 11 β-epimer of moxestrol
binds with higher affinity than the 11 α-form [31]. The α-orientation of
groups in that region of the ligand suggest some stereochemical restric-
tion in the receptor binding site. Recent studies investigating
2-phenylindole derivatives have suggested that substitution of a nitrogen
atom for the carbon atom in that position results in a compound with
significantly weaker activity [32]. Molecular comparisons of those
structures have not been reported, but it suggests that orientation of
the methyl is important in influencing the binding activity. Preliminary
results with the IB enantiomers demonstrated no difference in the binding
activity or nuclear occupancy and indicate that orientation of the ethyl
group corresponding to the C7-C8 region of the steroid is not restricted
by the binding site. This suggests that the binding mode of these
stilbene comounds is similar and that the binding site may have a border
which fits the upper region of the steroid nucleus in juxtaposition to
carbons 11, 12, 13, and 17. It appears that derivatives occupying the
lower edge of the steroid, such as carbons 4 and 6, do not decrease
activity to a great extent. This may be due to the fact that the ligand
binding site is open to that region of the molecule. Further work with
additional ligands is underway in an attempt to model the estrogen receptor binding site.

SUMMARY

Our initial approach in these studies was to simply determine what sites in the model of estrogen stimulation and tissue responsiveness were compromised by the different stilbene compounds. These studies have led to some interesting results, summarized below, concerning the estrogen receptor and estrogen uterine responsiveness. Hopefully, further investigations with these compounds may be even more informative to our understanding of estrogen action.

- Chemicals or compounds do not have to exhibit a planar structure to have high binding affinity (pseudo-DES isomers).

- Nuclear estrogen receptor occupancy is necessary but is not the only requisite needed for uterine stimulation or growth (pseudo-DES and indanestrol).

- Uterine tissue responses can be stimulated individually depending on the receptor ligand (indanyl DES compounds).

- Previously interrelated estrogen hormone responses can be dissociated suggesting alternative mechanism for estrogen stimulation of protein synthesis [PgR] and growth [DNA synthesis] (pseudo-DES and indenestrol A and B).

- The estrogen receptor exhibits selective stereochemistry in the ligand binding site. Only certain regions of the ligand have stereochemical influences on binding (indenestrol A and B enantiomers, pseudo-DES isomers).

ACKNOWLEDGMENTS

The authors would like to thank Thomas Golding, Michael Walker and Laura Benecki for their technical assistance and discussions; to Ms. Anna Lee Howard for her speed and excellence in typing this manuscript.

REFERENCES

1. K.S. Korach, M. Metzler, and J.A. McLachlan, Proc. Nat. Acad. Sci. 75, 468-471 (1978).
2. K.S. Korach in: Hormones and Cancer, E. Leavitt, ed. (Plenum Press, New York 1982) pp. 39-62.
3. K.S. Korach, M. Metzler, and J.A. McLachlan, J. Biol. Chem. 254, 8963-8968 (1979).
4. W.L. Duax, J.L. Griffin, C.M. Weeks, and K.S. Korach in: Environmental Health Perspectives: Structure Activity Correlations in Mechanism Studies in Predicative Toxicology, J.D. McKinney, ed. (In Press).
5. E.V. Jensen, T. Suzuki, T. Kawashima, W.E. Stumpf, P. Jungblutt, and E.R. DeSombre, Proc. Nat. Acad. Sci. 59, 632-638 (1968).
6. W.L. Duax, D.C. Swenson, P.D. Strong, K.S. Korach, J.A. McLachlan, and M. Metzler, Mol. Pharmacol. 26, 520-525 (1984).
7. J. Gorski, W. Welshons, and D. Sakai, Mol. Cell Endocr. 36, 11-15 (1984).
8. J.N. Anderson, E.J. Peck, Jr., and J.H. Clark, Endocrinology 96, 160-167 (1975).
9. J.H. Clark, Z. Paszko, and E.J. Peck, Jr., Endocrinology 100, 91-96 (1977).
10. K.S. Korach and E.B. Ford, Biochem. Biophys. Res. Comm. 83, 827-833 (1978).
11. K.S. Korach, C. Fox-Davies, and V. Baker, Endocrinology 106, 1900-1906 (1980).
12. H.M. Bolt, Pharmacol. Ther. 4, 155-181 (1979).
13. L.J. Fischer, J.L. Weissinger, D.E. Rickert, and K.L. Hintze, J. Toxicol. Environ. Hlth. 1, 587-606 (1976).
14. I. Nakamura, K. Hosokawa, H. Tamura, and T. Mirura, Bull. Environ. Cont. Tox. 17, 528-533, 1977.
15. J.H. Clark and E.J. Peck, Jr., Nature 260, 635-637, (1976).
16. J.H. Clark, B. Markaverich, S. Upchurch, H. Eriksson, and J.W. Hardin, Adv. Expt. Med. Biol. 117, 17-46 (1979).
17. B.M. Markaverich, S. Upchurch, S. McCormack, S.R. Glasser, and J.H. Clark, Biol. Reprod. 24, 171-181 (1981).
18. B.M. Markaverich, M. Williams, S. Upchurch, and J.H. Clark, Endocrinology 109, 62-69 (1981).
19. J.H. Clark and E.J. Peck, Jr., Female Sex Steroid Receptors and Function (Springer Verlag, New York 1979).
20. B.C. Moulton and K.L. Barker, Endocrinology 89, 1131-1136 (1971).
21. K.L. Barker, D.J. Adams, and T.M. Donohue, Jr. in: Cellular and Molecular Aspects of Implantation, S.R. Glasser and D.W. Bullock, eds. (Plenum Press, New York 1981) pp. 269-281.
22. C.W. Tabor and H. Tabor, Annu. Rev. Biochem. 45, 285-306 (1976).
23. E.A. Rorke, K.L. Kendra, and B.S. Katzenellenbogen, Mol. Cell. Endocrinol. 38, 31-38 (1984).
24. B.S. Katzenellenbogen, H.S. Iwamoto, D.F. Heiman, N.C Lan, and J.A. Katzenellenbogen, Mol. Cell Endocrinol. 10, 103-113 (1978).
25. V.E. Quarmby and K.S. Korach, Endocrinology 115, 687-697 (1984).
26. R.L. Eckert and B.S. Katzenellenbogen, Cancer Res. 42, 139-144 (1982).
27. K.S. Korach and C. Fox-Davies, 64th Endocrine Society Program, No. 622 (1982).
28. J. Harris and J. Gorski, Endocrinology 103, 240-245 (1978).
29. J.H. Clark, J.W. Hardin, H.A. Padykula, and C.A. Cardasis, Proc. Nat. Acad. Sci. 75, 2781-2784 (1978).
30. S.W. Landvatter and J.A. Katzenellenbogen, Mol. Pharmacol. 20, 43-51 (1981).
31. M.M. Bouton and J.P. Raynaud, Endocrinology 105, 509-515 (1979).

32. E. von Angerer, J. Prekajac, and J. Strohmeier, J. Med. Chem. 27, 1439-1447 (1984).
33. K.S. Korach, C. Fox-Davies, V.E. Quarmby, and M.H. Swaisgood, J. Biol. Chem. (In Press).

DISCUSSION

NAFTOLIN: This work is very illuminating; however, it does not invalidate prior and continuing work of Drs. James H. Clark, J. P. Raynaud, and others which indicates that such matters as nuclear residence time, association, and disassociation constants are important in estrogen action.

KORACH: I completely agree that our studies do not invalidate past work. Those studies you mentioned were completely correct for the type of steroidal compounds used (e.g., estriol). Although, as we have shown here, these DES compounds are unique enough in structure that they can be used as probes to examine individual responses which appear to be stimulated independently. In fact, those criteria you mentioned are also demonstrable by some of these DES compounds such as indanestrol or E-pseudo DES which have poor binding, short nuclear residency times, and weak biological activity.

MCLACHLAN: I would make a plea that we broaden our concept of estrogen interactions with cellular macromolecules to say "estrogen binding sites" rather than only referring to estrogen receptor. This takes into account other actions at various intracellular loci and helps keep our ideas of mechanisms of action sufficiently flexible.

KORACH: The concept of estrogen action in target cells and target tissue could be broadened to account for the newer observations concerning effects of estrogens on membranes, ribosomal components, etc. However, these types of interactions may not fall into the classical definitions of steroid (e.g., estrogen) receptor which we are familiar with, including "ligand specificity and related biological response." This definition, of course, separates the receptor, as defined, from a steroid binding protein. As more information is compiled on these other actions of estradiol, the definition may need to be restated, where the receptor is another binding protein which interacts in the nucleus in the course of its action.

CUNHA: Have you measured estrogen receptor (ER) in individual cell types and related ER level to actual biological response in individual cell types?

KORACH: We have measured estrogen receptor in epithelial cell components using receptor binding assays. By using modified procedures to stabilize the receptor, accurate measurements can be made. At the present, we have not applied those techniques to studies with the DES compounds. However, we do know from autoradiography studies that the DES compounds do stimulate mitotic and DNA synthetic responses in the same epithelial cell types as estradiol or steroidal estrogens in the ovariectomized animals.

RAYNAUD: Has the enantiomer 3S of Indenestrol weak or even antiestrogenic activity?

KORACH: We have only recently obtained sufficient quantities of the isolated pure enantiomers to study the estrogen receptor binding and nuclear receptor levels produced by in vivo treatment. In the future, we plan to assess the possible antiestrogenic properties of the enantiomers, but we have not done so as yet.

SONNENSCHEIN: The consensus of the previous two papers that I sense is that binding parameters to estrophilins is not a good criterion to measure the estrogenic potency of these compounds. Would you comment on this point?

KORACH: Binding parameters are still a good criterion for initial assessment of estrogenic potency, but they should not be used as the sole parameter. Biological activity, defined by whatever index you want to use, whether it is uterotropic stimulation, vaginal cornification or gonadotropin inhibition has to be assessed concomitantly. In the case of the common endogenous steroidal estrogens (estradiol, estrone, estriol), this relationship of receptor binding and/or nuclear residency to biological activity holds true. On the other hand, when you investigate other compounds such as triphenylethylene or stilbene compounds, this relationship is not necessarily obtained. This may suggest that there are additional mechanisms involved in stimulating these responses which are not accounted for by the receptor. One thing that is apparent is compounds which are very active biologically almost always bind to the receptor. There were some earlier cases where compounds did not bind to the receptor in vitro but were active in vivo. This was later shown to be due to metabolism to an active form. When the metabolite was tested, it was found to bind to the receptor. These observations are consistent with the receptor binding activity of the ligands.

MYERS: Receptor binding data as criteria for reflecting estrogenicity may be very misleading. Many types of compounds exhibit binding affinities close to that of estradiol-17β but lack in vivo activity. This type of compound has been described and discussed by endocrinologists. However, series of compounds that poorly compete with estradiol for cytosolic or nuclear estradiol receptors, yet are equal to estradiol in in vivo activity, are rarely discussed in terms of structure-activity relationships. The doisynolic acids and related "seco" steroid acids fall into the latter category.

KORACH: You are right. Most endocrinologists do discuss compounds in your first example where estriol is a good case. The stilbene compounds that I discussed here are additional examples. Compounds with these effects are important because their use allows the investigator to segregate various aspects of the hormone mechanism depending on their action for more detailed study. By comparing actions or responses with these compounds versus potent estrogens, we can ascertain how important the effect is to the overall mechanism and action. Your second point about the compounds with weak receptor binding but equal estrogenicity also is very interesting. These compounds, as I mentioned to Dr. Sonnenschein, were found to be active in vivo because of metabolism to an active form which binds the receptor. One of the best examples of this is the work from Drs. Kupfer and Bulger on methoxychlor. Other possibilities where metabolism of the compound is not an explanation involves examples where the compound actually causes an effect either in steroidogenic glands such as the adrenal or ovary to increase endogenous steroidogenesis resulting in a hormonal effect. In addition, the compound could also effect metabolism in such a way that the endogenous estrogens are not properly metabolized resulting in an effect. There are several alternative possibilities which have to be ruled out.

MEYERS: The chiral atoms of indenestrol A and B are allylic as well as benzylic, and should undergo quite rapid proton dissociation-reassociation. Like related chiral (α-carbon) ketones which racemize easily via the proton dissociation-reassociation route, these chiral indenestrols should undergo racemization relatively easily. Have you looked into this possibility in explaining your in vivo/in vitro data with the antipodal indenestrols? Have you run any deuterium/hydrogen exchange studies to examine the relative rates of proton dissociation?

KORACH: We have not performed any deuterium/hydrogen exchange reactions of these compounds. There is no discrepancy between the in vivo/in vitro data of the indenestrol A or B enantiomers. In those cases, where the enantiomer was a weak binder, it also resulted in poor nuclear receptor activity. The fact that the individual enantiomers of IA show the differences would argue against in vivo racemization. When the products of the treatments were reanalyzed, we obtained the same enantiomeric form which we had originally used, again suggesting the stability of the forms. Secondly, we have also followed the optical stability of the compounds in solution. This was also supported by Cram et al. who showed that optically active 1-t-butyl 3-methyl indene was optically stable except under conditions of very strong base.

NATURALLY OCCURRING NON-STEROIDAL ESTROGENS OF DIETARY ORIGIN

K.D.R. Setchell*
Clinical Mass Spectrometry Laboratory, Department of Pediatric Gastroenterology
and Nutrition, Children's Hospital Medical Center, Cincinnati, Ohio 45229, USA

INTRODUCTION

In 1954 Bradbury and White [1] listed 53 shown plants to possess estrogenic activity

as measured by their ability to initiate estrous in animals. Twenty years later over

3ↄ plants with this property were reported [2]. While the principal mammalian

estrogens, estradiol-17β and estrone have been shown to occur naturally in only a few

plants, the isoflavones, the coumestans and the resorcylic acid lactones (Fig. 1) are

the most commonly found classes of compounds identified with estrogenic activity.

Of more than twenty plant estrogens which have been found, many possess striking

similarities in structure to the synthetic and potent estrogen diethylstilbestrol (DES),

and this is particularly true for the isoflavones, many of which are regularly

consumed by man and animals. Table 1 lists some common foodstuffs consumed by

man with an indication of the active plant estrogens which have been recognized.

TABLE 1. Edible plants with recognized estrogenically active compounds.

Estrogens	Isoflavones	Coumestans	Resorcylic acid lactones	Others
liquorice	soyabean	alfalfa	oats	fennel
french bean	chick pea	soya sprouts	barley	carrot
date palm	cherry	cow pea	rye	anise
pomegranate		green beans	sesame	hops
apple		red beans	wheat	
		split peas	peas	

Compounds such as zearalenone and zearalenol which belong to the class of resorcylic

acid lactones are not intrinsic compounds of food plants but are secondary mould

metabolites of fungal spieces which generally accumulate on poorly stored grains and

seeds.

While the absolute levels of many of these estrogens may be low, it should be

emphasized that the overall consumption of several foods, particularly legumes, by

70

man is high and therefore the effects of chronic or long term exposure to such compounds may not be insignificant. This was amply illustrated from the problems of infertility in sheep, resulting from grazing in pastures rich in Trifolium subterraneum, a species of clover prevelant in Australia [3]. This particular species of clover is rich in the isoflavone formononetin, a weak estrogen. It was shown that bacterial metabolism of formononetin in the sheep's rumen led to the conversion of this isoflavone to equol, also a weak estrogen [3-5].Although the short term estrogenic effects of these isoflavones in sheep was reversible, prolonged grazing resulted in the infertility syndrome which became know as Clover Disease and led to permanant histological changes to the uterus and ovaries [6-8].

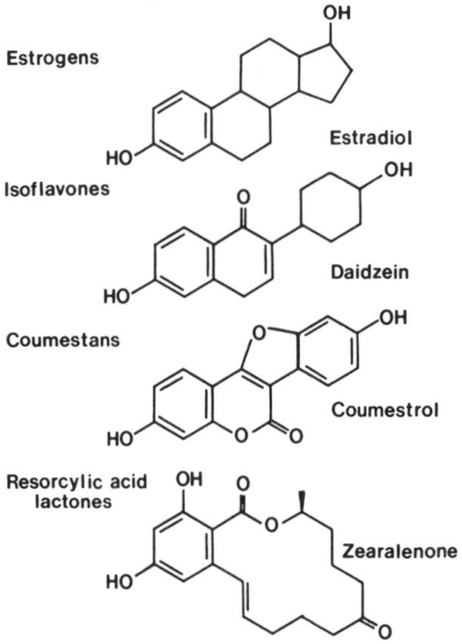

Fig. 1. Structures of naturally occurring classes of compounds with estrogenic activity.

In recent years, our own studies have shown that in addition to the presence of estrogens in biological fluids, there are many other phenolic compounds and that these are excreted in much higher concentrations than the classical steroidal estrogens [9-11].

Two of these compounds were identified as lignans (compounds with a 2,3-dibenzylbutane skeleton) and we assigned the trivial names enterolactone and enterodiol to these first mammalian lignans of novel structure [12]. The significantly higher levels of lignans excreted in the urine of vegetarians [13], the lower incidence of breast cancer in this type of population and the suggestion that these compounds may possess antiestrogenic acitivity lend support for a beneficial role for these compounds in hormonally related disease [12,14].

METHODOLOGY

The observations were made possible largely due to improvements in analytical techniques for these classes of compounds and particularly through the development and application of lipophilic gel chromatography for the isolation and purification of samples [15] and the use of high resolving capillary column gas chromatography and mass spectrometry (gc-ms) for their qualitative and quantitative determination.

A typical GLC urinary steroid profile of a healthy adult is shown in Fig. 2 and it is evident from this profile that the lignans enterolactone and enterodiol are excreted in amounts comparable to the major urinary neutral steroids. With the exception of the lignans, all of the steroids indicated are neutral compounds and because their concentrations far exceed those of the phenolic estrogens it is not possible to simutaneously determine estrogens in the presence of neutral steroids.

Sub-fractionation of the total hydrolysed biological extract using the lipophilic anion exchange gel, triethylaminohydroxypropyl Sephadex LH-20 (TEAP-LH-20) affords a means of isolating specifically phenolic compounds from neutral steroids,

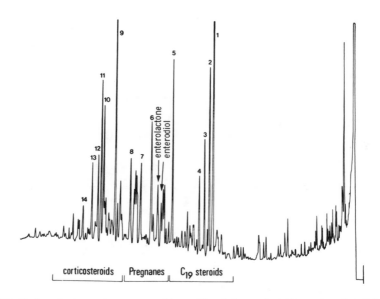

Fig. 2. A typical gas chromatographic profile of the methyloxime-trimethylsilyl ether derivatives of a steroid extract from the urine of a normal adult woman. Indicated is the position of entrolactone and enterodiol relative to the principal urinary steroids in the profiles. The sample was analysed using a 25 m open tubular glass capillary column coated with silicone OV-1 and the principal steroids indicated are: 1. androsterone; 2. aetiocholanolone; 3. dehydroepiandrosterone; 4. 11-oxoandrosterone; 5. 11β-hydroxyandrosterone; 6. pregnanetriol; 7. androstenetriol; 8. pregnane-3,16,20-triol; 9. tetrahydrocortisone; 10. tetrahydrocortisol; 11. allo-tetrahydrocortisol; 12. α-cortolone; 13. β-cortolone + β-cortol; 14. α-cortol

(Fig. 3) [15] thus allowing a greater concentration of the sample thereby assisting detection and identification.

Furthermore, use of DEAE-Sephadex offers a further means of isolating diphenolic compounds from mono-phenolics [16], thereby permitting the isolation of diphenolic isoflavonoid compounds from the monophenolic endogenous estrogens (Fig. 3).

Using these procedures and gc-ms, a general analytical scheme (Fig. 4) was adopted for the determination of these compounds which gave detection limits of approximately μg/day or the equivalent of 1 pg/ml urine.

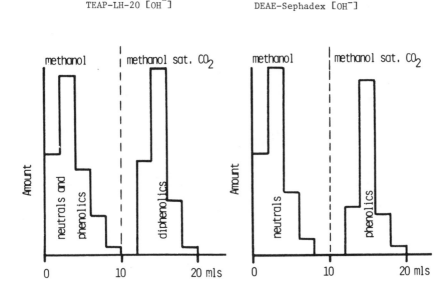

Fig. 3. Separation of neutral, phenolic and diphenolic compounds using lipophilic gel chromatography on two different gels.

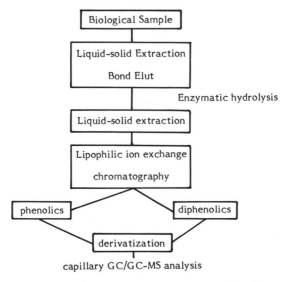

Fig. 4. General analytical scheme for the determination of phenolic compounds in biological samples.

Studies of lignans and equol in man and animals

In studies designed to elucidate the biosynthetic pathways and origins of the two newly discovered lignans, the rat proved an ideal animal model [16,17]. In addition to the presence of enterolactone and enterodiol, greater quantities of another diphenolic compound was found [16]. The mass spectrum of the trimethylsilyl ether derivative showed a molecular ion at mass m/z 386 and a fragmentation pattern consistent with the isoflavone equol [11]. This was confirmed by nmr specroscopy and comparison with the authentic compound [11].

The absence of equol in samples from germ free animals fed an identical diet to normal rats was indicative of a bacterial origin for this compound and its presence in high concentrations in portal venous blood and bile provided evidence that equol, in common the natural estrogens, undergoes an efficient enterohepatic circulation [16]. When the normal diet of the rat was replaced by a semi-synthetic diet, equol excretion rapidly declined to almost undetectable levels and excretion was restored when the normal diet was re-introduced [18].

Pelleted food contains a significant proportion (10% by weight) of soy protein and thus when soya protein alone was added to a semi-synthetic diet equol excretion increased markedly to the extent of 100μg equol excreted/g soya protein fed; excretion was also shown to be dose dependent [18].

These observations were particularly interesting in view of the fact that uterotrophic effects which had been previously described in rats fed commercially prepared rat cake containing soya meal [19]. These estrogenic effects however, had been attributed to the presence of the two isoflavones, daidzein and genistein [20], previously identified in soya-bean products [21-23], however, our failure to detect significant levels of daidzein or genistein in the urine relative to equol, indicates that the estrogenic effects reported earlier in the rat were most probably induced by equol formed by the bacterial conversion of precursor isoflavones in soya [18].

Our studies in man revealed for the first time, that equol was present in urine. This weak estrogens was first described as a minor steroid metabolite of mares' urine [24]. Levels of equol in the urine of adults consuming a diet with no obvious source of soy protein ranged from 0-80 μg/day [25], which was similar to the range also reported by Adlercreutz et al [18, 26], suggesting that soya may not necessarily be the only food product responsible for the presence of equol in man.

In view of our observations in rats fed soya meal and because of the increasing use of soya protein products for human consumption, the effects of soya-bean ingestion in adults was examined [25].

Fig. 5. shows typical glc profiles of the urinary phenolic compounds excreted before and 3 days after soya ingestion. Prior to soya ingestion, the amounts of equol were virtually undetectable but after soya consumption, equol was the major phenolic steroid present in urine.

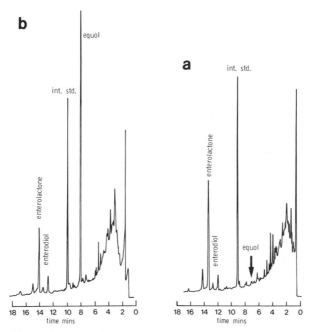

Fig. 5. Capillary column gas chromatographic profile of phenolic compounds excreted in the urine of a normal adult (a) before soy ingestion, (b) 3 days after soy ingestion. The internal standard is 5α-androstene-3β-17β and gas chromatography of the trimethylsilyl ethers was carried out on a 25 metre silicone SE-30 column using isothermal operation at 250 C.

Meals were prepared which consisted of 40g of textured soya, cooked according to the manufacturers specification and substituted for animal meat in the diet. Soya was taken at one meal time each day for 5 consecutive days.

Levels of equol following soya reached 3-7 mg/day, representing in most instances an increase of 500-1000 fold. In two of six subjects studied there was little response to the challenge of soya [25]. This inability to respond is not sex dependent and is presumed to be due either to an absence of the bacterial enzymes responsible for the conversion of isoflavone precursors to equol, or because of variations in gut-transit time, pH or redox potential, all of which are know to vary depending upon the type of diet. Experiments in vitro with fecal bacteria established that equol was formed from soya protein, [25], and confirmed that equol did not naturally occur in soya bean but was formed by the metabolism of precursor phytoestrogens which are present in soya-bean [18].

Equol is therefore by definition not strictly a plant estrogen, but nevertheless is clearly important given the increasing use of soya protein products as a food source.

The analysis of soybean has been carried out by many groups of workers, originally by Walz in 1931 [21]. Such analyses has revealed the presence of relatively large amounts of several isoflavones, including daidzein, daidzin, genistein, genistin, glycitin-7β-glucoside and glycitin. (Table 2)

TABLE II. Isoflavone content of soya products.

Sample	Daidzein (mg/100g)	Daidzin (mg/100g)	Genistein (mg/100g)	Genistin (mg/100g)	Ref.
Soya-bean meal	48.0	62.0	40.0	127.0	[47]
	2.2	11.0	4.0	102.0	[48]
	14.5	56.7	18.7	81.3	[49]
	17.8	42.0	108.0	151.0	[50]
Soya-bean flakes	5.6	59.6	6.7	215.0	[51]
	2.5	114.0	4.4	188.5	[30]
Soya-bean flour	48.0	77.0	46.0	154.0	[47]
Soya-bean cake*	35.0	–	21.3	–	[52]

*6.3 mg/100g formononetin also reported.

Most of these isoflavones are present as the highly polar glucoside conjugate, however as we have shown this does not prevent their absorption since the sugar moiety is readily hydrolysed either by the low gastric pH or by bacterial glucosidases in the gut [18] thereby releasing the unconjugated isoflavone for further metabolism.

In addition to equol in human urine, daidzein has also been identified [18,27), and a minor metabolite O'desmethylangolensin was recently described [28].

Many factors will effect the isoflavone content of soy products and despite a claim that the defating process removes active plant estrogens [29], work by Eldridge and Kwolek [30] and ourselves [18], indicates that this is not the case. Indeed, in three separate preparations of soy protein analysed we found daidzein to be present in abundance, although little genistein was present.

Since as little as 8 mg of genistein and 10 mg of daidzein are sufficient to intitiate uterotrophic effects in mice [31] it is not surprising that the relatively large amounts of isoflavones present in soy protein and clover will readily explain the previously observed estrogenic effects in animals. Furthermore, it should be noted that in addition to isoflavones, soya- bean also contains significant quantities of the more potent estrogen coumestrol.

While it is difficult to be accurate about the relative activities of these plant estrogens, it is clear that they show less activity than the natural estrogens, estradiol-17β and much less than the potent and synthetic estrogen diethylstilbestrol [32-35]. Despite the weaker estrogenic activity of the isoflavones marked estrogenic, effects have been observed in animals consuming diets containing phytoestrogens and therefore it might not be unexpected for similar responses to occur in man.

Biological Implications of Phytoestrogens

In spite of the controversy that surrounds the exogenous addition of estrogens such as diethylstilbestrol (DES) as a growth promoter in animals and its contamination in food [36-38], relatively little consideration appears to have been given to the contribution of naturally occurring plant estrogens in the diet.

Indeed, while the potency of DES far exceeds that of either the endogenous estrogens or the phytoestrogens, the amounts consumed of the latter are significantly greater. The effects of plant estrogens in man should however be of some concern, particularly since it has been suggested that soya might be as beneficial a growth promoter as DES in animals [20]. For example, the concentrations of phytoestrogens in soy, calculated to match 0.5ppb of DES are well within the concentration range of consumed soya products.

Akin to the effects of phytoestrogens in animals, the weak estrogenic activity of equol and other phytoestrogens may induce similar actions in humans. The higher levels of equol and lignans found in the urine of vegetarians [13,26] may help to explain the increased frequency of menstral cycle disorders in this group of women. Furthermore, we have demonstrated that in vitro equol will inhibit prostaglandin synthesis (R.W. Kelly, K.D.R. Setchell, M. Axelson, unpublished data) and such effects may be important given that enzymes responsible for prostaglandin production and metabolism are abundant within the reproductive tissue and are dependent upon steroid hormones, e.g. estrogens stimulate prostaglandin production.

While considering the weak estrogen effects of phytoestrogens, it is worth highlighting the recent finding that extracts of bourbon whisky given to rats produced significant uterotrophic effects with depression of plasma LH levels; effects which were dose dependent [39].

Feminisation including gynecamestia are frequent clinical symptoms of chronic alcoholism and attempts to explain the mechanism of action have largely focussed on the effects of ethanol. This study showed the effects to occur in the absence of the ethanol, ie. with the residue alone and it was suggested that phytoestrogens may be responsible for these actions [39].

Epidemiological studies have demostrated a lower incidence of breast cancer in women in countries consuming a vegetarian or semi-vegetarian type diet [40-42], yet while estrogerns are held to be important in tumor cell growth [43], the mechanism by which diet may influence breast cancer is still unclear.

The fact that several phytoestrogens have been demonstrated to inhibit the binding of estradiol to uterine cytosol receptors indicates that a steroid nucleus is not essential for such binding. Structurally the distance between the C-3 and C-l7 hydroxyl groups of estradiol is similar to that of the two hydroxyl groups on the aromatic rings of equol and other phytoestrogens, a factor which is important for strong binding to the estrogen receptor.

The effect of equol in binding to the receptor in the nucleus but failing to stimulate DNA synthesis to the same degree as estradiol is indicative of an antiestrogenic role for this phytoestrogen [35]. However, while data on equol are lacking, other phytoestrogens have been shown to bind to estrogen receptors in human breast cancer cells [34].

Exposure to high levels of phytoestrogens which we have demonstrated can occur following the ingestion of soya-bean products [18,25], suggests that any antiestrogenic effect of these compounds may be beneficial with respect to breast cancer development or during its treatment and requires examination, given the increasing use of soya-based foods and the important relationship between diet and disease [40].

Soy has been used as an alternative to drugs for the lowering of cholesterol levels in subjects with hyperlipidemias [44,45]. Diets containing high soya protein have been shown to effectively lower serum cholesterol levels and to increase bile acid excretion in man and animals with hypercholesterolemia. While the mechanism of this action is unclear [46] it is possible that it might be explained in the basis of phytoestrogen content of soy rather than the protein fraction because estrogens play a role in the complex metabolism and interaction of lipoproteins and cholesterol regulation.

Soya formula milks for infant feeding have seen greatly increased use over the last five years, yet the potential implications of the long-term exposure of the infant to the phytoestrogens which are present in soya based products appears to have been overlooked. Although the gut is sterile at birth, it rapidly develops a bacterial flora and whether equol is formed by the infants remains to be determined. Nevertheless, the phytoestrogens daidzein and genistein which are present in soya-bean are probably reabsorbed from the gut, as in adults, and presumably these would be capable of exerting estrogenic effects. Since the newborn infant will be subjected to chronic exposure to soya milk, in some cases for up to 2 years this situation could be considered analogous to the sheep grazing on clover. In recent years a reputed "epidemic" of cases of premature sexual development in children of Puerto Rico has been described and is highlighted in this meeting. While the causative agent has not been identified, compounds such as phytoestrogens may be of importance and should not be discounted merely because of their relatively weak estrogenic activity.

To place these findings in perspective, Table 3 lists typical values for the urinary excretion of natural estrogens, lignans and phytoestrogens in the normal adult and in vegetarians.

TABLE III. Levels of estrogens, lignans and phytoestrogens in urine (nmol/day).

		Normal adults	Vegetarians
Estrogens:	Estrone Estradiol Estriol	200	
Lignans:	Enterolactone Enterodiol	1000-3000 200-500	27,600 20,000
Phytoestrogens:	Equol Daidzein	0-300 0-300	20,000
After soya-bean ingestion:	Equol	110,000-25,000	

Despite the lower biological acitivity of these compounds compared with estradiol-17β it is difficult to believe that some biological effects do not occur when these levels are so high. In the future greater consideration should be given to the role of naturally occurring estrogens in our food and of the role of bacterial flora in the metabolism of exogenous compounds which are ingested in our diet.

REFERENCES

1. R.B. Bradbury and D.E. White, Oestrogens and related substances in plants. Vitamins, Hormones 12, 207-233 (1954).

2. N.R. Farnsworth, A.S. Bingel, G.A. Cordell, F.A. Crane, and H.H.S. Fong, Potential value of plants as sources of new antifertility agents II. J Pharm Sci 64, 717-754 (1975).

3. D.A. Shutt, The effects of plant oestrogens of dietary origin. Endeavour 35, 110-113 (1980).

4. A.W.H. Braden, N.K. Hart, and J.A. Lamberton, The oestrogenic activity and metabolism of certain isoflavones in sheep. Aust J Agric Res 18, 335-348 (1967).

5. D.A. Shutt and A.W.H. Braden, The significance of equol in relation to the oestrogenic responses in sheep ingesting clover with a high formononetin content. Aust J Agric Res 19, 545-553 (1968)

6. H.W. Bennetts, E.J.Underwood, and F.L. Sheir, A specific breeding problem of sheep on subterranean clover pastures in Western Australia. Aust Vet J 22, 2-12 (1946)

7. G.R. Moule, A.W.H. Braden, and D.R. Lamond, The significance of oestrogens in pasture plants in relation to animal production. Anim Breed Abstr 31, 139-157 (1963)

8. F.H.W. Morley, A. Axelsen, D. Bennett, Effects of grazing red clover (Trifolium pratense) during the joining season on ewe fertility. Proc Aust Soc Animal Prod 5, 58-61 (1964).

9. K.D.R. Setchell, A.M. Lawson, F.L. Mitchell, H. Adlercreutz, D.N. Kirk, M. Axelson, Lignans in man and animal species. Nature 287, 740-742 (1980).

10. K.D.R. Setchell, A.M. Lawson, E. Conway, N.F. Taylor, D.N. Kirk, G. Cooley, R.D. Farrant, S. Wynn, and M. Axelson, The definitive identification of the lignans trans-2,3-bis(3-hydroxybenzyl)butyrolactone and 2,3(bis(3-hydroxybenzyl)-butane-1,4-diol in human and animal urine. Biochem J 197, 447-458 (1981).

11. M. Axelson, D.N. Kirk, R.D. Farrant, G. Cooley, A.M. Lawson, K.D.R. Setchell, The identification of the weak oestrogen equol[7-hydroxy-3-(4'-hydroxyphenyl)chroman] in human urine. Biochem J 201, 353-357 (1982).

12. K.D.R. Setchell, A.M. Lawson, S.P. Borriello, R. Harkness, H. Gordon, D.M.L. Morgan, D.N. Kirk, H. Adlercreutz, and M. Axelson, Lignan formation in man-microbial involvement and possible roles in relation to cancer. Lancet 2, 4-8 (1981).

13. H. Adlercreutz, T. Fotsis, R. Heikkinen, J.T. Dwyer, B.R. Goldin, S.L. Gorbach, A.M. Lawson, and K.D.R. Setchell, Diet and urinary excretion of lignans in female subjects. Med Biol 59, 259-261 (1981).

14. H. Adlercreutz, Does fiber-rich food containing animal lignan precursors protect against both colon and breast cancer? An extension of the "Fiber Hypothesis". Gastroenterology 86, 761-766 (1984).

15. J. Sjovall, and M. Axelson, Newer approaches to the isolation, identification and quantitative of steroids in biological materials. Vitamins, Hormones 39, 31-144 (1982).

16. M. Axelson and K.D.R. Setchell, The excretion of lignans in rats-Evidence for an intestinal bacterial source for this new group of compounds. FEBS Lett 123, 337-342 (1981).

17. M. Axelson, J. Sjovall, B.E. Gustafsson, K.D.R. Setchell, Origin of lignans in mammals and identification of a precursor from plants. Nature 298, 659-660 (1982).

18. M. Axelson, J. Sjovall, B.E. Gustafsson, K.D.R. Setchell, Soya-a dietary source of the non-steroidal oestrogen equol in humans and animals. J. Endocrinol 102, 49-56 (1984).

19. H.M. Drane, D.S.P. Patterson, B.A. Roberts, and N. Saba, The chance discovery of oestrogenic activity in laboratory rat cake. Food Cosmet Toxicol 13, 491-492 (1975).
20. H.M. Drane, D.S.P., Patterson, B.A.Roberts, and N. Saba, Oestrogenic Activity of soya-bean products. Food Cosmet Toxicol 18, 425-426 (1980).
21. E. Walz, Isoflavon-und saponin-glucoside in Soja hispida. Justus Liebigs Annln Chem 489, 118-155 (1931).
22. M.W. Carter, W.W.G. Smart Jr, and G. Matrone, Estimation of estrogenic activity of genistein obtained from soybean meal. Proc Soc Exp Biol Med 84, 506-507 (1953).
23. E. Cheng, C.D. Story, L. Yoder, W.H. Hale, and W. Burroughs, Estrogenic activity of isoflavone derivatives extracted and prepared from soybean oil meal. Science 118, 164-165 (1953).
24. G.F. Marrian, and G.A.D. Haselwood, CXLV, Equol, a new inactive phenol isolated from the ketohydroxyestrin fraction of mares urine. Biochem J 26, 1226-1232 (1932).
25. K.D.R. Setchell, S.P. Borriello, P. Hulme, D.N. Kirk, and M. Axelson, Non-steroidal oestrogens of dietary origin: possible roles in hormone dependent disease. Am J Clin Nutr 40, 569-578 (1984).
26. H. Adlercreutz, T. Fotsis, R. Heikkinen, J.T. Dwyer, M. Woods, B.R. Goldin and S.L. Gorbach, Excretion of the lignans enterolactone and enterodiol and of equol in omnivorous and vegetarian post-menopausal women and in women with breast cancer. Lancet 2, 1295-1299 (1982).
27. C. Bannwart, T. Fotsis, R. Heikkinen, and H. Adlercreutz, Identification of isoflavonic phytoestrogen daidzein in human urine. Clin Chim Acta 136, 165-172 (1983).
28. C. Bannwart, H. Adlercreutz, T. Fotsis, K. Wahala, T. Hase, and G. Brunow, Identification of O-desmethylangolensin, a metabolite of daidzein and of matairesinol, one likely plant precursor of the animal lignan enterolactone, in human urine. Finn Chem Lett, 120-125 (1984).
29. A.N. Booth, E.M. Bickoff, and G.O. Kohler, Oestrogen-like activity in vegetable oils and milk by-products. Science 131, 1807-1808 (1960).
30. A.C. Eldridge and W.F. Kwolek, Soya-bean isoflavones: effect of environment and variety on composition. J Agriculture and Food Chemistry 30, 353-355 (1983).
31. M. Stob, Naturally occurring food toxicants: Oestrogens in: Handbook of Naturally Occurring Food Toxicants. M. Rechcigl Jr. ed. (Boca Raton, Florida, 1983) (RC Press) pp. 81-100.
32. D.A. Shutt and R.I. Cox, Steroid and phytoestrogen binding to sheep uterine receptor in vitro. J Endocrinol 52, 299-310 (1972).
33. M. Shemesh, H.R. Lindner, and N. Ayalon, Affinity of rabbit uterine oestradiol receptor for phyto-oestrogens and its use in a competitive protein binding radioassay for plasma coumesterol. J Reprod Fertil 29, 1-9 (1972).
34. K. Verdeal, R.R. Brown, J. Richardson, and D.S. Ryan, Affinity of phytoestrogens for estradiol-binding proteins and effect of coumesterol on growth of 7,12-dimethylbenz(a)anthracene induced rat mammary tumours. J Natl Cancer Inst 64, 285-290 (1980).
35. B.Y. Tang and N.R. Adams, The effect of equol on oestrogen receptors and on synthesis of DNA and protein in the immature rat uterus. J Endocrinol 85, 291-297 (1980).
36. O.G. Fitzhugh, Appraisal of the safety of residues of veterinary drugs and their metabolites in edible animal tissues. Ann NY Acad Sci 111, 665-670 (1964).
37. T.H. Jukes, Diethylstibesterol in beef production: What is the risk to consumers. Prev. Med 5, 438-453 (1976).
38. T.H. Jukes, Estrogens in beefsteaks, JAMA 229, 1920-1921 (1974).
39. J.S. Gavaler, E. Rosenblum, D.H. Van Thiel, C. Pohl, J. Gavaler, and D. McCullough, Estrogenicity of alcoholic beverages. Science (In press).

40. Diet Nutrition and Cancer. Committee on Diet Nutrition and Cancer, Assembly of Life Sciences, National Research Canine. Washington DC: National Academy Press (1982).

41. A.B. Miller, Role of nutrition in the etiology of breast cancer. Cancer 39, 2704-2708 (1977).

42. E.L. Wynder, Dietary Factors related to breast cancer. 46, 899-904 (1980).

43. C. Huggins, G. Briziasell, H. Saton Jr., Rapid induction of mammary carcinoma in the rat and the influence of hormones on the tumours. J Exp Med 109, 25-41 (1959).

44. C.R. Sirtori, E. Agradi, F. Conti, O. Montero, and E. Gatti, Soybean protein diet in the treatment of type-II hyperlipoproteinaemia. Lancet I, 275-277 (1977).

45. M.J. Gibney, Hypocholesterolaemic effect of soya-bean proteins. Proc Nutr Soc 41, 19-26 (1982).

46. T.F. Schweizer, A.R. Bekhechi, B. Koellreutter, S. Reimann, D. Pometta, and B.A. Bron, Metabolic effects of dietary fiber from dehulled soybeans in humans. Amer J Clin Nutr 38, 1-11 (1983).

47. A.C. Eldridge, Determination of isoflavones in soybean flours, protein concentrates and isolates. J Agri and Food Chem 30, 353-355 (1982).

48. P.A. Murphy, Phytoestrogen content of processed soybean products. Food Tech (Champaign) 60-64 (1982).

49. H. Pettersson and K.H. Kiessling, Liquid chromatographic determination of the plant oestrogens coumestrol and isoflavones in animal feed. J Asso Official Analy Chem 67, 503-506 (1984).

50. D.E. Pratt, and P.M. Birac, Source of antioxidant activity of soybeans and soy products. J Food Sci 44, 1720-1722 (1979).

51. A. Seo and C.V. Morr, Improved high-performance liquid chromatographic analysis of phenolic acids and isoflavonoids from soybean protein products. J Agri Food Chem 32, 530-533 (1984).

52. H.R. Lindner, Occurrence of anabolic agents in plants and their importance. Envir Qual Safety Supp 5, 151-158 (1976).

DISCUSSION

NAFTOLIN: Please tell us whether antibiotics will affect the amounts of these estrogens furnished by gut metabolism.

SETCHELL: Yes, antibiotics will abolish the production of these dipheno- lic compounds. This was demonstrated from the effects seen with the wide spectrum antibiotic oxytetracyclin where lignan absorption was rapidly abolished. The bacteria responsible for their production appear to be anaerobic.

NAFTOLIN: Is there a difference in the timing of puberty in vegetarian versus ominiverous people?

SETCHELL: I do not know whether there is any evidence for differences in the timing of onset of puberty between vegetarians and omnivores.

NAFTOLIN: Does a vegetarian diet effect the occurrence of osteoporosis in agonadal subjects?

SETCHELL: I do not know the answer to this question.

SIITERI: Hypoestrogenicity in humans is associated with obesity and high fat diets, e.g., puberty earlier in heavy girls, osteoporosis less severe in obese women, more severe in thin.

NEW: It seems unlikely that phytoestrogen ingestion influences the age of puberty since the age of menarche is the same all over the world despite some countries having a strictly vegetarian diet (for example, Buddhist countries). Furthermore, infants fed soya formulas from birth for family history of allergy or other reasons show disappearance of neonatal breast development frequently observed in the newborn. This soya ingestion does not prevent the normal disappearance of breast tissue in the newborn. This suggests that the phytoestrogens in soya formulas fed to newborns are not highly estrogenic.

SIITERI: What are blood levels of equol?

SETCHELL: Blood levels of equol are very low and at the ng/ml level in the few samples we have analyzed. We are presently developing a RIA technique for their measurement in human serum to facilitate the analysis of a larger number of samples than is possible by GC/MS techniques.

JONES: What effect do phytoestrogens have on sex hormone binding globulin (SHBG)? Do phytoestrogens bind to albumin?

SETCHELL: We have not studied this aspect of biological effects.

JORDAN: Do you have any biological data to classify the activity of enterolactone?

SETCHELL: We have carried out an extensive number of studies to assess the biological activity of the lignans, particularly since this group of compounds has diverse activities. We have shown enterolactone to have anti-mitotic and antiviral activity but at concentrations which are above physiological levels. It is not strongly estrogenic, but I understand that Dr. James H. Clark has shown it will bind to the antiestrogen receptor. I believe it may be weakly estrogenic; but at the time we tested for estrogenicity, we had insufficient authentic compound to complete testing at high levels. Waters and Knowles (J. Reprod. Fert. 66, 379, 1982) have shown effects indicating it may be antiestrogenic. More recently we have shown that enterolactone is a potent inhibitor of the cholesterol-7α-hydroxylase and acyl-CoA: cholesterol acyl transferase enzymes inhibit--implying that it may be important as a protection against colon carcinogenesis. We have studied the effects on increased lignan levels in the rat with DMH-induced colorectal cancer and the indications are that it may have a significant protective effect against tumor formation in this model--this is unpublished data and as yet incomplete work.

JORDAN: You mentioned that the phytoestrogens could be antiestrogens. Do you have evidence for that?

SETCHELL: This is taken from published data by several groups of workers and cited in our previous publications.

KUPFER: The observation by you and Kelly that equol inhibits uterine prostaglandin (PG) synthesis is interesting, particularly in view of the fact that Kelly demonstrated that 2-hydroxy-estradiol stimulates prostaglandin biosynthesis. This raises the question whether antiestrogens inhibit PG synthesis? Also, has anyone observed a decrease in urinary excretion of this in vegetarian women who have high levels of equol?

SETCHELL: To my knowledge, I know of no published work where prostaglandins and equol have been examined in vegetarians.

DEGEN: What was the concentration at which you found equol inhibition of prostaglandin biosynthesis? This is surprising since equol has a phenolic group and various estrogens which we have tested undergo cooxidation by prostaglandin synthase and during this reaction stimulate prostaglandin synthesis. However, at higher concentrations, we find inhibition of prostaglandin synthase. Could this be the reason for this observation that equol inhibits PG-synthesis?

SETCHELL: I do not recollect the figures for the concentrations of equol tested. However, they were in a similar molar concentration to that of aspirin.

DEGEN: Aspirin-like concentrations of equol are relatively high compared to other compounds such as indomethacin, and you may find our opposite (stimulatory) effect on prostaglandin synthase when you test equol at low concentrations. Also, antiestrogens such as tamoxifen have been found to inhibit prostaglandin synthase catalyzed cooxidation of DES and in another in vitro assay as mentioned earlier by Dr. J. P. Raynaud.

ADLERCREUTZ: With regard to the biological activity of the lignans, Waters and Knowles showed by in vivo experiments in rats that enterolactone in amounts of 0.2 µg/kg inhibited the effect of estradiol on labeled thymidine uptake in uterine cells. Enterolactone at high concentration inhibits binding of estradiol to the estrogen receptor and to the rat liver cytosol type II receptor; it is doubtful whether these effects have biological significance. These experiments were carried out by Dr. James H. Clark. Furthermore, Dr. Shirata Fujiki made some experiments showing that enterolactone has a weak anti-tumor promoting activity. In collaboration with Dr. Vickery, we found slight inhibition of placental transfer of enterolactone; the effect is about 70% of that of flavone. The lignans are also weak anti-oxidants.

I would like to answer some of the many questions asked about lignans and isoflavonic phytoestrogens. I cannot discuss them all, and, in fact, some of the results will be presented during the poster session.

The first question was whether these phytoestrogens may be protective with regard to osteoporosis and whether vegetarians have less osteoporosis. In fact, vegetarians tend to have more osteoporosis, which may be the result of their lower estrogen levels. Lactovegetarians do not excrete much isoflavonic estrogens because they get their supply of proteins from milk products. Macrobiotics excrete large amounts of equol in urine. In collaboration with Dr. Sherwood Gorbach in Boston, we are studying the excretion of lignans, estrogens, and phytoestrogens in different groups of women on various habitual diets. At present, we do not have sufficient data to show whether the macrobiotic women eating a lot of soy products containing equol precursors have less osteoporosis than the lactovegetarians.

The second question I would like to answer was about lignan and SHBG. In a preliminary computer analysis of our data, we found a positive correlation between urinary excretion of enterolactone and serum SHBG and a negative correlation between urinary enterolactone and serum free testosterone and estradiol in women. Vegetarians have higher SHBG and a higher excretion of the lignans. Whether lignans stimulate SHBG synthesis in the liver remains to be elucidated. Some other compound in vegetarian diets may have the effect, but we are working on the hypothesis that lignans may interfere with estrogen and perhaps also androgen metabolism.

Morphological Analysis of Chlordecone (Kepone) Action in Different Mouse Organs: Choroid Plexus in Adult Males and Vaginal Epithelium in Suckling Neonates.

Victor P. Eroschenko
Department of Biological Sciences, University of Idaho, Moscow, Idaho 83843

INTRODUCTION

Estrogens are important internal hormones that stimulate the growth and development of the female sex organs in the vertebrates. Under normal conditions, estrogens are synthesized in the ovaries in response to pituitary hormones. In sexually mature animals, there exists a balance between estrogen synthesis, metabolism, and clearance. However, this balance can be altered experimentally in a research laboratory or inadvertently in the environment. In that case, excessive intake of estrogenic compounds may impair the reproductive capabilities in both sexes of the species.

Numerous contaminants presently found in our environment exhibit estrogenic action. Daily intake by animals or humans of such estrogenic compounds becomes highly possible and consequently, increased incidence of reproductive failure may occur. Among environmental pollutants that exhibit estrogenic action are organochlorine insecticides chlordecone (Kepone), DDT and its derivatives or metabolites, and industrial contaminants polychlorinated biphenyls (PCB's). Although these compounds differ chemically from one another as well as from steroidal estrogens, they mimic estrogenic actions in the reproductive tracts of laboratory animals by binding with estrogen receptors [1, 2, 3, 4]. These estrogen receptors appear to bind not only natural estrogens with high affinity and specificity but also structurally unrelated compounds such as organochlorine insecticides and synthetic chemicals [5]. This indicates that a wide range of estrogenic compounds with class and structural diversity may influence the structure and function of estrogen-sensitive cells in exposed species. Although environmental pollutants are generally weaker than steroidal estrogens, chronic exposure to even small amounts may eventually increase the body burdens of animals or humans to illicit an estrogenic response. In the recent past, the inadvertent exposure of industrial workers to insecticide chlordecone during its manufacture and the subsequent reproductive impairments illustrate the cumulative action of one such environmental pollutant with weak estrogenic potency [6].

Over the years, our research concerned the study of chlordecone and its estrogenic effects on the reproductive organs in birds and mammals. Although chlordecone is no longer manufactured or applied for pest control and does not pose an immediate health hazard, interest in its mechanism of action in different mammalian systems remains high. This could partly be due to the fact that chlordecone exhibits estrogenic action and that key toxicological findings of chlordecone effects were first reported in humans and subsequently confirmed in laboratory animals [6]. Due to its chemical stability and high resistance to physical degradation or biological metabolism, chlordecone may remain in the environment indefinitely as an environmental estrogen.

The estrogenicity of chlordecone and its detrimental effects on reproductive systems have been well documented in neonatal and adult females. However, information about the passage of chlordecone in milk and its influence on developing reproductive organs in the suckling neonates remains very limited. Chlordecone was detected in human milk in the southeastern states where photodegradation of mirex to chlordecone appears the contamination source [7, 8]. In addition to impairing the reproductive functions in different species, including man, chlordecone also affected the mammalian nervous system. As a result of industrial accident numerous chlordecone-poisoned workers exhibited neurological disorders, tremors, headaches and elevated cerebrospinal fluid (CSF) pressure in absence of any intracranial mass [9]. The apparently detrimental effects of chlordecone on the cerebrospinal fluid-producing cells, the choroid plexus, have not been previously examined.

The intent of this paper is to review our recent experimental data concerning chlordecone mechanism of action in two different but important mammalian systems. In the first experiment, we examined the effects of chlordecone on the male mouse choroid plexus in order to elucidate the possible causes of elevated cerebrospinal fluid pressure reported in chlordecone-poisoned workers [9]. In the second experiment, we determined whether treating lactating dams with large doses of chlordecone would contaminate the milk in sufficient quantities to influence the development of the reproductive tract in suckling female offspring. In both experiments, the recorded changes induced by chlordecone were examined with ultrastructural means and then compared to changes induced by estradiol 17β.

METHODS AND RESULTS

Changes in the Choroid Plexus of Adult Male Mice in Response to
Estradiol and Chlordecone

Five groups of adult male mice received 15 daily intraperitoneal injections of either 10.0 μg estradiol-17β or 100.0, 250.0, 500.0 or 1,000.0 μg chlordecone suspended in sesame oil. The mice in the control group were injected with the vehicle only. Chlordecone-treated males exhibited tremors and neuromuscular disorders similar to those reported in chlordecone-poisoned workers [9]. Mortality rates varied after the treatments and were recorded in both estradiol- and chlordecone-treated groups (Table 1).

Table 1. *Variable Mortality Rate in Adult Male Mice After Treat-*
ment with Different Estradiol and Chlordecone Doses.

Group**	Dose (µg/0.1cc)	Mortality Rate (%)
C	Oil	0.0
E	10.0	13.0
K	100.0	0.0
K	250.0	33.0
K	500.0	27.0
K	1,000.0	50.0

Each group consisted of 15 mice treated for 15 days.
**C=Control; E=Estradiol; K=Chlordecone*

At the end of 15 injections, all mice were terminated, the choroid plexus removed from the fourth ventricles, fixed in situ by immersion and examined ultrastructurally. The choroid plexus from control males consisted of a convoluted structure with the uniform cell surfaces profusely covered with microvilli. Some microvilli exhibited either bulbous tips or periperhal expansions (Fig. 1) and appeared very similar to that described previously [10].

Treatment of males with either estradiol or chlordecone produced dramatic and abnormal morphological changes on the choroid plexus cell surfaces with chlordecone inducing dose-dependent alterations. The lowest chlordecone dose (100.0 µg) did not induce any visible cell surface changes. However, in mice treated with 250.0 µg chlordecone the surfaces of choroid plexus cells exhibited either decreased number or complete lack of microvilli. In addition the cells exhibited membrane pitting. The two highest chlordecone doses (500.0 and 1,000.0 µg) induced complete microvilli elimination or denudation resulting in bare cell surfaces. In addition, the cell surfaces appeared uneven, with the cell membranes exhibiting pitting or disruption (Fig. 2).

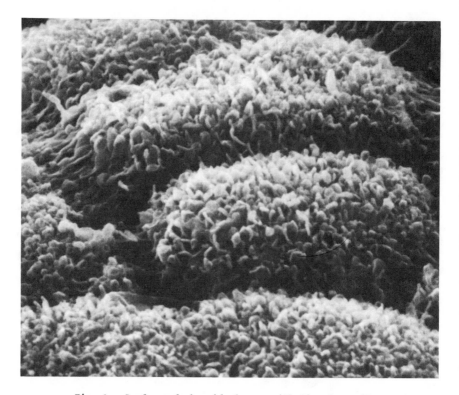

Fig. 1.　Surface of choroid plexus epithelium from oil-
treated control mouse illustrating microvilli
density.　9,000 x

Treatment of male mice with 10.0 μg estradiol-17β for the same duration
produced similar changes in the choroid plexus epithelium that were recorded
with the two highest chlordecone doses.　All cells lacked microvilli, the cell
membranes exhibited increased pitting or disruption and the cell surfaces were
covered with increased debris (Fig. 3).

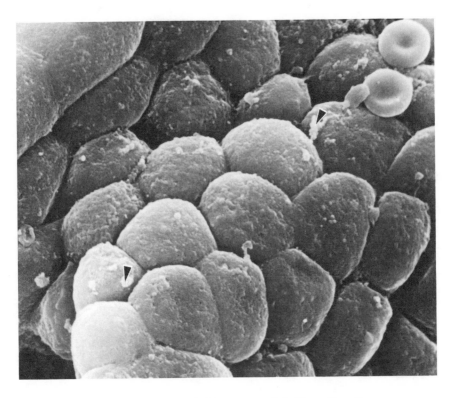

*Fig. 2 Surface of choroid plexus epithelium after 15
injections of 1,000 μg chlordecone. Note the
absence of microvilli, membrane pitting and surface debris (arrows). 4,000 x*

Changes in the Vaginal Epithelium of Suckling Neonatal Mice in Response to
Estradiol and Chlordecone Passage in Milk

Pregnant mice were kept in individual cages until parturition. Within 24

hours of birth, the lactating dams with their litters were assigned to

different treatment groups. All lactating dams received 9 daily

intraperitoneal injections containing the following chemicals: sesame oil, or

10.0, 20.0, or 40.0 μg estradiol-17β, or 250.0, 500.0 or 1,000.0 μg

92

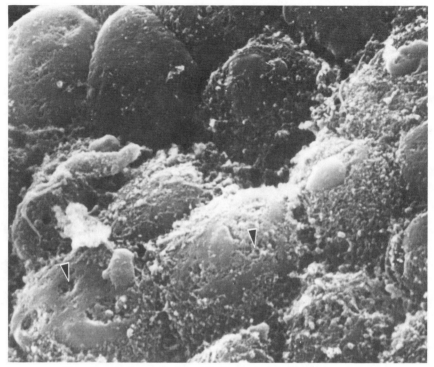

Fig. 3. Surface of choroid plexus epithelium after 15
injections of 10.0 µg estradiol. Microvilli
elimination, membrane pitting (arrows) and
surface debris were similar to changes induced
by chlordecone (Fig. 2). 4,200 x

insecticide chlordecone. All treated dams were allowed to nurse their pups.

At 12 days of age, selected female offspring from each litter were sacrificed,

the   reproductive   tract   weight   measured   and   vaginas   prepared   for

ultramicroscopic examination.

The dose-dependent increase in the suckling neonate reproductive tract

weights, the stimulatory surface alterations and the keratinization in the

vaginal canals indicated that the chemicals injected into the lactating dams

contaminated the ingested milk (Table 2).

Table 2. Administration of 10 Intraperitoneal Injections of
Estradiol 17-β or Chlordecone to Lactating Dams and
Their Effects on 12-day-old Female Reproductive Tract
Weight (RTW) and Vaginal Keratinization (VK).

Group*	(μg) Dose**	No. Pups	RTW (mg)***	VK (%)
C	Oil	6	19.9	0.0
E	10.0	6	25.4	0.0
E	20.0	9	28.2	44.0
E	40.0	5	28.3	60.0
K	250.0	5	22.2	0.0
K	500.0	6	26.3	50.0
K	1,000.0	6	29.8	83.0

*C=Control; E=Estradiol; K=Chlordecone
**All chemicals were administered in 0.1cc sesame oil to all
the lactating dams.
***All weights were significantly heavier (P<0.05%) than the
controls.

When the present data from Table 2 was compared to data in which smaller

estradiol or chlordecone doses were directly injected into neonatal mice [2,

11], there was a significant acceleration of the reproductive tract

development (Table 3).

Table 3. Effects of 10 Direct Intraperitoneal Injections of
Estradiol 17-β or Chlordecone on Neonatal Female Reproductive Tract Weights (RTW) and Vaginal Keratinization (VK).

Group*	Dose**	No. Neonates	RTW (mg)***	VK (%)
C	Oil	5	14.0	0.0
E	10.0	10	35.0	100.0
K	15.0	5	21.0	0.0
K	30.0	5	27.0	33.0
K	60.0	5	27.0	100.0
K	125.0	5	42.0	100.0

*C=Control; E=Estradiol; K=Chlordecone
**All chemicals were administered in 0.05cc sesame oil directly
to neonates.
***All weights were significantly heavier (P<0.05%) than the
controls.

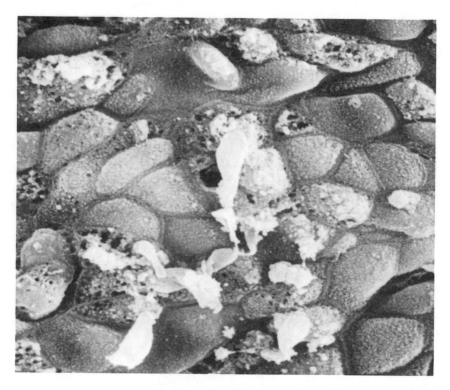

Fig. 4.   *Hypertrophy and mucification of vaginal cells in pups that ingested milk from dams treated with 250.0 µg chlordecone.   2,300 x*

Ultrastructural examination of vaginal canals in pups that were nursed by estradiol- or chlordecone-treated dams revealed that the heavier reproductive tract weights were due to stimulatory changes. The vaginal cell surfaces exhibited cellular hypertrophy, microvilli growth, cellular mucification, and release of secretory material into vaginal canals as debris.   Vaginal mucification was seen in offspring that ingested milk from dams treated with the lowest estradiol (10.0µg) or chlordecone (250.0 µg) doses (Fig.4). Advanced vaginal stimulation, cellular desquamation, and the exposure of underlying keratinized cells were recorded in pups that were nursed by dams treated with the highest two estradiol (20.0 and 40.0μg) or chlordecone (500.0 and 1,000.0 μg) doses (Fig. 5). The initial stimulatory changes in the vaginal canals were similar in pups that were nursed either by estradiol- or chlordecone-treated dams. However, distinct cell surface differences were recorded in keratinized vaginal canals. The surfaces of

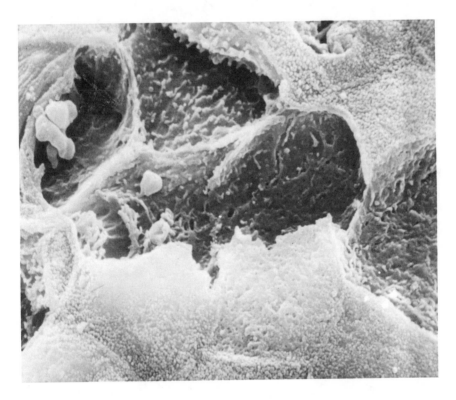

Fig. 5. Desquamation of surface cells and initial keratinization of underlying vaginal cells in pups that ingested milk from dams treated with 500.0 μg chlordecone. 5,100 x

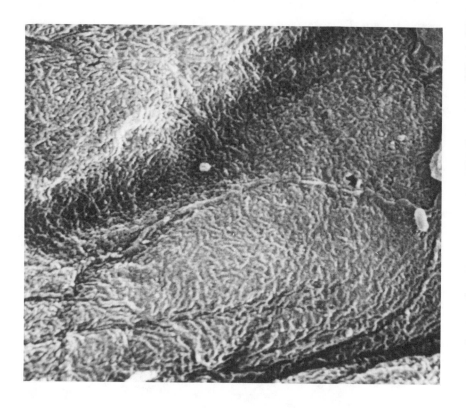

Fig. 6.   Keratinized vaginal cells with prominent, complex microridge patterns in pups that ingested
milk from dams treated with 20.0 or 40.0 ug
estradiol.   4,500 x

keratinized vaginal cells in pups nursed by estradiol-treated dams were

covered by prominent and complex, interdigitating pattern of microridges (Fig.

6). On the other hand, the surfaces of the keratinized vaginal cells in pups

nursed by chlordecone-treated dams were smoother and exhibited less pronounced

microridge patterns (Fig. 7).   These smoother cell surface features were

highly characteristic of chlordecone influence and were recorded in every

female that exhibited vaginal keratinization.

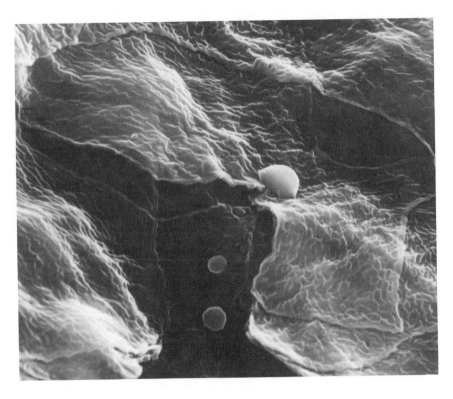

Fig. 7.   *Keratinized vaginal cells with smoother surfaces
and decreased microridges patterns in pups that
ingested milk from dams treated with 1,000 µg
chlordecone. 4,500 x*

DISCUSSION AND CONCLUSIONS

We have previously reported that in undeveloped avian and mammalian

reproductive organs, chlordecone action closely resembled that of estradiol by

binding to estrogen receptors. In the the avian oviducts, chlordecone induced

cell proliferation and stimulated the development of Golgi complex,

endoplasmic reticulum, ribosomes and protein synthesis [12]. In addition to

similar stimulatory influences resembling typical steroidal estrogens, chlordecone also produced cellular abnormalities in the undeveloped mammalian reproductive tracts and impaired reproductive functions in neonatally-treated adults [1, 2].

The cellular abnormalities induced by chlordecone in the choroid plexus of adult mice indicated that the chlordecone mechanism of action in these cells was again similar to estradiol. This could be due to a possible affinity between the injected chemicals and some cytoplasmic component of the choroid plexus cells. Further examination of the choroid plexus cells revealed increased intracellular damage, cytoplasmic and organelle degeneration, plasmalemma rupture and expulsion of the cytoplasmic contents into ventricular lumina. The only difference between estradiol and chlordecone action in the choroid cells was the mitochondrial damage in chlordecone-treated males [13], a characteristic feature of chlordecone toxicity.

The recorded damage in the choroid plexus cells is possibly due to the specific estrogenic toxicity of chlordecone and estradiol. The amount of chlordecone required to produce the same damage in the choroid plexus cells was significantly more than estradiol. The observed chlordecone weakness is in agreement with its action recorded in the mammalian reproductive organs which indicated that chlordecone potency was much less than that of estradiol [4, 14]. However, due to its prolonged action and long half-life, chlordecone may be as potent or as toxic as estradiol to sensitive cells after chronic exposure.

Other chemicals such as acetazolamide which lowers CSF secretion and which is not related to estradiol or chlordecone also reduced or eliminated microvilli on the mouse choroid plexus cells. Such surface changes were believed to represent inhibitory effects of the chemical on CSF production

[15, 16]. In the undeveloped reproductive tracts, chlordecone and estradiol induced similar stimulatory changes. In the male mouse choroid plexus, chlordecone and estradiol induced similar inhibitory as well as abnormal changes. Damage to choroid plexus microvilli could alter the established cell functions for CSF production since it was shown that in rat choroid plexus, Mg 2^+-dependent Na^+, K^+ and ATPase pumps are located on the microvilli [17]. Recently it was shown that chlordecone inhibited oxidative phosphorylation and membrane transport system in different cells of the body [18]. It is possible that chronic industrial exposure to chlordecone may have damaged the membrane transport system and/or the choroid plexus cells in the poisoned workers and altered the balance between CSF production and absorption. The consequence of such damage could have elevated CSF pressure and caused headaches [9].

Our studies with treated lactating dams show that both estradiol and chlordecone were excreted in milk in sufficient quantities to induce accelerated reproductive tract maturation in the suckling offspring. This indicates the importance of lactation in nursing females for eliminating chemical contaminants. Furthermore, the exposure of nursing infants to chemical contaminants may be potentially more hazardous than the prenatal or adult exposure since lactation represents an early nutritional stage during which the developing offspring remain totally dependent on milk.

The degree of vaginal development and frequency of vaginal keratinization observed in the offspring nursed by dams treated with either estradiol or chlordecone doses was not as advanced as that recorded in neonatal mice treated directly but with much lesser doses of the same chemicals [2]. The excreted concentrations of estradiol or chlordecone in milk were apparently less which is in agreement with earlier reports that indicate that lactating rats excrete about 52.0% of the injected chlordecone in milk [19]. Based on previous experiments in which prenatal or neonatal treatment of rodents with either estradiol or chlordecone produced persistent vaginal cornification and anovulation in adults [1, 20, 21], we anticipate similar reproductive impairments in the adult offspring exposed neonatally to estradiol or chlordecone-contaminated milk. This would be in addition to possible reproductive tract abnormalities that may occur in mice that ingested chlordecone-contaminated milk. The expression of chlordecone's estrogenicity remains different from that of estradiol. The surfaces of all keratinized cells in this and previous experiments [2] lacked the well-developed ridges and which resembled those seen in adult mice treated prenatally with diethylstilbestrol [22], instead of those in mice treated with estradiol. At this time, the significance of this structural variation is not known, however, prenatal exposures to DES have been associated with genital tract lesions and abnormalities in female mice [23].

Although chlordecone has been detected in human milk in those regions where mirex photodegrades to chlordecone [7] no information is currently available concerning chlordecone action in women or in human infants. At the present time, chlordecone no longer poses a health hazard. However, there are numerous other chemical contaminants and industrial pollutants in our surrounding environment that exhibit similar estrogenic activity. Consequently, these chemicals may constitute an estrogenic hazard to the exposed species. Studying the mechanism of chlordecone action in different avian and mammalian systems has provided the scientific community with useful information that can be used in predicting the possible actions of other environmental agents that exhibit estrogenic potencies.

ACKNOWLEDGEMENTS

The author acknowledges and expresses appreciation to Mr. James M. Schumacker, Junior medical student at the University of Washington, for permission to use the micrographs pertaining to choroid plexus study. Appreciation is also expressed to Laurel Mickelsen for manuscript preparation.

REFERENCES

1. Gellert, R.J. (1978) Environ. Res. 16, 131-138.
2. Eroschenko, V.P. (1982) Biol. Reprod. 26, 707-720.
3. Bulger, W.H. and Kupfer, D. in Reproductive Toxicology, D. R. Mattison, ed (Alan R. Liss, Inc., New York, 1983) pp. 163-173.
4. Hammond, B., Katzenellenbogen, B.S. Krauthammer, V. and McConnell, J. (1979) Proc. Natl. Acad. Sci. USA. 76, 6641-6645.
5. Katzenellenbogen, J.A., Katzenellenbogen, B.S., Tatee, T., Robertson, D.W. and Landvatter, S.W. in Estrogens in the Environment, J.A. McLachlan, ed (Elsevier/North Holland, New York, 1980) pp. 33-51.
6. Guzelian, P.S. (1982) Ann. Rev. Pharmacol. Toxicol. 22, 89-113.
7. National Research Council (1978) Wash. D.C. Natl. Acad. Sci.
8. Carlson, D.A., Konyha, K.D., Wheeler, W.B., Marshall, G.P. and Zaylskie, R.G. (1976) Science 194, 939-941.
9. Sanborn, G.E. and Selhorst, J.B. (1979) Neurology 29, 1222-1227.
10. Peters, A., Sanford, L. and Webster, H. in The Fine Structures of the Nervous System (W.B. Saunder, Philadelphia 1976) pp.280-294.
11. Eroschenko, V.P. and Mousa, M.A. (1979) Toxicol. Appl. Pharmacol. 49, 151-159.
12. Eroschenko, V.P. and Palmiter, R.D. in Estrogens in the Environment, J.A. McLachlan, ed (Elsevier/North Holland, New York 1980) pp. 305-325.
13. Schumacker, J.M. and Eroschenko, V.P. (1985) Toxicology (In Press).
14. Bulger, W.H., Muccitelli, R.M. and Kupfer, D. (1979) Molec. Pharmacol. 15, 515-514.
15. Azzam, N.A.., Choudbury, S.R. and Donohue, J.M. (1978) J. Anat. 127, 333-342.
16. Collins, P. and Moriss, G.M. (1975) J. Anat. 120, 571-579.
17. Masuzawa, T., Ohta, T., Kawamura, K., Nakahara, N. and Sato, F. (1984) Brain Research 302, 357-362.
18. Desaiah, D. (1982) Neurotoxicology 3, 103-110.
19. Kavlock, R.J., Chernoff, N., Rogers, E. and Whitehouse, D. (1980) 14, 227-235.
20. Kimura, T. (1975) Endocrinol. Japon. 22, 497-502.
21. Gellert, R.J. and Wilson, C. (1979) Environ. Res. 18, 437-443.
22. Lamb, J.C. IV, Newbold, R.R. and McLachlan, J.A. (1979) J. Toxicol. Environ. Health 5, 599-603.
23. McLachlan, J.A. (1977) J. Toxicol. Environ. Health 2, 527-537.

DISCUSSION

MCLACHLAN: Have you used lower doses of estradiol in the neonatal mouse to get a better estimate of the developmental estrogenicity of Kepone? Your data implies only a six-fold difference in potency, but estradiol might be at least 10 times more potent. What about low dose, long-term effects?

EROSCHENKO: In most of our work, we used variable concentrations of Kepone (from low to very high). In order to compare the effects of different Kepone doses on morphological changes in the neonatal reproductive tracts prior to sexual maturation, we used estradiol doses that would produce quick responses. It is true that the changes recorded in these tracts with estradiol at 12 days of age were there much earlier. However, to "catch" up with Kepone's slow action, a larger interval of time was allowed. As a result, the estimate of Kepone's estrogenicity in terms of morphological changes during the 12 days of its action probably does not reflect its true potency since estradiol completed its action before Kepone. Kepone's potency was better shown with in vivo and in vitro studies using the receptor-mediated cell functions. These studies showed that Kepone potency was 1000 to 5000 times less than that of estradiol. The low dose, long-term studies with Kepone show dose-dependent reproductive impairments in adult animals treated with the chemical neonatally. Anovulation and appearance of persistent vaginal keratinization appeared earlier in females that were treated with larger doses of Kepone. These data illustrate that, although Kepone may have a lower potency than estradiol, it is, nevertheless, a very long acting estrogen-like compound. In birds, a dose as low as 10 ppm would have no effect on eggshell strength and thickness until the animal consumed the diet for over 200 days. After that time, similar eggshell weakness and decreased eggshell thickness were recorded that appeared much earlier in those birds which consumed diets with either 80 or 160 ppm Kepone. This data illustrates the bioaccumulative action of Kepone in exposed animals and its ability to exert eventual detrimental action on sensitive organs if it is allowed to influence the system for a prolonged interval of time.

MEYERS: Mirex is identical to Kepone except Mirex has no carbonyl function. Mirex also has no estrogenic activity; Kepone does. What has been done to learn about the origin of the estrogenic activity associated with Kepone? What is the role played by the carbonyl group? What is the chemistry (metabolism) associated with Kepone that might be responsible for its estrogenic activity? I have found very little in the literature in this regard.

EROSCHENKO: The estrogenic action of Kepone has been investigated at the subcellular level in both birds and mammals. It appears that Kepone action is mediated through its affinity for and combination with estrogen receptors in both avian and mammalian reproductive tracts. Although Kepone exhibits estrogenicity, it is much less active than estradiol. I do not know what role carbonyl group plays in Kepone's estrogenicity. Mirex, which is not estrogenic, has two bridge head chlorine atoms which are replaced by a carbonyl group in Kepone. Estrogen receptor affinity and the estrogenic activity of Kepone is probably due to its hydrate form and, therefore, depend on one or both of its hydroxyl substituents. Mirex is a completely chlorinated analog and lacks estrogenic action in female reproductive organs. The major Kepone metabolite is a stable, reduced form of Kepone, called Kepone alcohol, which was first isolated from human stool. There is strong evidence that the site of bioreduction of Kepone is human liver. Thus, hepatic bioreduction of Kepone followed by glucuronide conjugation of the alcohol metabolite is the major metabolic pathway of Kepone in man. I do not have any information on specific estrogenicity of this Kepone metabolite.

FORSBERG: You compare the effects of Kepone and estradiol. What about similarities or differences between these molecules in affinity to alpha-fetoprotein?

EROSCHENKO: I am not aware of any studies concerning Kepone and its affinity for alpha-fetoprotein.

FORSBERG: Have you looked at ovarian morphology in Kepone-treated animals?

EROSCHENKO: I have examined ovaries from mice neonatally treated with Kepone. Approximately 30 days later, most of the ovaries were without recent corpora lutea. This agrees with other Kepone studies that report anovulation and persistent vaginal estrus in mice or rats treated neonatally with Kepone. Whether Kepone actually damages both the ovarian cells and the neuroendocrine axis is not as clear. I suspect, however, that the effect of Kepone is primarily an inhibitory one on the neuroendocrine axis which in turn inhibits the ovarian functions. If the ovaries were to be removed from the Kepone-treated animals and transplanted into untreated, castrated hosts, they should eventually exhibit normal cyclicity since the inhibitory effects of Kepone would now be removed from the ovaries. In a similar fashion, transplanting normal ovaries into Kepone-treated hosts would probably result in anovulation and cessation of ovarian functions due to Kepone's inhibitory action on the neuroendocrine axis.

NAFTOLIN: Do antiestrogens block Kepone's effects?

EROSCHENKO: Antiestrogens such as tamoxifen bind to estrogen receptors and consequently, inhibit or block Kepone-mediated induction of protein synthesis. This has been especially well demonstrated in immature avian oviducts.

NAFTOLIN: Kepone's actions at membranes could be direct, nongenomic effects.

EROSCHENKO: This can be especially true in the membranes of the choroid plexus which are dramatically altered by estradiol and Kepone action.

Analysis and Characterization of Estrogenic Xenobiotics

and Natural Products

ANALYSIS AND CHARACTERIZATION OF
ESTROGENIC XENOBIOTICS AND NATURAL PRODUCTS

Alice K. Robison, Venkat R. Mukku, and George M. Stancel

Department of Medicine, Washington University School of Medicine,
St. Louis, MO. (A.K.R.) , and Department of Pharmacology,
The University of Texas Medical School at Houston,
Houston, TX. (V.R.M. and G.M.S.)

INTRODUCTION

The analysis and characterization of estrogenic xenobiotics has historically been carried out in a fashion similar to the study of ovarian estrogens. The initial observation that a given xenobiotic possessed estrogenic activity was often made at the "organ" level following administration of the xenobiotic to an experimental animal; sometimes these observations were accidental. In some cases the xenobiotic was initially administered as one component of a mixture. Once an estrogenic effect was observed the active compound was typically purified and tested for it's ability to interact with an estrogen receptor. Structure-activity relationships have usually been determined by studying both biological responses and receptor binding interactions. These studies have often been expanded to "catalog" the effects of the xenobiotic in other organs and animal models; to examine the effects of the compound at the cellular level; and ultimately to elucidate the molecular basis of the xenobiotic's estrogenic activity.

This approach is fairly typical for a compound with estrogenic activity. In addition, however, an overall understanding of a xenobiotic estrogen poses several other considerations. For example: (1) these compounds are usually studied following acute administration of high doses, rather than by chronic exposure to low doses which may be a more appropriate paradigm for the environmental scientist; (2) xenobiotics may have pharmacological and toxicological activities unrelated to their estrogenic activity; (3) these compounds may undergo extensive metabolism in vivo, may alter their own metabolism following repeated in vivo exposure, and may alter the metabolism of other xenobiotics as well as ovarian estrogens; and (4) xenobiotics may have pharmacokinetic properties markedly different than ovarian estrogens which have relatively short plasma half-lives in mammalian species. For these and other reasons the study of estrogens present in the environment must include, but not be limited to, the thinking and approaches used to study ovarian estrogens.

The plethora of compounds reported to exhibit estrogenic activity and the numerous studies of each preclude an extensive review here. Rather, we will focus on a single compound, o,p'-DDT, as a historical prototype of a xenobiotic estrogen. We will attempt to briefly review major studies on this environmental estrogen, and point out questions unanswered at present. Hopefully this brief review will provide a framework to understand the approaches used to characterize an estrogen and the techniques available for such studies.

BACKGROUND

The first indication that DDT had estrogenic activity was reported by Burlington and Linderman [1]. They noted that daily injections of DDT inhibited testicular growth and comb development in cockerels and suggested the pesticide might be working as an estrogen. Subsequent studies on the biological effects of DDT have been numerous; they have included laboratory animal experiments involving acute and chronic exposures, field studies of animal populations, and epidemiological surveys of human populations. In many cases, effects which were observed, particularly in animal experiments using high doses, were interpreted as being associated with changes in the hormonal state of the animal. However early results were often conflicting, variously assigning estrogenic, antiestrogenic or antiandrogenic mechanisms for DDT action (see [2]). Some factors leading to confusing observations have been: 1) Studies were conducted with technical grade DDT preparations which varied in content and proportions of constituents, 2) Some DDT congeners are potent inducers of hepatic mixed function oxidases (MFOs); increased MFO activity leads to degradation of endogenous steroid hormones as well as of DDT itself. Additonally, some of the DDT-like compounds are more readily metabolized than others by the MFO system, 3) o,p'-DDT, a major contaminant of technical DDT possesses both estrogenic properties and the ability to induce MFO's, thus yielding a "mixed bag" of results [3], and 4). Other environmental chemicals with estrogenic and/or MFO stimulating properties, such as mycotoxins, phytoestrogens, and pesticide residues may have been present in animal feed and quarters.

ESTROGENIC EFFECTS OF DDT ON THE REPRODUCTIVE SYSTEM

As noted above the earliest report of an effect of DDT on reproductive systems was made by Burlington and Linderman [1]. The discovery that technical DDT has estrogenic effects in mammals was made accidentally by Levin, Welch and Conney [4], who attempted to use it to diminish the uterotropic activity of administered estradiol (by induction of MFOs in rats), but instead observed increased uterine weights. These studies were extended by Welch et al. [5] who showed that o,p'-DDT, technical DDT and methoxychlor, but not p,p'-DDT, caused increased uterine weights, increased ^{14}C-glucose incorporation into macromolecules and decreased uterine uptake of $^3H-E_2$. Bitman et al [6] showed that o,p'-DDT caused increased glycogen content of rat uteri and increased oviduct weight in 2 species of birds.

Numerous estrogenic effects of o,p'-DDT and other organochlorine pesticides have since been demonstrated by various investigators. These include precocious puberty and persistent vaginal estrus following neonatal administration of DDT to rats [7,8]; interference with reproduction in mice [5,9,10,11]; inhibition of LH [but not FSH] release by the pituitary of rats [12]; increases in glycolytic and hexose monophosphate shunt enzyme activity in rat uteri [13]; induction of rat uterine ornithine decarboxylase activity [14]; induction of "Induced Protein" synthesis in rat uteri [15]; induction of the progesterone receptor [16]; and stimulation of uterine DNA synthesis [17].

These examples and the many other reported studies of DDT's estrogenic activity might seem at first glance like "beating a dead horse". It is important to remember, however that the term "estrogen" is a generic designation. The observation that a given compound produces one specific estrogenic effect is by no means a guarantee it will produce all the effects of an ovarian estrogen such as 17β-estradiol. A particularly clear example of this is provided by Clark's work that 17β-estradiol and estriol, two very similar estrogens can elicit comparable or divergent estrogenic effects depending upon the specific parameter measured and the mode of administration [18].

In a similar vein, low doses of Kepone, which do not elicit estrogenic effects when administered acutely, produce constant estrus and a uterine response when administered for 7-10 weeks [19]. Again, this observation indicates that conclusions based upon a single response or single exposure regimen cannot always be generalized.

ESTROGEN-RECEPTOR INTERACTIONS

In the 1960's the pioneering studies of Jensen and Gorski revealed the presence of specific cytosolic receptors (R_c) in estrogen target tissues, and suggested a two-step mechanism of estrogen action [20]. In this mechanism the estrogen was postulated to interact with the R_c, and the resultant complex was thought to translocate to the nucleus of the target cell. Clark's group [21] subsequently developed a nuclear-exchange assay which permitted a quantitation of the amount of nuclear estrogen receptor (R_n) translocated by various estrogens. These studies provided a framework and the experimental techniques for investigating the interaction of DDT with the estrogen receptor system.

To test the assumption that interactions with the cytoplasmic estrogen receptor (R_c) are involved in subsequent estrogenic actions, several investigators have examined DDT's ability to interact with the R_c. Nelson [22] was the first to show that o,p'-DDT could competitively inhibit $^3H\text{-}E_2$ binding to rat uterine cytosol in a concentration-dependent manner. In an in vitro binding assay, he showed that o,p'-DDT had 1/2000 the relative binding affinity of diethylstilbesterol (DES), a compound which is similar to E_2 in its affinity for the R_c. In comparing several chlorinated hydrocarbons to o,p'-DDT, he found that the ability to inhibit $^3H\text{-}E_2$ binding in vitro correlated well with the ability to produce an in vivo estrogenic response (increased uterine wet weight). In order of decreasing potency in the binding assay the compounds were: o,p'-DDT;technical methoxychlor; o,p'-DDD; o.p'-DDE; Arochlor 1221;methoxychlor;m,p'-DDD; Arochlor 1254;p.p'-DDT;p,p'-DDD=p,p'-DDE.

Other groups studied o,p'-DDT's ability to interact with the uterine estrogen receptor using sucrose density gradient analysis [23,24]. Kupfer and Bulger [24], in addition to confirming Nelson's results, showed by Scatchard analysis that DDT did not reduce the number of R_c binding sites. They also demonstrated for the first time that in vivo exposure to o,p'-DDT resulted in translocation of the R_c to the nucleus. In a logical extension of their uterine R_c studies, Kupfer and Bulger [25] showed that o,p'-DDT could compete with E_2 for in vitro binding to estrogen receptors from human mammary and uterine tumors. Similarly, Mason and Schulte [26] demonstrated that o,p'-DDT could compete with E_2 for binding to estrogen receptors from a DMBA-induced rat mammary tumor.

Recently, several studies have shown a very strong correlation between levels of R_n and uterine responses in vivo [27] and in vitro [28] following administration of o,p'-DDT.

Taken together these studies provide reasonable correlative evidence that the estrogenic effects of the pesticide result from its interaction with the estrogen receptor system. Binding studies in cell-free systems thus seem to provide a reasonable screening test to predict whether a xenobiotic might exhibit estrogenic activity.

IDENTITY OF THE ACTIVE COMPOUND

DDT is extensively metabolized, thus raising the question of whether o,p'-DDT itself and/or other metabolites are responsible for the estrogenic effects observed following in vivo administration of the pesticide. This question was raised by Welch et al [4], who showed a decreased uterotropic response to DDT following carbon tetrachloride administration. Bitman and Cecil [29] suggested that active estrogens are derived from o,p'-DDT by metabolic conversion to a hydroxylated metabolite, and demonstrated in a later study [30] that 3-hydroxy-o,p'-DDT was more potent than the parent o,p'-DDT when uterine glycogen levels were measured 18 hr after injection into immature rats. In the same test the 4-methoxy and 5-hydroxy derivatives were equipotent with o,p'-DDT. Of these compounds, only the 3-hydroxymetabolite was previously identified in the feces of rat and chicken following oral administration of o,p'-DDT [31,32].

Several investigators have provided indirect evidence that o,p'-DDT itself is an active estrogen. Nelson et al [33] showed that an in vitro incubation of rat liver microsomes with o,p'-DDT did not change the compound's ability to inhibit ^{3}H-E$_{2}$ binding to rat uterine R$_{c}$. This finding was confirmed and extended by Kupfer and Bulger [34], who incubated DDT with uteri in the presence and absence of rat liver microsomes, followed by determination of R$_{c}$ and R$_{n}$ levels by exchange assay. No change in receptor distribution followed these microsomal incubations. Finally, Stancel et al. [15] and Robison et al. [28] demonstrated that either in vivo or in vitro exposure of uteri to DDT resulted in similar stimulation of Induced Protein synthesis.

These studies establish that o,p'-DDT itself possesses estrogenic activity, but do not unequivocally prove that estrogenic effects observed in vivo result from the unmodified pesticide. The definitive experiment would follow o,p'-DDT's uptake and localization in the uterine cell nucleus directly, after both in vivo administration and in vitro incubation, followed by positive identification of the compounds associated with the R_n.

EFFECTS OF DDT ON ESTROGEN RESPONSIVE TUMORS

Most studies to date have used responses of normal tissues as an index of the estrogenicity of DDT. As noted above, however, several groups have demonstrated that o,p'-DDT interacts with estrogen receptors from uterine and mammary tumors. It seemed logical, therefore, to investigate the ability of o,p'-DDT to support the growth of estrogen responsive tumors. We have recently shown that o,p'-DDT supports the growth of a rat mammary tumor, MT2, to the same extent as estradiol (Robison, et al., submitted), thus indicating that DDT can in fact support the growth of at least one such tumor. Similar studies showed that the pesticide did not support the growth of an estrogen responsive kidney tumor, H-301, in the hamster under similar conditions. At present we do not understand the different responses of these two tumor models to DDT, and without further studies we cannot rule out the possibility that the lack of a response with the H-301 cells is due to trivial reasons, or that the response of the MT2 cells is unique for estrogen responsive tumors. Again, these results point to the necessity of examining a number of systems before generalized conclusions can be drawn.

SUMMARY

o,p'-DDT elicits a variety of estrogenic responses in several species. Most such studies have monitored estrogenic effects in normal tissues, but recent results suggest that the pesticide may be able to support the in vivo growth of at least one estrogen responsive tumor. There is substantial evidence that these effects are mediated by the interaction of the pesticide with the classical estrogen receptor systems; although this evidence is largely based on correlations between responses and receptor

114

binding. While o,p'-DDT probably possesses inherent estrogenic activity, it is unclear whether the unmodified pesticide is entirely responsible for the many effects observed in vivo.

ACKNOWLEDGEMENTS

We gratefully acknowledge the technical assistance of J. Ireland and D. Spalding and the support of the National Institute of Child Health and Human Development (HD-08615) for studies performed in our laboratory. We also thank R. Dotson for help preparing this manuscript.

REFERENCES

1.   H. Burlington, and V.F. Linderman, Proc. Soc. Exp. Biol. 74, 48-51 (1950).
2.   D. Kupfer, Crit. Rev. Toxicol., 4, 83-124 (1975).
3.   D. Kupfer, and W.H. Bulger, Estrogens in the Environment, J.A., ed. McLachlan (Elsevier/North-Holland, N.Y. 1980) pp. 239-263.
4.   R.M. Welch, W. Levin, and A.H. Conney, A.H., Toxicol. Appl. Pharmacol. 14, 358-367 (1969).
5.   R.M. Welch, W. Levin, R. Kuntzman, M. Jacobson, and A.H. Conney, Toxicol. Appl. Pharmacol. 19, 234-240 (1970).
6.   J. Bitman, H.C. Cecil, S.J. Harris, and G.F. Fries, Science, 162, 371-372 (1968).
7.   T. R. Wrenn, J.R. Wood, G.F. Fries, and J. Bitman, Bull. Environ. Contam. Toxicol 5, 61-73 (1971).
8.   R.J. Gellert, W.L. Heinrichs, and R. Swerdloff, Neuroendocrinology 16, 84-94 (1974).
9.   J.J. Huber, Toxicol. Appl. Pharmacol. 7, 516-523 (1965).
10. G.W. Ware, and E.J. Good, Toxicol. Appl. Pharmacol, 10, 54-67 (1967).
11. M.L. Keplinger, W.B. Deichmann, and F. Sala, Pesticides Symposia, W.B. Deichmann, ed., (Halos and Assoc., Miami, 1970) pp. 125-138.
12. R.J. Gellert, W.L. Heinrichs, and R.S. Swerdloff, Endocrinology 91, 1095-1101 (1972).
13. R.L. Singhal, J.R.E. Valadares, and W.S. Schwark, Biochem. Pharmacol. 19, 2145-2151 (1970).
14. W.H. Bulger, and D. Kupfer, Fed. Proc. 34, 810-816 (1975).
15. G.M. Stancel, J.S. Ireland, V.R. Mukku, and A.K. Robison, Life Sciences 27, 1111-1117 (1980).
16. R.R. Mason, and G.J. Schulte, Res. Comm. Chem. Path. Pharmacol., 29, 281-290 (1980).
17. J.S. Ireland, V.R. Mukku, A.K. Robinson, and G.M. Stancel, Biochem. Pharmacol. 29, 1469-1474 (1984).
18. J.H. Clark, and E.J. Peck, Jr., Female Sex Steroids (Springer-Verlag, New York 1979).
19. B. Hamond, B.S. Katzenellenbogen, N., Krauthammer, and J., McConnell, Proc. Natl. Acad. Sci. 76, 664-6645 (1979).
20. E.V. Jensen, and E.R. DeSombre, Ann. Rev. Biochem. 41, 203-230 (1972).
21. J. Anderson, J.H. Clark, and E.J. Peck Jr., Biochem. J., 126, 561-567 (1972).
22. J.A. Nelson, Biochem. Pharmacol. 23, 447-451 (1974).
23. M.S. Forster, E.L. Wilder, and W.L. Heinrichs, Biochem. Pharmacol. 24, 777-1780 (1975).
24. D. Kupfer, and W. H. Bulger, Pesticide Biochem. Physiol., 6, 561-570 (1976).
25. D. Kupfer, and W.H. Bulger, Res. Comm. Chem. Pathol. Pharmacol. 16, 451-462 (1977).
26. R.R. Mason, and G.J. Schulte, Res. Comm. Chem. Pathol. Pharmacol., 33, 119-128 (1981).
27. A.K. Robison, and G.M. Stancel, Life Sciences, 31, 2479-2484 (1982).
28. A.K. Robison, V.R. Mukku, D.M. Spalding, and G.M. Stancel, Toxicol. Appl. Pharmacol. 76, 537-543 (1984).
29. J. Bitman, H.C. Cecil, J. Agric. Food Chem. 18, 1108-2224 (1970).
30. J. Bitman, H.C. Cecil, S.J. Harris, and V.J. Feil, J. Agric. Food Chem. 26, 149-151 (1978).
31. V.J. Feil, C.H. Lamoureux, E. Styrovoky, R.G. Zaylskie, E.J. Thacker, and G.M. Holman, J. Agric. Food Chem. 21, 1072-1078 (1973).
32. V.J. Feil, V.H. Lamoureux, and R.G. Saylskie, J. Agric. Food Chem. 23, 382-388 (1975).
33. J.A. Nelson, R.F. Struck, and R. James, J. Toxicol, and Environ. Health, 4, 325-339 (1978).
34. D. Kupfer, and W.H. Bulger, Life Sciences 25, 975-984 (1979).

116

Chemical Analysis and Characterization of Estrogens

Jack D. Henion, Thomas R. Covey, Dominique R. Silvestre, and Kevin K.
Cuddy, Drug Testing and Toxicology, New York State College of Veterinary
Medicine, Cornell University, 925 Warren Drive, Ithaca, New York 14850

ABSTRACT

The ultratrace determination of diethylstilbestrol
(DES) and zeranol in bovine liver tissue is used to
compare the analytical capability of several modern
analytical techniques. These include the use of solid
phase extraction techniques and tritium labeling for
sample cleanup and recovery studies combined with ECD GC
with fused silica capillary columns for sensitive and
selective screening purposes. Unequivocal identification
of the analytes is described using selected ion monitoring
(SIM) capillary GC/MS, DLI micro-LC/MS, and tandem mass
spectrometry with LC/MS (LC/MS/MS). The limit of identification using selected reaction monitoring (SRM) LC/MS/MS
was approximately 250ppt for DES and zeranol.

INTRODUCTION

The determination of toxic or forbidden organic compounds at the trace
level in complex biological matrices represents a challenging problem in
analytical chemistry. In what has been called the "search for zero"
analysts are increasingly faced with the problem of both detection and
identification of analytes at ultra trace levels that seemed impossible
just a few years ago. Usually it is an easier task to "detect" a foreign
substance than it is to identify it. The simple detection scheme does not
have stringent criteria placed upon it as does the identification process.
In other words, the detection of an analyte usually results from a
relatively simple screening procedure which is not driven by severe
constraints. There is less confidence in a screening result and as such it
may be in error.
    Due to the increasing importance of regulatory constraints for certain
toxic or suspect compounds, it has become essential that these compounds be
unequivocally identified when they are "detected" in tissues of animals
used for human consumption. This is no small task since it requires modern
analytical equipment and highly competent personnel. It
also increasingly requires refined sample work up methodologies which may
deviate from classical techniques. These and the intrinsic problems of
ultratrace analysis create a considerable challenge for the analyst.
    Recently there has been renewed interest in several important
synthetic estrogens. Two important substances are diethylstilbestrol (DES)
[1,2], the popular but now illegal growth promoter used in the bovine, and
zeranol, which has been recently implicated in premature tellarche in
Puerto Rico [3]. The zero tolerance level of DES in edible tissues resulting from the Delaney Clause [4] and the search for possible ultratrace
levels of zeranol in small volumes of infant plasma [5] have thrust
involved analysts to press some of their analytical techniques beyond the
practical limits. Therefore, concerned analysts are addressing these
problems by equipping their laboratories with state-of-the-art equipment
and developing improved methods for both screening and confirmatory
purposes.

The three areas of importance for the ultratrace analysis of biological samples include sample workup, screening, and confirmation of the analyte. The preferred sample workup method should utilize limited sample and allow high sample throughput such that up to 50 samples per day may be analyzed. The desirable screening method must be both as sensitive and specific as possible to preclude unnecessary efforts spent trying to confirm a false positive. Finally, the confirmatory technique should be both ultra sensitive (sub part per billion, ppb) and unequivocal. These analytical attributes are possible today, but they are easier said than done.

It would appear that a preferred approach to ultratrace sample workup involves minimizing both the number of times that a sample is handled and the amount of sample utilized. The old adage of using more sample in order to obtain more analyte is not practical when one considers the large sized glassware required and the correspondingly high levels of endogenous background recovered from such large amounts of extracted sample. Instead, it appears that careful, optimized treatment of one to five grams of biological sample with minimal sample transfer steps may provide improved detection limits and higher sample throughput. Specifically, modern solid phase extraction techniques [6] coupled with successive elution steps from specially designed miniature chromatographic columns allows one to achieve adequate cleanup of the sample for subsequent analyses. The most important gains from this approach include both higher recovery and sample throughput and the elimination of a large portion of the endogenous background matrix.

The speed of the improved screening techniques must parallel that of the sample workup procedure. In addition, the screening procedure must be both as sensitive and specific as possible. Finally, it should require relatively inexpensive equipment or supplies, and be performed by non technical personnel. These criteria are a tall order because such capabilities are not often available per these requirements. Other than the technique of radioimmuno assay (RIA) the only analytical techniques that may meet these requirements are thin layer chromatography (TLC) and capillary gas chromatography (GC) with electron capture detection (ECD). The latter GC technique offers the ultimate in separation efficiency and sensitivity, but unfortunately is rather costly and requires experienced personnel for its operation. However, it does provide the best analytical performance for screening purposes.

Finally, the confirmatory step is the most important stage in the analytical scheme for those samples which were deemed positive in the screening step and may be subject to legal scrutiny [7]. There is little disagreement that mass spectrometry is required for unequivocal confirmation of organic analytes. Mass spectral confirmation requires a clean, unambiguous mass spectrum which agrees in all respects with an authentic sample of the suspect analyte. Unfortunately, the analysis of complex biological samples often can result in mass spectra which contain interferent ions due to endogenous materials from the sample matrix. To minimize this possibility we must use high resolution capillary chromatographic columns coupled to the mass spectrometer (GC/MS). Under optimized conditions, such coupling offers remarkable separation and resolution of the analyte from the sample interfering components. In addition we can utilize a selective ionization technique such as negative chemical ionization (NCI) to increase our ability to detect the analyte of interest at the expense of matrix components.

Recently, the unique capabilities of the mass spectrometer as an HPLC detector have offered new analytical horsepower to our ability to analyze biological samples. The technique of HPLC is extremely useful for separating biological matrix interferents from analytes of interest. In addition, this technique requires no elevated temperatures as does the GC so there is less possibility of thermal degradation of trace analytes which can often occur in the latter. Thus combined HPLC/MS (LC/MS) could offer

significant opportunities for the ultratrace analysis of important analytes
in biological samples [8].

Finally, a recent advance in mass spectrometry has provided the
technique of tandem mass spectrometry (MS/MS) [9]. This modern analytical
technique reduces the problem of the mixed mass spectra noted above. The
MS/MS technique allows one to specifically focus on the ions particular to
the analyte of interest even when it is in the presence of interfering
material. Thus MS/MS provides a final "separation" after either GC or HPLC
separation of materials introduced into the mass spectrometer. We have
recently investigated the merits of both solid probe MS/MS and LC/MS/MS
applied to the characterization of estrogens in complex biological
matrices.

This paper will review recent studies which utilize each of the
analytical techniques mentioned above. Most of our effort has focused on
the isolation and ultratrace determination of DES and zeranol in bovine
liver tissue [10]. Appropriate internal standards have been utilized
whenever possible and analyzed tissues have contained the analyte by either
fortification or actual administration. This survey of results will serve
as an introduction to the implementation of some new approaches to
ultratrace analysis and represents a progress report of work underway.

EXPERIMENTAL

Sample Workup

The isolation of estrogenic substances from tissue matrices utilized
solid phase extraction procedures and a so-called micro technique which
required no more than 5 grams of tissue [10]. The details of this
procedure are not the focus of this paper since they will be published
elsewhere. Basically, the tissue homogenate was hydrolzed overnight with
-glucuronidase, extracted with acetonitrile and transferred to a small
DuPont anion exchange (Type AS) extraction cartridge. Up to 12 of these
cartridges may be placed into the carrousel of a DuPont Prep I sample
preparation device (DuPont Clinical Systems, Wilmington, DE.) and treated
to successive pH and solvent washes. By appropriate control of pH both the
ion exchange and reversed phase chromatographic characteristics of the type
AS cartridges may be utilized without any sample transfer steps. In this
way a sequence of elution solvents, centrifugations, and excess solvent
removal may be accomplished without any transfer of the sample from one
container to another. We believe this is an important aspect of ultratrace
analysis since a considerable amount of the analyte is generally lost or
decomposed in multiple sample transfers. With the aid of tritium labeled
internal standards the overall recovery of DES and zeranol from liver
tissue using this procedure ranged from 70 - 85% at the 100 ppt level. The
extract from this sample work up was collected in a 100ul conical
Reactivial (Pierce Chemical Co., Rockford, IL.) and subjected to the
analytical techniques described below.

Capillary GC with ECD detection

The tissue extract was derivatized with heptafluorobutyric Acid
anhydride (HFBA) by a modified procedure [10] for subsequent capillary GC
analysis using an ECD detector. The gas chromatograph was a Carlo Erba
Mega Series HRGC model 5160-10 equipped with a heated split/splitless
injector operated in the splitless mode. The column was a Hewlett-Packard
narrow bore fused silica capillary coated with a crosslinked 5% phenyl
methyl silicone (200um i.d. x 25 m) connected directly to a ECD 40 electron
capture detector (Erba Instruments). The samples were injected in hexane
solution and the chromatograms were recorded on a Spectra-Physics SP4270

Chromatography Integrator. A typical temperature program was initial oven temperature held for 2 minutes at 65 degrees, then programmed at 20 degrees per minute to 220 degrees where it was held for 15 minutes followed by a 5 degrees per minute program to 285 degrees. The temperature was held at 285 degrees for 5 minutes and then heated ballistically to 300 degrees to clear the column of less volatile components before making the next injection at the initial column temperature.

SIM Capillary GC/MS

A Hewlett-Packard Model 5970 Mass Selective Detector (MSD) equipped with a direct capillary interface, 5% phenyl methyl silicone 0.200mm id x 15m fused silica capillary, (Hewlett-Packard Co.) a HP 5790 capillary gas chromatograph and a MSD Workstation with associated software was used for the capillary GC/MS results reported in this work. Samples were injected either as HFBA derivatives exactly as described above for capillary GC screening, or by co-injection of trimethylsilylation reagents and underivatized tissue extracts to form trimethylsilyl (TMS) derivatives of the analyte. The preferred silyating reagent mixture was a 2% solution of TSIM in BSTFA (Pierce Chemical Co.) co-injected with a hexane solution of the tissue extract. This reagent mixture was particularly effective at providing quantitative derivatization of all three active hydrogens on zeranol. The flash heater derivatization procedure precludes the HFBA off-line derivatization step and yields derivatives whose molecular weights are within the mass range of the MSD mass spectrometer.

For the ultratrace determination of DES and zeranol the technique of selected ion monitoring (SIM) was used wherein up to six unique ions including the molecular ion were monitored. The corresponding ions of the internal standard were also monitored after verification that there were no interfering ions appearing in the control extract of tissue. The criteria for SIM GC/MS confirmation of the corresponding estrogens in tissue extracts included correct relative abundances of the selected ions with the correct capillary retention time for authentic standards of the corresponding analytes. These criteria were met for all ultratrace analyses reported in this work.

Direct liquid introduction micro-LC/MS

Direct Liquid Introduction (DLI) LC/MS introduces either a portion or all of the liquid effluent from a HPLC instrument directly into the chemical ionization (CI) source of a CI mass spectrometer [11]. For trace analysis it is only practical to direct the entire HPLC effluent into the mass spectrometer, but the high vacuum requirements of the latter makes this impractical in many instances. One way to readily accomplish this task is by using micro HPLC columns with effluent flow rates in the neighborhood of 20-50uL/min. With these reduced flow rates it is possible to accomplish micro-LC/MS with ppb detection limits using SIM techniques.

The micro-LC/MS system used in this work included a Brownlee Labs Micropump (Brownlee Laboratories, Santa Clara, CA) equipped with a Rheodyne Model 7520 micro loop injector (Rheodyne Inc., Cotati, CA), and a home-packed C-18 five micron particle silica microbore column (1mm i.d.. x 25cm) using hexane/isopropanol (96/4) as the mobile phase. The exit of the microbore column was connected directly to a DLI micro-LC/MS diaphragm probe interface [12] which was inserted into the solid probe inlet of a Hewlett-Packard 5985B GC/MS equipped with a liquid nitrogen cryopump. The LC/MS experiments were conducted in the SIM mode wherein selected ions of both DES (DO-DES) and its internal standard, octadeutero-DES (D8-DES), were monitored. The crude liver extract was analyzed by micro-LC/MS without any prior derivatization.

LC/MS and LC/MS/MS

In order to utilize conventional HPLC flow rates, very short run
times, and tandem mass spectrometry we have investigated the use of short,
three micron HPLC columns for ultratrace analysis of estrogens in
biological samples. The system used included two model 6000A pumps, a
M-660 solvent programmer, a model 440 UV detector (Waters Assoc., Milfred,
MA) equipped with a Rheodyne model 7510 injector and a three micron C-18
"fast" HPLC column (4.6mm i.d. x 3cm) from Perkin Elmer (Perkin Elmer
Corp., Norwalk, CN). The mobile phase was 70/30 methanol/water. The exit
of the UV detector was connected to a heated nebulizer LC/MS probe which
was inserted into the atmospheric pressure chemical ionization (APCI)
source of a TAGA 6000E triple quadrupole mass spectrometer (Sciex, In.,
Thornhill, Ontario, Canada). HPLC flow rates of one milliliter per minute
could be continually introduced into the APCI source under either LC/MS or
LC/MS/MS conditions. The mass spectrometer could be operated in either the
full scan or selected reaction monitoring (SRM) mode in the LC/MS/MS
experiment.[9]

RESULTS AND DISCUSSION

Sample workup for the results which follow was done in the same manner
as described above and utilized the polystyrene anion exchange cartridges
for solid phase extraction of liver tissue homogenate. Since the details
of this sample purification procedure have been described in detail
elsewhere [10], the procedure will not be described here. The recoveries
using the current optimized method for zeranol and DES respectively were
70% and 80% overall as determined by tritium labeled recovery studies at
the 100 ppt level.

Figure 1AB shows the capillary ECD gas chromatogram of HFBA
derivatized bovine liver extract. The upper GC trace was obtained from a
control liver (Figure 1A), and the lower GC trace resulted from the
extraction of a liver homogenate fortified with 50 ppb zeranol (Figure 1B).
Considerable effort was expended to optimise the yield of the HFBA
derivatization and the chromatography of the derivatized extract.
Fortunately the zeranol HFBA derivatives elute in a region of the
chromatogram where there is little matrix interference. However, the
practical detection limit (5 ppb) is not as good as desired and the
analysis time of 35 minutes is too long for high sample throughput. In
addition, the two ECD peaks observed for zeranol in Figure 1B indicates
that the derivatization is not quantitative. In spite of these
shortcomings ECD capillary GC can provide a reliable indication of whether
a tissue extract may contain zeranol.

Screening for DES in tissue extracts can be combined with quantitative
analysis. We have utilized a stable isotope form of the drug, D8-DES, as
an internal standard for quantitative GC/ECD. Figure 2 shows an ECD
capillary GC chromatogram of a 1ng standard mixture of cis/trans DO-DES and
D8-DES. This chromatogram demonstrates that the deuterated analog of DES
can be nearly baseline resolved by this chromatographic system and offers a
unique way to complement the screening and quantitative determination of
DES in tissue extracts. Thus a standard solution of D8-DES could be added
to a suspect tissue extract and the appearance of the corresponding GC
"doublet" for D8-DES/DO-DES at the appropriate retention time could provide
evidence of both the presence and quantity of DES in a suspect tissue
extract.

The detection of DES in a fortified homogenate extract by ECD
capillary GC is shown in Figure 3AB. The upper GC chromatogram (Figure 3A)
shows the chromatogram of a derivatized control tissue extract while Figure
3B shows the capillary GC chromatogram of the extract from a tissue
homogenate fortified with 1 ppb of D8/DO DES. The detection limit for DES with

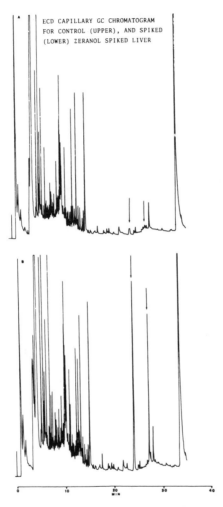

ECD CAPILLARY GC CHROMATOGRAM
FOR CONTROL (UPPER), AND SPIKED
(LOWER) ZERANOL SPIKED LIVER

Figure 1.   A) ECD capillary GC chromatogram of the HFBA derivatized extract
from control bovine liver homogenate. B) ECD capillary GC
chromatogram of the HFBA derivatized extract from a bovine liver
homogenate spiked with 50 ppb zeranol. Note that a peak at 24
min and 27 min retention time for both the di- and tri- HFBA
derivative of zeranol are obtained due to the non quantitative
nature of this derivatization.

ECD detection is considerably better than that for zeranol described above.
Figure 3B readily reveals the presence of the 1 ppb level of DES in the
chromatogram without significant interference from endogenous materials.
Thus, with the exception of the 19 minute retention of DES which limits the
sample throughput somewhat, this analytical technique offers significant
improvement over conventional methods of screening for DES in tissues.

122

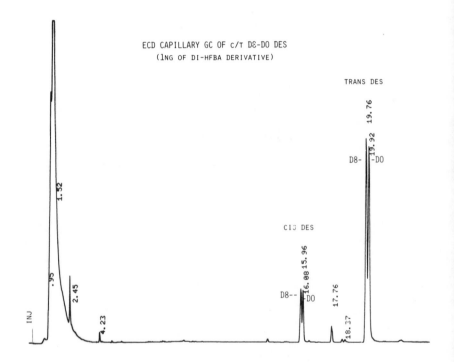

ECD CAPILLARY GC OF c/T D8-DO DES
(1NG OF DI-HFBA DERIVATIVE)

TRANS DES

Figure 2.   ECD capillary GC chromatogram of the di-HFBA derivative of
standard cis/trans D8/DO DES.

Figure 4 shows the standard curve for DES spiked into bovine liver
tissue homogenate at levels ranging from 1 ppb - 4 ppb. The internal
standard used was D8-DES added to the tissue homogenate at the 1 ppb level.
Each point on the curve represents the mean of triplicate ECD peak height
ratios of DO DES/D8-DES obtained as described above. The correlation
coefficient for the three points on the standard curve was 0.999 and
suggests that reliable quantitative determination of DES in liver tissue is
possible within the concentration range defined by the data in Figure 4.
These preliminary results encourage further documentation of this
quantitative capability over a wider concentration range.

Since the chosen screening technique serves only to focus the
analyst's attention upon the samples which may contain the suspected
foreign substance, an unambiguous technique must be utilized for final
confirmation. Mass spectrometry combined with capillary GC is the
technique of choice for this purpose. Figure 5 shows the selected ion
monitoring (SIM) capillary GC/MS results obtained from the analysis of calf
liver extracts which were derivatized with HFBA. The SIM capillary GC/MS

chromatogram shown in Figure 5A was obtained from the analysis of a control calf liver. The ions m/z 447, 631 and 660 were selected as unique ions for

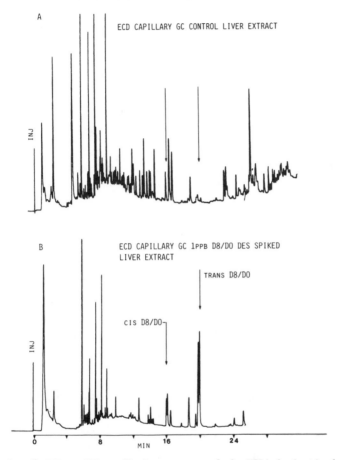

Figure 3. A) ECD capillary GC chromatogram of the HFBA derivatized extract from control bovine liver homogenate. B) ECD capillary GC chromatogram of the HFBA derivatized extract from a bovine liver homogenate spiked with 1ppb cis/trans D8/D0 DES.

DES. The GC/MS data system utilized for this work confined the choice of ions to a maximum of three ions when SIM of six ions would have been preferrable. The data shown in Figure 5B were obtained in the same manner from the extract of a tissue homogenate which had been fortified with 100 ppt of DES. The di-HFBA derivative for both the cis and trans isomers of DES are observed at 6.4 and 7.4 min retention times for the 100 ppt levels of these analytes. The data show that there are no significant interferences observed in the retention time region where these ions of the analyte occur. The ion abundance ratios were in good agreement with those observed for authentic standards of these compounds (not shown here). Thus

124

SIM capillary GC/MS determination of cis/trans DES in tissue matrices may
be accomplished within 10 minute time frames at sub ppb levels.

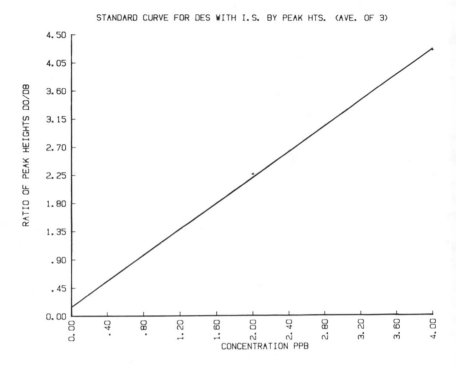

STANDARD CURVE FOR DES WITH I.S. BY PEAK HTS. (AVE. OF 3)

Figure 4.   ECD capillary GC standard curve for DES in bovine liver from
            1ppb-4ppb. The points on the curve were means from triplicate
            injections of each sample.

The identification of zeranol in tissue extracts may be similarly
accomplished by SIM capillary GC/MS. Figure 6AB shows the corresponding
GC/MS analysis for a control mature bovine liver extract (Figure 6A) and an
extract obtained from a tissue homogenate fortified with 0.1 ppb zeranol
(Figure 6B). Note that this control liver sample appears to contain about
10 ppt of zeranol presumably due to the widespread legal use of zeranol.
In this example the TMS derivative is produced by co-injecting the sample
with a trimethylsilylating reagent into the heated GC injector. The
tri-TMS derivative of molecular weight 538 is quantitatively produced by
this procedure and six unique higher mass ions of the zeranol TMS
derivative were monitored in the SIM experiment. These experiments allow
one to unequivocally identify zeranol in tissue extracts down to at least
the 0.1 ppb level in a relatively straightforward manner.
       The total ion current chromatogram (TIC) obtained from a tissue
homogenate fortified with 0.5 ppb zeranol under full scan capillary GC/MS
is shown in Figure 7A. The signal measured at the time corresponding to
the analyte retention (11.22 min) produces a full scan mass spectrum that

is a mixed spectrum which is inadequate for confirmation of zeranol. In
contrast, the SIM selected ion current chromatogram for the same sample is

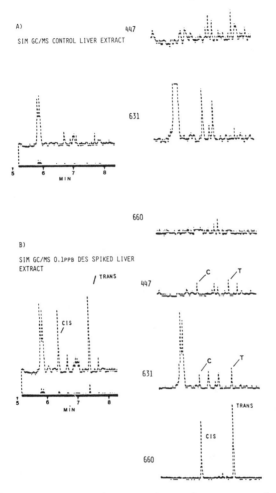

Figure 5. A) SIM capillary GC/MS ion current chromatogram of the HFBA
derivatized extract from control bovine liver homogenate. The
GC/MS was set to monitor m/z 447,631, and 660 ions. B) SIM
capillary GC/MS ion current chromatograms of the HFBA
derivatized extract from a bovine liver homogenate spiked with
.1ppb cis/trans DES.

shown in Figure 7B. The selected ions of m/z 379.2, 389.2, 433.2, 453.2,
523.4 and 538.4 for the zeranol tri-trimethylsilyl derivative were combined
to give the ion current chromatogram shown in Figure 7B. This latter
chromatogram shows much less interference and clearly displays the 11.22
min peak for 0.5 ppb zeranol. Thus SIM is preferrable to full scan

126

capillary GC/MS in these experiments due to increased sensitivity and increased specificity for the analyte of interest.

Although the GC/MS technique described above offers a viable approach to confirming estrogens such as DES and zeranol, the necessary derivatization procedures and the unavoidable elevated temperatures of the gas chromatograph can produce some undesirable problems. In addition, the

A) SIM GC/MS CONTROL LIVER EXTRACT

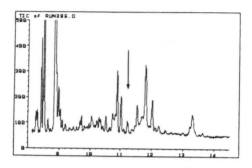

B) SIM GC/MS,1PPB ZERANOL SPIKED LIVER EXTRACT

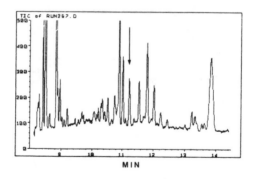

MIN

Figure 6.   A) SIM capillary GC/MS ion current chromatogram of the trimethylsilyl derivatized extract from control bovine liver homogenate. This selected ion current chromatogram is the composite of the six selected ions. B) SIM capillary GC/MS selected ion current chromatogram of the same six ions of the trimethylsilyl derivatized extract from a bovine liver homogenate spiked with 0.1ppb zeranol.

capillary GC chromatograms are often rather long which limits the sample throughput of the analysis. An alternative to this approach would be the use of HPLC as the chromatographic inlet device to the mass spectrometer. In principle, analytes could be determined by HPLC in shorter time periods without derivatization and without unnecessary extended exposure to elevated temperatures as in gas chromatography. Thus, LC/MS determination of estrogens in tissue extracts would appear to be a desirable goal.

An example of this approach is shown in Figure 8. These data show the utility of the DLI micro-LC/MS technique when used to analyze the liver extract obtained from a bovine calf which had received a 10 mg dose of DES

FULL SCAN CAPILLARY GC/MS OF 0.5PPB ZERANOL TISSUE EXTRACT

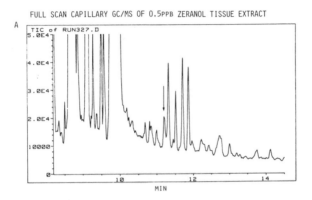

SIM CAPILLARY GC/MS OF 0.5PPB ZERANOL TISSUE EXTRACT

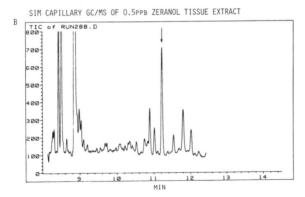

Figure 7. A) Full scan capillary GC/MS TIC of a trimethylsilyl derivatized extract from a bovine liver homogenate spiked with 0.5ppb zeranol. B) SIM capillary GC/MS selected ion current chromatogram of the trimethylsilyl derivatized extract from the same 0.5ppb zeranol spiked bovine liver homogenate shown in Figure 7A.

ten days prior to its sacrifice. The DLI micro-LC/MS data in Figure 8A show the selected ion current profiles for the (M+1) ions of parent cis/trans DES (m/z 269), the D8-DES internal standard (m/z 277), and another commercial anabolic E,E-dienestrol (m/z 267) in a spiked liver extract. One advantage of the DLI micro-LC/MS approach was that separation of trans DES and dienestrol which is a very difficult task using capillary GC/MS. Normal phase micro HPLC readily achieved this separation, however. Figure 8B shows a quantitative estimation of DES in an administration calf liver. Peak areas of the unlabeled DES are 80% of the labeled internal standard. The relative peak areas appear distorted due to software normalization on the most abundant peak in the chromatogram. Although LC/MS has not enjoyed widespread implementation, the benefits of the technique may change this situation in the future.

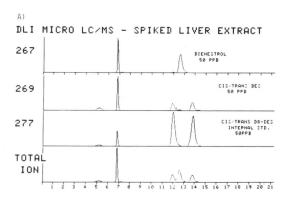

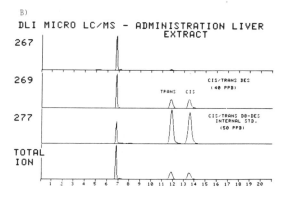

Figure 8. A) SIM DLI micro-LC/MS ion current profiles of an underivatized extract of a bovine liver homogenate spiked with 50ppb each of cis/trans DO DES, cis/trans D8 DES, and E,E-dienestrol. B) SIM DLI micro-LC/MS ion current profiles of an underivatized extract of a bovine liver homogenate obtained from a calf which had been sacrificed 10 days after the administration of 10mg DES. The liver tissue homogenate was spiked with 50ppb cis/trans D8 DES prior to extraction.

129

Finally, in a continuing effort to achieve rapid sample analysis with
high sensitivity and specificity, we have evaluated so-called "fast" HPLC
as an inlet system for tandem mass spectrometry. The focus of this
approach is to combine automated solid phase sample cleanup techniques with
LC/MS/MS. In this way the complex biological extract may be further
chromatographed by a short, high efficiency HPLC column. Components which
co-elute with the analyte of interest may be separated in a final stage by
the tandem mass spectrometer. The approach taken is demonstrated in the
examples which follow.

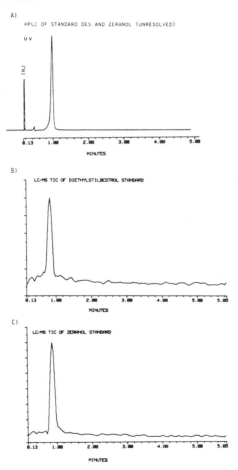

Figure 9. A) HPLC determination of a mixed standard of DES and zeranol (50
ng each). B) APCI LC/MS TIC of 50 ng standard DES. C) APCI
LC/MS TIC of 50 ng standard zeranol.

The HPLC conditions were optimized for short retention times and high
sample throughput while chromatographic resolution was deliberately
sacrificed. Using the tandem mass spectrometer (MS/MS) as a detector,

130

co-eluting components in an HPLC peak can be readily resolved. Figure 9A
shows the UV trace of a 50ng mixture of DES and zeranol, demonstrating the
lack of chromatographic resolution under these fast HPLC conditions (1
minute). Figures 9B and C show the corresponding total ion current traces
(TIC) for the APCI LC/MS determination of 50ng standard DES and zeranol.
The APCI LC/MS data shown in Figure 10 show the UV and LC/MS detection of
DES in the extract of a spiked liver homogenate. The peak at about 0.8 min
retention time observed in the UV chromatogram shown in Figure 8A was
thought to be due to the 10ppb spike of DES but the complexity of the
chromatogram made its identity uncertain. The APCI LC/MS TIC shown in
Figure 10B shows little indication for a peak corresponding to the
suspected 10ppb spike of DES known to be present in this liver extract.
The limited chromatographic separation afforded by the short three micron
HPLC column does not adequately resolve the DES from interfering

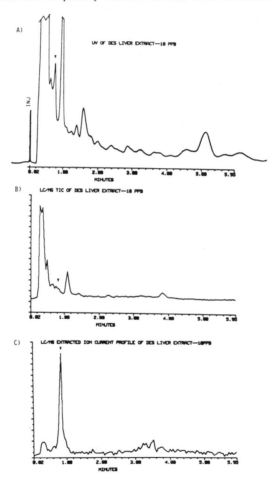

Figure 10. A) HPLC UV chromatogram of the extract of a bovine liver
homogenate spiked with 10ppb DES. B) APCI LC/MS TIC of the
extract described in A. C) APCI LC/MS EICP of the extract
described in A and B.

components. However, when an extracted ion current profile (EICP) for the (M+1) ion of DES is viewed as shown in Figure 10C, the 10ppb level of DES is readily detected. Although this information can be very useful, one requires more mass spectral information for identification purposes such as either a full scan mass spectrum or SIM data of several ions unique to the analyte of interest.

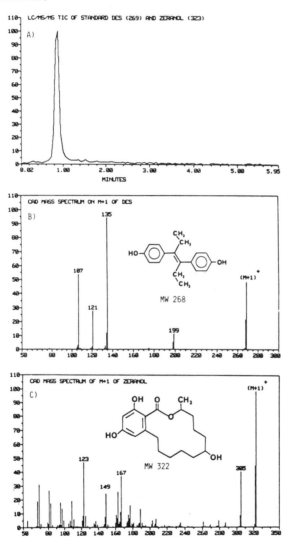

Figure 11. A) APCI LC/MS/MS TIC of the unresolved standard mixture of DES and zeranol described in Figure 9A above. B) APCI LC/MS/MS full scan mass spectrum of the (M+1) ion of standard DES present in the TIC shown in A. C) APCI LC/MS/MS full scan mass spectrum of the (M+1) ion of standard zeranol present in the TIC shown in A.

LC/MS/MS determination of trace analytes can provide the final
necessary analytical information for unequivocal determination of
ultratrace levels of compounds such as DES and zeranol. This technique
benefits from the tandem mass spectrometer's ability to focus unique ions
characteristic of the analyte and then induce fragmentation of that ion to
a family of daughter ions unique to the structure of the analyte. This
so-called collisionally activated dissociation (CAD) [9] experiment allows
identification of an analyte while in the presence of other analytes.

The ability to identify a component by MS/MS while in the presence of
another analyte is shown in Figure 11A where the LC/MS/MS TIC of standard
DES and zeranol are shown chromatographically unresolved as before (cf
Figure 9). The (CAD) experiment of the corresponding (M+1) ions at m/z 269
and m/z 323 of DES and zeranol respectively produces the full scan CAD mass
spectra shown in Figure 11A and 11C respectively. These mass spectra
correspond exactly to those of pure standards and allow facile
identification of these compounds even though they elute unresolved from
the HPLC column.

When one has biological extracts with analytes such as DES and zeranol
present at the 1-10ppb level the above full scan CAD experiments can
provide identification of these analytes. However, for ultratrace analyses
the technique of selected reaction monitoring (SRM) in the LC/MS/MS mode
may be more appropriate for identification purposes [9]. For example, the
SRM LC/MS/MS determination of low nanogram levels of DES and zeranol is
shown in Figure 12A and 12B respectively. In these experiments the tandem
mass spectrometer was set to alternately focus the (M+1) ions of both DES
and zeranol into the central quadrupole collision region and then drive the
third quadrupole mass filter to monitor five selected fragment ions unique
to each analyte. Both Figure 12A and 12B show duplicate injections of 0.5,
0.75, 1.00, and 2.00 ng of DES and zeranol respectively at exactly one
minute intervals. Thus the short three micron HPLC column provides rapid
elution of these standard materials and the SRM LC/MS/MS experiment allows
detection and identification of these compounds at sub nanogram levels.

Figures 13A and 13B show the SRM LC/MS/MS determination of zeranol and
DES respectively in extracts of spiked liver homogenate at levels of 0.25,
0.375, 0.5, and 1.0 ppb. These samples were injected at one minute
intervals onto the HPLC system while the tandem mass spectrometer
continuously monitored the total HPLC effluent. The data shown in Figure
13AB show expected signal increases for the various levels of spiked
analyte and demonstrate that an initial injection of control extract showed
no evidence of zeranol or DES.

The UV chromatogram shown in Figure 14A was obtained from one minute
injections of extracts from spiked liver homogenates containing 0.0, 0.25,
0.375, 0.5, and 1.0 ppb of zeranol. The short HPLC column effectively
resolved the components eluting with low k' [13] values from the lower
levels of components eluting in the vacinity of the k' for zeranol.
However, there is still considerable interference from co-eluting material
with zeranol which would render LC/MS or related techniques ineffective.
Only the mixture analysis capability [9] of tandem mass spectrometry
combined with the sensitivity and specificity of SRM LC/MS/MS can
effectively and rapidly provide analytical data such as those shown in
Figure 14. It should be noted that Figure 14B shows the analysis and
identification of zeranol in four samples plus one control within five
minutes. Thus the technique of LC/MS/MS, albeit expensive and complex, can
provide rapid sample throughput.

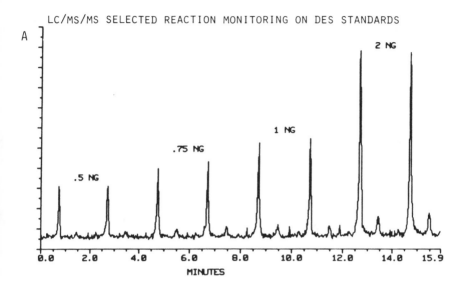

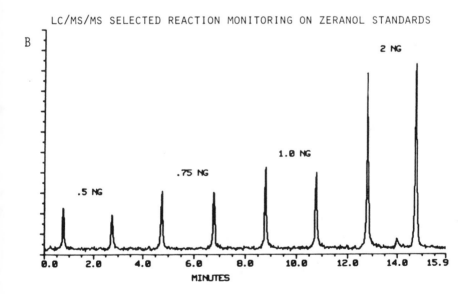

Figure 12. A) APCI LC/MS/MS selected reaction monitoring ion current chromatograms from duplicate one minute injections of 0.5, 0.75, 1.0, and 2.0ng of standard DES. B) APCI LC/MS selected reaction monitoring ion current chromatograms from duplicate one minute injections of 0.5, 0.75, 1.0, and 2.0ng of standard zeranol.

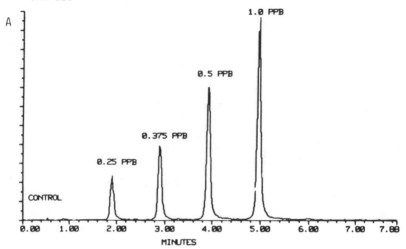

LC/MS/MS SELECTED REACTION MONITORING OF ZERANOL SPIKED LIVER SAMPLES

A

1.0 PPB

0.5 PPB

0.375 PPB

0.25 PPB

CONTROL

0.00   1.00   2.00   3.00   4.00   5.00   6.00   7.00 7.88
MINUTES

LC/MS/MS SELECTED REACTION MONITORING OF DES SPIKED LIVER SAMPLES

B

1.0 PPB

.5 PPB

.375 PPB

CONTROL   .25 PPB

0.00   1.00   2.00   3.00   4.00   5.00   6.00   7.00 7.88
MINUTES

Figure 13. A) APCI LC/MS/MS selected reaction monitoring ion current
chromatograms from successive one minute injections of extract
from bovine liver homogenate spiked with 0.0, 0.25, 0.375, 0.5,
and 1.0ppb zeranol. B) APCI LC/MS/MS selected reaction
monitoring ion current chromatograms from successive one minute
injections of extracts of bovine liver homogenate spiked with
0.0, 0.25, 0.375, 0.5, and 1.0ppb DES.

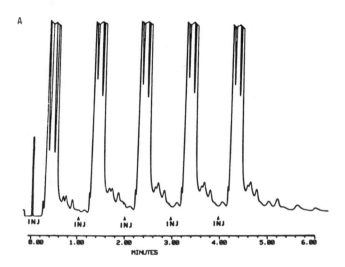

SIMULTANEOUS UV CHROMATOGRAM OF ZERANOL SPIKED LIVER SAMPLES (AUFS=0.2)

A

INJ   INJ   INJ   INJ   INJ

0.00   1.00   2.00   3.00   4.00   5.00   6.00
MINUTES

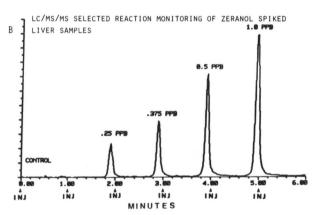

LC/MS/MS SELECTED REACTION MONITORING OF ZERANOL SPIKED
B   LIVER SAMPLES   1.0 PPB

0.5 PPB

.375 PPB

.25 PPB

CONTROL

0.00   1.00   2.00   3.00   4.00   5.00   6.00
INJ   INJ   INJ   INJ   INJ   INJ
            MINUTES

Figure 14.   A) HPLC UV chromatogram from successive one minute injections
from extracts of bovine liver homogenate spiked with 0.0, 0.25,
0.375, 0.5, and 1.0ppb zeranol.   B) APCI LC/MS/MS selected
reaction monitoring ion current chromatograms from the same
sequence of zeranol injections shown in A.

SUMMARY AND CONCLUSIONS

   This analytical review presents preliminary results from a comparative
study of several techniques used for the determination of DES and zeranol
at ultratrace levels in liver tissues. The approach differs from other

reports in that it considers the entire analytical problem from sample
preparation to analyte confirmation with an emphasis on new analytical
techniques and the problems related to low ppb to sub ppb identification.
The optimized solid phase extraction procedure facilitates high performance
from ECD capillary GC screening in addition to the confirmatory procedures
of SIM cappillary GC/MS, micro-LC/MS, APCI LC/MS, and LC/MS/MS. Although
SIM capillary GC/MS has been reported for the confirmation of DES in
tissues [14], the various approaches to LC/MS have not been evaluated for
these purposes. Since HPLC techniques offer several advantages for the
analysis of complex biological samples, the sensitivity and specificity of
mass spectrometry merit attempts to utilize these two techniques in
combination. This report attempts to present some of the analytical
possibilities that may be afforded by this approach.

The results from this work suggest that our current techniques and
equipment are capable of detecting and unequivocally identifying DES and
zeranol at tissue levels down to 100 ppt using small sample sizes (1-5 gram
tissue) while maintaining high sample throughput (40-50 samples/day).
Although either SIM capillary GC/MS or SRM LC/MS/MS may be utilized to
achieve these detection limits, if one requires rapid sample analysis the
latter technique is preferred. It seems unlikely that capillary GC
techniques will ever offer sample throughput capability for real world
samples that "fast" HPLC is capable of providing. Thus, one could expect
to see more effort expended to utilize the unique combination of short run
times of HPLC and rapid scanning capability of mass spectrometry in the
future. That LC/MS has "come of age" is suported by the increasing
interest and success of, for example, thermospray LC/MS [15,16]. It is
only a matter of time before the cost and ease of use of LC/MS will reach
the point that this uniquely capable technique will be as common as GC/MS.

ACKNOWLEDGEMENTS

We thank T. Mallinson for valuable sample preparation and recovery
studies, and M.K. Hoffman of the USDA for helpful suggestions,
contributions and discussions.

CREDITS

We thank the United States Department of Agruculture for financial
support of this work.

REFERENCES

1. M. Metzler, "The Metabolism of Diethylstilbestrol", CRC Crit. Rev.
    Biochem., 10 171-212 (1981).
2. J.A. McLachlan, K.S. Korach, R.R. Newbold, G.H. Degen,
    "Diethylstilbestrol and other Estrogens in the Environment", Fund.
    Appl. Toxicol. Oct; 4 (5): 686-91 (1984).
3. Food Chemical News, "USDA Puerto Rican Meat Screening will Include
    Pesticides, Antibiotics", p.10, Feb. 25, (1985).
4. Regulatory Aspects of Carcinogenisis and Food Additives: The Delaney
    Clause, F. Coulston, Ed., J.G. Martin, "The Delaney Clause: An Idea
    Whose Time has Come For a Change", 121-389, Academic Press, New York,
    (1979).
5. M.K. Hoffman, Personal Communication. (1984).
6. B.A. Bildingmeyer "Guidelines for proper usage of solid phase
    extraction devices", LC Mag., 2, 578-580, (1984).
7. J.A. Sphon, "Use of Mass Spectrometry for Confirmation of Animal Drug
    Residues", J. Assoc. Off. Anal. Chem., 61 1247-52 (1978).

8. D.S. Skrabalak, T.R. Covey and J.D. Henion,"Qualitative Detection of Chorticosteroids in Equine Biological Fluids and the Comparison of Relative Dexamethasone Metabolite/Dexamethasone Concentration in Equine Urine by Micro-Liquid Chromatography Mass Spectrometry", J. Chromatogr., 315 359-372 (1984).
9. Tandem Mass Spectrometry, F.W. McLafferty, Ed., (John Wiley & Sons, Inc., 1983).
10. T.R. Covey, G.A. Maylin, and J.D. Henion, "Quantitative SIM GC/MS of Diethylstilbestrol in Bovine Liver", Biomed. Mass Spectrom., In Press (1985).
11. J.B. Crowther, T.R. Covey, D. Silvestre, and J.D. Henion, "Direct Liquid Introduction LC/MS:Four Different Approaches", LC Mag., 3 240-254 (1985).
12. C. Eckers, D.S. Skrabalak, and J.D. Henion, "On-line Direct Liquid Introduction Interface for Micro-Liquid Chromatography/Mass Spectrometry: Application to Drug Analysis", Clin. Chem., 28 1882-1886 (1982).
13. L.R. Snyder and J.J. Kirkland, "Introduction to Modern Liquid Chromatography", Chapt. 2., (John Wiley & Sons), (1979).
14. L.G.M. Th. Tuinstra, W.A. Traag, H.J. Keukens, and R.J. Van Mazijk, "Procedure for the Gas Chromatographic-Mass Spectrometric Confirmation of some Exogenous Growth Promoting Compounds in the urine of Cattle", J. Chromatogr., 279 533-542 (1983).
15. C.R. Blakley and M.L. Vestal, "Thermospray Interface for Liquid Chromatography/Mass Spectrometry", Anal. Chem., 55 750-754 (1983).
16. T.R. Covey, J.B. Crowther, E.A. Dewey, and J.D. Henion, "Thermospray Liquid Chromatography/Mass Spectrometry Determination of Drugs and Their Metabolites in Biological Fluids", Anal. Chem., 57 474-481 (1985).

DISCUSSION

SETCHELL: This was a very nice presentation. One obvious extension of this work must surely be to attempt to use LC/MS analysis of the intact glucuronide conjugates of these metabolites, thereby eliminating a time-consuming hydrolysis step. Our experiences with fast atom bombardment for the analysis of intact steroid conjugates indicate that these compounds should be very amenable to the LC/MS thermospray interface. Have you considered this option?

HENION: Yes. We have looked at several commercially available glucuronide conjugates and published their thermospray LC/MS mass spectra. We have not as yet commenced isolation of glucuronide conjugates from biological samples. This is a very exciting area which I believe LC/MS is ideally suited.

SETCHELL: What is the minimum amount of tissue you believe one could use to assay for these compounds? Have you sufficient sensitivity to look at small quantities (e.g., human tissue)?

HENION: The present method requires 1 g of tissue when DES or zearanol is present at the 100 ppt level. Perhaps future improvements will allow identification with as little as 0.1 g of tissue.

O'NEILL: If you were going to look for evidence of zearanol in children affected by premature sexual development, where would you look: (a) urine, (b) whole blood, (c) red cells, (d) plasma, (e) other.

HENION: I would analyze the urine and plasma.

KUPFER: Can one distinguish isomers which have different abundances of the same fragment (i.e., ratio of fragments is different) but which separate on LC by only a few seconds?

HENION: If the isomers really have the same mass spectrum and they co-elute chromatographically, the isomers cannot be distinguished. If the relative abundances of common fragments were different by, for example, 30% or more, then carefully run S/M GC/MS or LC/MS could probably distinguish the isomers.

KUPFER: For isomers which do not separate on LC, could one use different volatility of the isomers to separate them in the mass spec and then identify them?

HENION: No. Fractional volatilization made in the ion source of co-eluting components is not practical.

PAREKH: What was the level of zearanol in control slaughter house liver samples? Have you analyzed any other tissue sample?

HENION: Zearanol was observed in several livers at approximately 20 ppt, the detection limit of the assay. Zearalenone was found in most samples tested at levels ranging from 50 ppt to 2 ppt. We have confined the analysis thus far to bovine liver.

FOTSIS: What is the within and between assay precision of your method when used in the quantitation of samples?

HENION: I do not have the actual precision numbers with me, but the correlation coefficient for all our work so far has consistently been 0.999 for DES from liver tested.

FOTSIS: Do you have any problems from contamination of the mass spectrometer from biological samples?

HENION: Of course, any use of a GC/MS with real samples contributes to getting the instrument dirty and less sensitive. However, the sample work-up procedure used and the significantly reduced matrix recovery provides extract residues which do not significantly contaminate the mass spectrometer. By injecting known spiked samples during the course of an analysis sequence, we can monitor the performance and response of the mass spectrometer. Basically, contamination is not a problem for either our GC/MS S/M or SEM LC/MS/MS work.

FOTSIS: What is the detection limit of your method when used for the quantitation of biological samples?

HENION: We have a limit of quantitation down to the 100 ppt level at the present time for DES and zearanol by S/M GC/MS.

BIOCHEMICAL ANALYSIS OF ESTROGENS

D.C. COLLINS AND P.I. MUSEY

V.A. Medical Center and Department of Medicine, Emory University
School of Medicine, Atlanta, Georgia

INTRODUCTION

In recent years, considerable interest has developed in the measurement of estrogens in meat and milk. Without sensitive and reliable procedures, it is difficult to monitor the use of illegal anabolic agents and exposure to environmental estrogens. Several major problems confound any effort to develop a general procedure for measuring all compounds which have estrogenic activity. One problem is the wide variety of compounds which can show estrogenic activity, such as the natural steroidal estrogens, diethylstilbesterol, as well as a wide range of plant estrogens and synthetic chemicals. A second problem is the low levels of estrogen that are normally present in tissue and milk samples and the difficulty in extracting these small amounts of estrogen from the meat and milk matrix.

We have used the following approach to develop a screening procedure to test meat and milk samples for the presence of natural or environmental estrogens. First, the estrogens are extracted from the meat or milk matrix utilizing an appropriate extraction procedure. Subsequently, the estrogenic activity of the compound is quantitated by measuring its interaction with estrogen receptors from rat uteri. If significant estrogenic activity is indicated, the compound should be measured by a more specific procedure for further identification. If no significant estrogenic activity is present, it is assumed that no estrogens are present in the particular sample. In this paper, we report our initial experience in attempting to set up a biochemical procedure for measurement of estrogen activity in milk and meat samples.

MATERIALS AND METHODS

Materials

Celite 545 (Johns Manville); polyethylene transfer jumbo bulb pipettes (Falcon Plastics); reagent grade solvents were purchased from Fisher Scientific Co. Iso-octane, benzene and methanol were glass distilled and used within a week. $2,4,6,7,16,17-^3$H-Estradiol-17β (151 Ci/mMole) and $16\alpha-^{125}$I-estradiol-17β (^{125}I-E$_2$, 2200 Ci/mMole) were purchased from New England Nuclear Corp., Boston, Massachusetts. Unlabeled estrogens, estradiol-17β, diethylstilbestrol (DES) and zearalenol were purchased from Sigma Chemical Co., St. Louis, Missouri. A solid phase extraction system and C_{18} extraction cartridges were purchased from American Scientific Products Co. or Waters Associates, Milford, Massachusetts (3 ml cartridges from Baker or standard size (Ca 5 ml) from Waters). Twenty-one day old female rats were obtained from Charles Rivers Co.

Preparation of Meat Samples

Two methods were used to prepare meat samples. Small samples (1-2 gm) of beef, pork or chicken (including both lean and fat) were pulverized in liquid nitrogen. The pulverized samples were transferred to test tubes and homogenized in methanol with 4 x 10 seconds bursts from a polytron homogenizer. An internal standard of ^{3}H-estradiol-17β (10-20,000 cpm) was added at this stage to monitor method recovery. The homogenate was transferred to a large (50 ml) screw cap test tube with successive methanol washings of tube and polytron blade shaft. Prolonged homogenization was necessary with tough muscular tissues to achieve a fine and uniform homogenate. The homogenization was carried out in an ice cold bath to prevent flask ignition of methanol. The homogenate was then mechanically extracted for at least 2 hr on a reciprocating shaker or for 30 min on a vortex mixer.

The alcoholic extract was kept overnight at -20°C to complete protein and neutral fat precipitation and then centrifuged at 5000 x g at 4°C. The methanolic extract was evaporated to dryness in vacuo using a flask evaporator. The extract was redissolved in 25 ml 10% aqueous methanol and applied to a C_{18} solid phase chromatographic column. These columns generally retain small molecules such as estrogens and estrogen conjugates while allowing large molecules such as proteins to be eluted in the aqueous phase. The "estrogen" fraction was eluted with 25 ml methanol, evaporated to dryness in vacuo and resuspended in 1 ml of methanol. Aliquots were taken for the estrogen assay or were subject to further purification by celite chromatography.

Processing of Milk Sample

Twenty five ml aliquots of milk samples were extracted with 300 ml methanol by shaking vigorously (10-15 min) in a 500 ml separatory flask, then stored at -20°C for 1-2 hr. The extraction (vigorous shaking) was repeated two more times followed by overnight storage of the mixture at -20°C. The mixture was filtered through a 0.45 micron nylon membrane filter, evaporated to dryness in vacuo, then resuspended in 20-30 ml of

10% aqueous methanol and applied to a solid cartridge as described above. The organic extract was evaporated and resuspended in a small volume of methanol for estrogen assay or further purification by celite partition chromatography.

Celite Partition Chromatography

Some samples were further purified with celite chromatography [1]. Celite 545 was prepared and small 1 gm columns were packed after thoroughly mixing 0.5 ml ethylene glycol (stationary phase) with a spatula for 20 min, followed by excess iso-octane (mobile phase) as previously described [1]. Columns were packed in transfer pipettes with glass wool to plug the tip. Aliquots of the extract to be chromatographed (equivalent to 1 gm of tissue or 5 ml of milk) were absorbed on 0.2 gm celite. The celite was then transferred to the top of the 1 gm column. The tube was washed with 20 µl of methanol, followed by two 1 ml aliquots of the mobile phase and applied to the celite column. The column was eluted successively with 4 ml each of iso-octane; 100%, 20%, 40%, 60%, 80% benzene in iso-octane, then 16 ml 100% benzene.

The eluates were pooled and evaporated in 13 x 100 test tubes. The evaporated eluate sometimes leaves a sticky residue or traces of ethylene glycol. These compounds interfered in the receptor assay and must be removed by solid phase extraction. The residue was redissolved by vortexing in 0.4 ml methanol, then by successive addition of 0.6 ml and 3 ml of distilled water. This was followed by extraction through a C_{18} cartridge and elution with HPLC grade methanol. The alcoholic extract was aliquoted into four parts; one part was counted for radioactivity to assess recovery while the remaining triplicates were dried in 12 x 75 cm test tubes and used for the receptor assay.

Rat Uterine Cytosol Bioassay of Estrogens

Rat uterine-cytosol receptors for estrogens were prepared according to methods previously described with some modifications [2,3]. Batches of twelve 21-25 day old female rats were sacrificed by rapid decapitation and their uteri removed, cleaned of fat and homogenized in 4 vol cold (4°C) TEM buffer (1% Tris, 0.5% EDTA and 0.01% monothioglycerol). The homogenate was centrifuged at 1,000 g for 30 min at 4°C and the precipitate discarded. The lipid pad was lifted from the top and the supernatant decanted and centrifuged at 100,000 g for 1 hr at 4°C. The supernatant (cytosol fraction) was decanted and the protein concentration determined by the method of Bradford [4]. The final protein concentration was adjusted to 2.0-2.5 mg/ml with TEM buffer.

Varying volumes (10-200 µl) of the cytosol were titrated against 16α-^{125}I-estradiol (12-20,000 c/m) and the volume giving approximately 50% displacement was used in subsequent assays. The cytosol was stored in 3-5 ml aliquots at -80°C until needed. The preparation remains stable for 4-6 weeks.

The cytosol preparation was used in a competitive protein binding assay ("receptor assay") for estradiol-17β as previously described [3-5]. A standard curve with estradiol-17β ranging from 10-1000 pg/tube was established. Samples and unknowns were vortexed and incubated overnight at 4°C. Separation of bound and free estrogen was carried out by incubation with 1.0 ml Dextran-coated charcoal as previously described at 4°C [5]. Quantitation of unknowns was based on the percent ^{125}I-estradiol-17β bound and expressed as estradiol-17β mass equivalents.

Quality control standards (low and high) were included in each assay run. The assay values from these standards were used to calculate inter- and intra-assay coefficient of variation [5].

Meat and Milk Controls

Samples of chicken, beef and pork and milk were obtained from a supermarket. These samples were homogenized and/or extracted as described above and standard amounts of estradiol-17β added. Two standard levels (low - 50 pg and high - 200 pg) were used.

Several endogenous estrogen samples were prepared by feeding diethylstilbesterol, estrone, xearalenol or estriol to chickens. These animals were sacrificed and their tissues used as control samples to test the viability of the assay procedure.

RESULTS AND DISCUSSION

The purification steps outlined are based on the removal of proteins and other interfering substances and leaving the small organic molecules, including the estrogens. Table 1 summarizes our experience with recovery using the extraction procedures described above. These results indicate that there is a large variability in the recovery from meat samples. This suggests that extraction from meat samples is more difficult and may be dependent upon the composition of the particular meat sample. In general, tissue containing large amounts of fat yield lower recoveries.

Table 1. Recovery of ^{3}H-estradiol-17β from extraction procedures described above. All types of meat (chicken, pork and beef) were calculated together.

Sample Type	Number of Extractions	Mean Recovery ± SD	Range
meat	144	57 ± 29.5	38 - 88
milk	81	53 ± 6.8	35 - 65

A review of the data indicates an abnormal distribution of the recovery with a large number of the samples clustered either near the maximum or minimum recovery with relatively few near the mean recovery. The distribution of the recovery of ^{3}H-estradiol-17β was much nearer to a Gaussian distribution, resulting in much less variability around the mean.

The results of recovery from the laboratory standards prepared by adding known amounts of estradiol-17β to homogenized meat samples and analyzing the samples using the uterine estrogen receptor assay are shown in Table 2. These results suggest that the recovery of estradiol-17β from the meat samples can be expected to give reliable results in at least controlled circumstances.

Table 2. Results of six analyses of known amounts of estradiol-17β to a homogenized meat sample.

Analytical Run	Triplicate Values for Amount of Estradiol Added	
	50 pg/gm	200 pg/gm
1	51, 52, 52	241, 236, 237
2	46, 39, 45	245, 245, 239
3	45, 51, 51	228, 233, 273
4	42, 49, 50	234, 245, 235
5	50, 44, 46	232, 233, 228
6	44, 53, 50	240, 238, 236
Mean ± SD	48 ± 4.0	239 ± 10.0

The analysis of samples taken from chickens fed either estrone, estriol, diethylstilbesterol (DES) or a placebo are shown in Table 3. Analysis of these results suggests that the interassay variation is very large in comparison to the intra-assay variance. The interassay variance accounts for 75% of the total variance. The mean intra-assay variance is less than 20% whereas the mean interassay variance is over 70%.

Table 3. Precision of estrogen values obtained from measurements taken
from chickens fed various estrogens. Different samples from the same
chicken were run in each assay.

Estrogen	N	Mean	Observed Min	Observed Max	Coefficient of Variation Intra-assay	Coefficient of Variation Interassay
DES	9	1583	1012	2346	28.50	52.49
Placebo	9	1092	587	2032	10.05	98.34
Estrone	9	2411	544	5361	21.06	96.73
Zearalenol	6	886	637	1160	8.69	93.22
Estriol	12	3059	1156	5755	19.69	94.60

N = number of samples in triplicate

While the method appeared feasible and the intra-assay variance was
acceptable as a semi-quantitative assay to detect estradiol-17β, the
results from the estrogen fed chickens were extremely variable.
Furthermore, there did not appear to be any differences in values in the
estrogen-fed and placebo-fed chickens. It has been suggested that the
large interassay variance may result from the different characteristics
of individual tissue samples interfering with the receptor assay. This
suggests that either the extraction or the assay procedure needs to be
modified to solve this problem before reliable results independent of
the quality of the tissue sample can be obtained. We are currently
carrying out studies in our laboratory to resolve these problems.

REFERENCES

1. J.R.K. Preedy and E.H. Aitken, J. Biol. Chem., 236, 1300 (1961).

2. S.G. Korenman, L.E. Perin and T.P. McCallum, J. Clin. Endocrinol.
Metab.,29, 876 (1969).

3. L. Erb, B.L. Lasley, N.M. Czekala, S.L. Montfort and A.B. Bercovitz,
Steroids, 39, 33 (1982).

4. M. Bradford, Anal. Biochem., 72, 248 (1976).

5. K. Wright, D.C. Collins and J.R.K. Preedy, J. Clin. Endocrinol.
Metab.,47, 1084 (1978).

DISCUSSION

NAFTOLIN: Lipoidal estrogens have been proposed by Hochberg and colleagues as biologically active compounds which could explain the difference between estrogens measurable by methods such as you have described and those measured by biological action such as vaginal cornification. Could you comment on the importance of these compounds and your ability to include them in your analysis?

COLLINS: The method described would detect these compounds if they bind to the estrogen receptor. However, they may not survive the extraction procedure since they are very nonpolar and may be lost with the lipid fraction. We have no data on this point.

COVEY: With respect to your comments regarding problems with interference from lipid materials in extracts--we have developed a 3-phase solvent extraction system consisting of water, dichloromethane (DCM), acetonitrile, and hexane. The middle acetonitrile/DCM layer isolates estrogens with lipids in the hexane layer. Application of this extract to a polystyrene strong anion exchanger gives additional ion exchange and reverse phase clean-up of the sample for analysis.

COLLINS: That is a very interesting approach; we would be interested in trying it in our system.

DOES ESTROGEN-INDUCED GENOTOXICITY REQUIRE RECEPTOR-MEDIATED EVENTS?

ROBERT H. PURDY*, NEIL J. MACLUSKY** AND FREDERICK NAFTOLIN**
*Department of Organic Chemistry, Southwest Foundation for Biomedical
Research, San Antonio, TX 78284; **Department of Obstetrics and Gynecology,
Yale University School of Medicine, New Haven, CT 06510

INTRODUCTION

The metabolism and mechanism of action of estrogens in inducing
physiologic events have become increasingly understood, with evidence that
many estrogen actions on sex steroid sensitive tissues require initial
binding of the estrogen to specific receptors and subsequent interaction of
the ligand-receptor complex with the genome [1,2,3]. While carcinogenic
actions of estrogens may also require interaction with the genome, it is
not known whether this pathologic process is dependent upon classical
receptor mechanisms or whether a bioactivated metabolite of the estrogen is
involved, perhaps by actions which do not require receptors. Recently, we
have focused our attention upon the metabolic hydroxylation of the phenolic
ring in steroidal and nonsteroidal estrogens as a bioactivation step in the
development of estrogen-induced genotoxicity underlying estrogen-mediated
carcinogenesis. In this report we provide our data, obtained with diethylstilbestrol and various steroidal estrogens, which compare the biological
activity of these hormones and derivatives with their ability to enhance
the mutagenicity of an established mammary carcinogen or induce the neoplastic transformation of mammalian cells. Our findings of a dissociation
between estrogenic potency and genotoxic activity support the possibility
that bioactivation of estrogens to catechol metabolites is a feature of the
genotoxicity of estrogens, and raises the question of the requirement for
this step in estrogen-related carcinogenesis.

METHODS

Competition Binding to Uterine Cytosol Estrogen Receptors

Adult female rats (250-300 g) were ovariectomized under ether anes-
thesia 5-7 days before use. The animals were killed by decapitation and
their uteri removed and placed on a chilled glass plate for dissection.
All subsequent procedures were performed at 0-4°C. Fat and connective
tissue were removed and the uteri minced finely with scissors. The minced
tissue was homogenized using a motorized ground glass homogenizer in buffer
containing 10 mM Tris-HCl, 1.5 mM EDTA, 1 mM dithiothreitol and 10% (v/v)
glycerol, pH 7.4 (TEGD buffer), using 5 ml buffer per uterus. The

homogenate was centrifuged at 105,000 x g for 1 h. The supernatant (cytosol) was decanted, divided into 1 ml aliquots and either used immediately or stored frozen at -40°C for up to 3 weeks before use. Results obtained with fresh and frozen cytosols were indistinguishable.

For competition studies, cytosol preparations were diluted 5-fold with TEGD buffer and 200 µl aliquots were incubated with 1 nM [2,4,6,7-^{3}H]estradiol in the presence and absence of each of the unlabeled test ligands. The test compounds were dissolved in TEGD buffer (100 µl) at final concentrations ranging from 10^{-10}M to 10^{-6}M. Incubations were performed for either 15 h at 0-4°C or 4.5 h at 25°C. Aliquots (100 µl) of the incubates were then chromatographed on Sephadex LH-20 microcolumns to separate the bound estradiol [4]. Data were analyzed using a nonlinear least squares curve fit computer program [5] adapted to an Apple II microcomputer [6] and expressed in terms of relative binding affinity compared with estradiol [7].

Uterotrophic Activity

In vivo estrogenic potency of the different estrogens was assessed using the uterotrophic response of the immature rat, as previously described by Franks et al. [8]. Weanling female rats (22 days of age) were given 100 µl subcutaneous injections of the test steroid dissolved in a vehicle containing 10% ethanol in sesame oil. The total dose was divided equally between six injections, spaced 12 h apart. Control animals received injections of the ethanol-oil vehicle. Twelve hours after the last injection (25 days of age), the animals were killed by decapitation. The uteri were removed, cleaned of adhering fat and mesentery, drained of luminal fluid, and weighed. Dose-response curves for compounds inducing a significant increase in uterine wet weight were analyzed by a nonlinear least-squares procedure [5].

Mutagenesis assay

Rat liver activating systems (S-9) were prepared following administration of 2-acetylaminofluorene (AAF, 22.3 mg/kg i.p. in corn oil, 24 h induction) or Aroclor 1254 (500 mg/kg i.p. in corn oil, 5 day induction) to male Sprague-Dawley rats to induce hepatic mixed-function oxidase activity. Assays for histidine reversion of S. typhimurium strain TA 98 were performed according to Maron and Ames [9]. To the molten top agar (2 ml containing 50 µM L-histidine, 50 µM L-biotin and 77 mM NaCl) was added strain TA 98 (0.1 ml containing 2 x 10^8 bacteria), the compound to be tested in dimethylsulfoxide (0.1 ml), and the S-9 preparation (0.5 ml containing 1.5-2.2 mg protein) in 0.1 M sodium phosphate buffer (pH 7.4) containing 4 mM NADP, 5 mM glucose-6-phosphate, 8 mM $MgCl_2$, and 3 mM KCl. In assays with catechol estrogens, 18 mM L-ascorbic acid (50 µl) was also added to the above 2.7 ml mixture. The colonies of histidine revertants on three or more replicate plates were scored using a Biotran II automatic colony counter (New Brunswick Scientific, Edison, NJ) after 48-72 h incubation at 37°C in the dark. The spontaneous reversion rate varied between 40 and 50 colonies per plate.

Metabolism of [^{3}H]DES

The [ring-^{3}H]DES (28 mCi/mmol, New England Nuclear, Boston, MA) was purified before use by HPLC on a LiChrosorb Diol column (5 µm, 0.46 x 50 cm, Rainin Instrument Co., Inc, Woburn, MA) equilibrated with 7.5% ethanol in heptane (v/v). After injection of the sample at a flow rate of 1.5 ml/min, a curvilinear gradient (No. 10, Waters model 273 gradient system, Waters Assoc., Milford, MA) was run over 1 h to 12.5% ethanol in heptane (v/v). [^{3}H]Z,Z-DES eluted at 13 min. The fractions containing the purified DES were evaporated under nitrogen at 24°C and dissolved in dimethylsulfoxide just prior to incubation. The incubation mixtures (5 ml) contained 20 mM phosphate, 3.1 mM $MgCl_2$, 5 mM glucose 6-phosphate, 0.8 mM NADPH, 0.3 ml/ml of a 5% Aroclor-induced S-9 fraction and 5 µg/ml [^{3}H]DES (0.54 µCi/ml), as described by Tsutsui et al. [10]. After incubation for periods of 10 min to 2 h, duplicate 200 µl aliquots were cooled to 0°C and extracted with ether (3 times with 2 ml). Aliquots (200 µl) were also cooled to 0°C, recovery standards (25 µg) of 3'-hydroxy-DES and 3'-hydroxy-Z,Z-dienestrol in tetrahydrofuran/aqueous 0.2% ascorbic acid (1/4, v/v) were added, and the solutions were extracted with ethyl acetate containing 1% acetic acid (3 times with 2 ml). The separate ether or ethyl acetate extracts were combined, evaporated under nitrogen, dissolved in 50 µl acetonitrile, and analyzed by HPLC.

HPLC analysis was performed using a 5 µm Ultrasphere ODS column (0.46 x 25 cm, Rainin) equilibrated with 33% acetonitrile, 1% acetic acid, and 66% water (v/v/v). After injection of the sample at a flow rate of 1.5 ml/min, a curvilinear gradient (No. 10, Waters gradient system) was run over 1 h to 48% acetonitrile, 1% acetic acid, and 51% water (v/v/v). The column effluent was monitored at 280 nm for the unlabeled recovery standards. The catechol standards eluted together at 15 min, Z,Z-DES at 33 min, and Z,Z-dienestrol at 45 min. The amount of radioactivity was measured using a Flo-One model HP radioactive flow detector (Radiomatic Instruments and Chemical Co., Tampa, FL).

Relative Rate of Catechol Estrogen Formation

Washed microsomes from male Sprague-Dawley rat livers and male Syrian hamster kidneys were prepared by differential centrifugation [11] and stored in 0.25 M sucrose at -70°C prior to use. Washed microsomes from about 2 x 10^9 nonconfluent Balb/c 3T3 cells were similarly prepared [12] and used immediately. Mushroom monophenol o-monooxygenase (tyrosinase, EC 1.14.18.1) was purchased from Sigma Chemical Co., St. Louis, MO. Protein concentration was determined by the method of Bradford [13].

The radioenzymatic assays for catechol formation were carried out under conditions where product formation was linear for 6 or 10 min. Incubations were performed with 50 μM estrogen dissolved in 5 μl dimethyl-sulfoxide using the stated amount of microsomal protein per aliquot (80 μl) in 0.5 ml 0.1 M HEPES buffer containing 100 Sigma units catechol-O-methyltransferase (EC 2.1.1.6, Sigma), 0.75 μM S-[methyl-^{3}H]adenosyl-L-methionine (7.5 μCi, New England Nuclear), 2 mM NADPH, 40 mM MgCl$_2$ and 0.33 mM L-ascorbic acid. After incubation at 37°C for intervals of 1-10 min, aliquots (80 μl) were withdrawn and added to 1 ml 0.05 M sodium borate buffer (pH 10) containing 20 μg recovery standards of the unlabeled catechol monomethyl ethers [14]. The radioactive monomethyl ethers were extracted with 6 ml heptane and the radioactivity in 0.5 ml aliquots was measured in duplicate. The remainder of the heptane extracts was evaporated and the products were identified by HPLC [14]. The controls were incubations using 50 μM 3-fluoro-17β-hydroxyestra-1,3,5(10)-triene, which is not a substrate for estrogen 2-/4-hydroxylase activity.

Neoplastic Transformation of Balb/c 3T3 Cells

The A-31-1-13 subclone of the Balb/c 3T3 embryo-derived mouse fibroblast cell line isolated by Kakunaga et al. [15] was used in the assays for cell transformation [16]. After 72 h treatment of the cells with five concentrations of estrogen (5-50 μM), in which least four concentrations had 20% or greater cell survival, the cells were washed twice with fresh medium and allowed to recover in fresh medium for 24 h. The cells were then harvested, counted using a hemocytometer, and plated for the determination of cloning efficiency and for the determination of transformation [16] using 10^4 cells per dish in 12 dishes. The cells were refed biweekly for about 4 weeks, when they were stained and examined [17]. Type III transformed foci [17] were transplanted to culture flasks for further characterization [12]. Assays included a solvent control of 0.25% dimethylsulfoxide and a positive control of 1 μM 3-methylcholanthrene. Transformation frequency was not calculated where cell survival was less than 20%.

150

RESULTS

Comutagenicity

Mutagenesis assays with 4 µg/plate 2-acetylaminofluorene (AAF) gave a background level of 50-55 histidine revertants/plate using an AAF-induced rat liver metabolic activating system with strain TA 98. In the presence of 2.5-50 µM ethinyl estradiol, estradiol, DES, and estrone, there was a significant enhancement of the mutagenicity of 4 µg AAF shown in Figure 1.

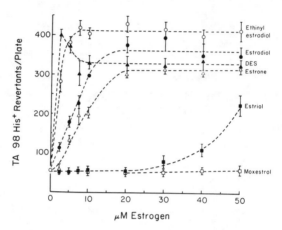

FIG. 1 Effect of estrogens on the mutagenicity of S. typhimurium strain TA 98. Mutagenicity assays with 4 µg AAF/plate were performed with 2.2 mg protein/plate of the AAF-induced S-9 preparation as described in Methods.

TABLE I. Enhancement of mutagenicity of AAF by estrogens, and relative rates of catechol estrogen formation using the AAF-induced microsomal activating system used in the mutagenicity assays[a].

Estrogen	Enhancement of mutation by				Catechol Formed[b]
	5 µM	10 µM	20 µM	50 µM	
Ethinyl estradiol	7.1	7.5	8.2	7.6	116 ± 6
Estradiol	3.4	5.5	7.1	6.4	136 ± 6
DES	7.1	6.2	6.1	6.1	44 ± 2
Estrone	2.5	3.7	5.6	6.0	118 ± 6
Estriol	1.0	1.0	1.0	4.3	16 ± 1
Moxestrol	1.0	1.0	1.0	1.0	< 3 ± 1

[a]Mutagenicity assays were performed as described by Purdy and Marshall [11] using 4 µg/plate AAF. The AAF-induced S-9 protein concentration was 2.2 mg/plate.

[b]Calculated from the initial rate of total catechol monomethyl ether formation as pmol product/min/mg microsomal protein ± s.e.

151

Estriol enhanced mutagenicity of AAF only at 40-50 µM. Moxestrol did not enhance the mutagenicity of AAF. The comparative enhancement of mutagenicity of AAF calculated in Table I does not parallel the rates of catechol estrogen formation for the active estrogens. The two inactive estrogens, moxestrol (11β-methoxyethinyl estradiol) and estriol were only marginal substrates for estrogen 2-/4-hydroxylation.

The role of catechol estrogen formation in this comutagenic effect was examined by comparing the effect of ethinyl estradiol versus that produced by its catechol. Assays were performed in the presence of 0.33 mM ascorbic acid to minimize nonenzymatic oxidation of the catechol which occurs in aqueous systems [18]. This concentration of ascorbic acid did not alter the enhancement of mutagenicity of AAF produced by ethinyl estradiol. The data shown in Figure 2 demonstrate that the maximal effect of 2-hydroxy-ethinyl estradiol occurred at 2.5 µM, whereas the enhancement by ethinyl estradiol was still increasing at 10 µM. In contrast to moxestrol (Figure 1), 10 µM 2-hydroxymoxestrol was as effective as 10 µM ethinyl estradiol in enhancing the mutagenicity of 4 µg AAF. Neither the estrogens nor their catechols were mutagenic by themselves in this system [11].

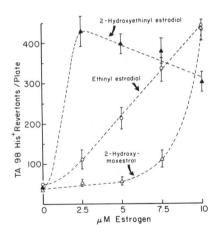

FIG. 2. Effect of 2-hydroxyethinyl estradiol, 2-hydroxymoxestrol, and ethinyl estradiol on the mutagenicity of strain TA 98 as described in FIG. 1 using 2.2 mg protein/plate of the S-9 preparation and 0.33 mM ascorbic acid. From Purdy and Marshall [11].

The data in Table I for catechol formation with DES as substrate implies that the 3'-hydroxy metabolite of DES was formed by the AAF-induced microsomal activating system and further converted to a mixture of its [³H]-labeled monomethyl ethers in the radioenzymatic assay. Using a similar Aroclor-induced liver activating system, which was also found to be effective in catalyzing estrogen enhanced mutagenicity of AAF [11], Tsutsui et al. [10] were unable to detect a significant amount of [¹⁴C]-labeled 3'-hydroxy DES after incubation of [monoethyl-2-¹⁴C]DES with this activating system for 2 h at 37°C. We repeated their incubation conditions using [ring-³H]DES, followed by either their extraction procedure with diethyl ether, or by the addition of catechol recovery standards of 3'-hydroxy derivatives of DES and Z,Z-dienestrol and extraction with ethyl acetate in the presence of ascorbic acid and 1% acetic acid. The results of the HPLC analysis of the radioactive metabolites recovered by these two extraction procedures are shown in Figure 3.

The major metabolite isolated by both extraction procedures was Z,Z-dienestrol, increasing to an average yield of about 28% of the extracted products after incubation for 2 h. The unlabeled recovery standards of the 3'-hydroxy derivatives of DES and Z,Z-dienestrol were not separated in this chromatographic system. With ether extraction, less than 1% of a mixture of the latter [³H]-labeled catechol products were recovered from 1-2 h incubations. However, the ethyl acetate extracts contained about 9% of one or both of these catechols as [³H]-labeled metabolities.

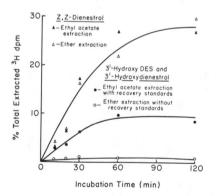

Incubation Time (min)

Fig. 3. Recovery of metabolites of [³H]DES after incubation with an Aroclor-induced rat liver activating system and separation of the ether extracts or the ethyl acetate extracts by HPLC. The ethyl acetate extractions were performed after addition of 25 μg each of unlabeled 3'-hydroxy derivatives of DES and Z,Z-dienestrol.

The recovery of [^{3}H]-DES decreased from 62% after 10 min to 14% after 1 h and 4% after 2 h incubation.

Alteration of Estrogen-induced Cell Transformation by D-ring Modification

DES and the steroidal estrogens, estrone and estradiol, have been shown to induce the neoplastic transformation of the A-31-1-13 subclone of nontumorigenic Balb/c 3T3 cells [12]. This fibroblast cell line, which does not have detectable high affinity estrogen receptors (ER), is particularly sensitive to polycyclic aromatic hydrocarbon-induced transformation [15]. In order to explore the effect of D-ring modification on estrogen-induced genotoxicity and binding to ER, we converted estrone to a mixture of its syn- and anti-methoxime derivatives, whose structures are shown below.

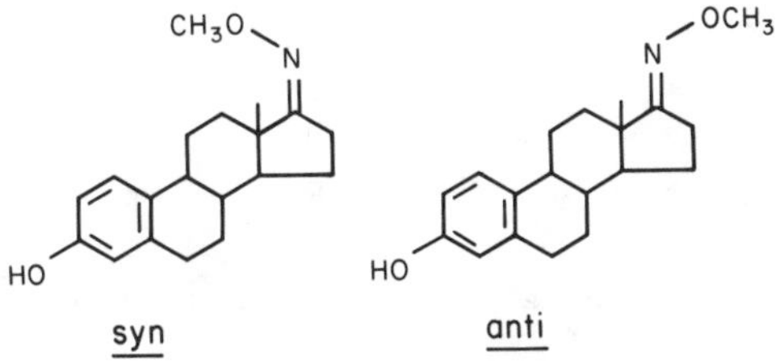

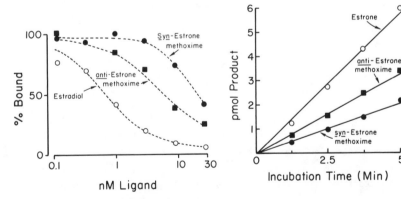

FIG. 4. Displacement curves for inhibition of [^{3}H]estradiol binding by unlabeled ligands using uterine cytosol from ovariectomized rats at 0°C.

FIG. 5. Radioenzymatic assay for catechol estrogen formation using microsomes (27.6 μg protein) from male Sprague-Dawley rat liver.

The 17-methoxime group [19] was chosen because of its chemical and biological stability and its relatively small size. These methoximes were separated and rigorously purified by HPLC to remove any residual estrone. The displacement curves for the binding of these methoximes compared to the binding of estradiol to rat uterine ER at 0°C is shown in Figure 4.

The relative rates of catechol estrogen formation from these methoximes with rat liver microsomes is shown in Figure 5. HPLC analysis showed that the [^{3}H]-labeled monomethyl ethers had the same retention times as the products obtained from incubation of the 2-hydroxy catechols of the substrates with catechol-O-methyltransferase and S-[methyl-^{3}H]adenosyl-L-methionine. Although the results in Table II show an apparent 3-fold difference in the relative rates of catechol estrogen formation between estrone and its syn-methoxime, it was found that there was a similar 2-fold difference between rates of monomethyl ether formation using 2-hydroxyestrone and the 2-hydroxy catechol of syn-estrone methoxime as standards. Therefore, the apparent rates shown in Figure 5 for the methoximes are misleading. The results of the calculated rates of catechol formation and relative binding affinity (RBA) are summarized in Table II.

TABLE II. Summary of relative binding affinity (RBA) and rate of catechol estrogen formation with male rat liver microsomes.

Compound	% RBA[a]		Catechol Formed[b]
	0-4°C	25°C	
Estradiol	[100]	[100]	51.1 ± 0.6
Estrone	11.1	1.0	39.4 ± 1.9
anti-Estrone methoxime	7.1	1.8	22.8 ± 0.5
syn-Estrone methoxime	2.3	0.8	13.8 ± 0.6

[a]Estradiol = 100%; calculated from data shown in FIG. 4 and competitive binding data at 25°C (not shown).

[b]Calculated from data shown in FIG. 5 as pmol product/min/mg protein ± s.e.

The syn-methoxime had a lower RBA than the anti-methoxime and was therefore compared to estrone for its ability to induce the neoplastic transformation of Balb/c 3T3 cells. The results of this genotoxicity study are shown in Table III.

TABLE III. Neoplastic transformation of subclone A-31-1-13 of Balb/c 3T3 cells by estrogens.

Compound	Conc. (μM)	Survival[a] (%)	Avg Type III foci per dish	Type III foci/10^4 survivors
DMSO Control (0.25%)		[100]	0.08	0.2
3-Methylcholanthrene	1	39	1.42	8.5
Estrone	5	83	0.33	0.9
	10	61	0.55	1.4
	20	34	0.58	4.0
	30	27	0.73	6.3
	40	28	0.64	5.3
	50	23	0.67	6.7
syn-Estrone methoxime	5	71	0.25	0.8
	10	67	0.55	1.9
	20	49	0.44	2.0
	30	32	0.64	4.6
	40	33	0.67	4.7
	50	31	0.55	4.1

[a]Average cloning efficiency for DMSO control (43%) taken as 100%.

The average of the transformation frequency (right hand column in Table III) minus the spontaneous background level (DMSO control) normalized to 10 μM concentration of estrogen was 1.48 ± 0.13 (s.e.) for estrone and 1.20 ± 0.14 (s.e.) for syn-estrone methoxime. Thus, there is no significant difference between the genotoxicity of estrone and its syn-methoxime in this assay system, despite the marked differences in their RBA.

Alteration of Estrogen-induced Cell Transformation by A-ring Modification

Fluorine-probe methodology has been employed in an effort to block or reduce the formation of 2-hydroxy and 4-hydroxy catechols of estradiol. The A-ring structures of the fluorinated derivatives of estradiol used in this study are shown below.

Estradiol   3-Fluoro Analog

4-Fluoroestradiol   2-Fluoroestradiol   2,4-Difluoroestradiol

The monofluorinated derivatives, 2-fluoro- and 4-fluoroestradiol, were first synthesized in 1956 by Zillig and Mueller [20]. The arrows indicate the expected positions of hydroxylation of these compounds at C-2 and C-4. The 3-fluoro analog [21] is not a substrate for A-ring hydroxylation since it is not a phenol. Appelman and Purdy recently synthesized 2,4-difluoroestradiol [22]. The binding of the 2-, 4- and 2,4-fluorinated derivatives of estradiol to ER is shown in Figure 6. The relative binding affinity of 4-fluoroestradiol is significantly greater than that of estradiol and the other compounds; summarized in Table IV.

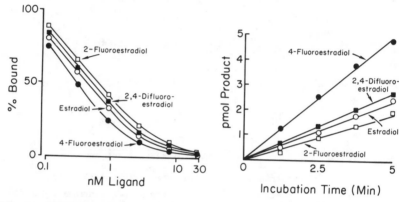

FIG. 6. Displacement curves for inhibition of [3H]estradiol binding by unlabeled ligands using uterine cytosol from ovariectomized rats at 0°C.

FIG. 7. Radioenzymatic assay for catechol estrogen formation using microsomes (100 μg protein) from male Syrian hamster kidney.

TABLE IV. Summary of relative binding affinity (RBA) and relative rates of catechol estrogen formation with mushroom monophenol o-monooxygenase and microsomes from the male Syrian kidney and Balb/c 3T3 cells.

| Compound | % RBA[a] | | Catechol Formation[b] | | |
	0-4°C	25°C	Mono-oxygenase	Hamster kidney	Balb cells
Estradiol	[100]	[100]	540	4.4	0.156
4-Fluoroestradiol	182	154	327	10.0	0.059
2-Fluoroestradiol	51	30	173	3.7	0.192
2,4-Difluoroestradiol	90	78	129	5.5	0.021

[a]Estradiol = 100%; calculated from data shown in Fig. 6 and competitive binding data at 25°C (not shown).
[b]Calculated from data shown in FIGS. 7 and 8 as pmol product/min/mg protein.

The uterotrophic response in immature rats to these estrogens was determined. The following effective dose for 50% maximum response of the uteri was calculated in nmol/kg ± s.e.: estradiol, 5.1 ± 1.7; 4-fluoro-estradiol, 4.4 ± 1.5; 2-fluoroestradiol, 21.0 ± 6.8; and 2,4-difluoroestradiol. 22.6 ± 7.3. Thus, estradiol and 4-fluoroestradiol were equipotent in vivo; 2-fluoroestradiol and 2,4-difluoroestradiol were equipotent but weaker uterotrophic agents.

Liehr recently employed both monofluoro-substituted estradiols and tetrafluorodiethylstilbestrol as probes to determine the carcinogenic and hormonal activities involved in estrogen-induced tumor formation in the kidney of the Syrian hamster [23,24,25]. Using microsomes from Syrian hamster kidneys we obtained the relative rates of catechol estrogen formation shown in Figure 7. The most active substrate in this series was the carcinogenic 4-fluoroestradiol [23], which was bioactivated to 4-fluoro-2-hydroxyestradiol at a 2.3-fold greater rate than the formation of 2-hydroxyestradiol from estradiol; summarized in Table IV. However, analysis of the radioactive monomethyl ethers by HPLC revealed that 2-fluoroestradiol and 2,4-difluoroestradiol had been defluorinated at C-2 to the 2-hydroxy catechols, since the retention times of the products corresponded to those of the monomethyl ethers of 2-hydroxyestradiol and 4-fluoro-2-hydroxyestradiol, respectively. The 3-fluoro analog of estradiol was not a substrate for estrogen 2-/4-hydroxylase activity in this system.

To obtain further evidence regarding the role of defluorination of A-ring substituted fluoroestradiols in the possible bioactivation of these compounds to catechol estrogens, we investigated their metabolism by microsomes from Balb cells and by mushroom monophenol o-monooxygenase (tyrosinase) [26]. The relative rates of catechol estrogen formation are shown in Figure 8.

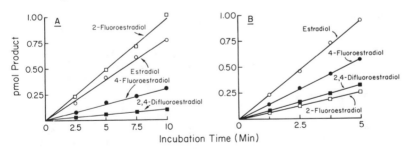

FIG. 8. Radioenzymatic assay for catechol estrogen formation using microsomes (494 μg protein) from Balb/c 3T3 cells in A and mushroom monophenol o-monooxygenase (2 μg protein) in B.

HPLC analyses of the products demonstrated that defluorination had occurred at C-2 of 2-fluoroestradiol and 2,4-difluoroestradiol in both cases. This was confirmed by treatment of the monomethyl ethers obtained from the radioenzymatic assay with diazomethane. From 2-fluoroestradiol we obtained a radioactive derivative which had the same retention time (23 min) by HPLC as authentic 2-methoxyestradiol 3-methyl ether. The products from 2,4-difluoroestradiol yielded a radioactive derivative with the retention time (21 min) of 4-fluoro-2-methoxyestradiol 3-methyl ether. However, the products from 4-fluoroestradiol also yielded a radioactive methylated derivative with the expected retention time of 4-fluoro-2-methoxyestradiol 3-methyl ether. Thus, no evidence was obtained for defluorination of 4-fluorestradiol. The relative rates of catechol estrogen formation using these fluorinated estrogens are reported in Table IV.

The genotoxicity of the fluorinated derivatives of estradiol was investigated using the Balb cell transformation assay. The results are shown in Table V.

TABLE V. Neoplastic transformation of subclone A-31-1-13 of Balb/c 3T3 cells by estrogens

Compound	Conc. (μM)	Survival[a] (%)	Avg Type III foci per dish	Type III foci/10^4 survivors
DMSO Control (0.25%)		[100]	0.09	0.2
3-Methylcholanthrene	1	68	1.63	5.3
2-Fluoroestradiol	2.5	106	1.18	2.5
	5	101	0.83	1.8
	10	68	1.25	4.1
	20	35	1.17	7.4
	25	23	1.00	9.7
	30	10	0.67	---
4-Fluoroestradiol	5	68	0.25	0.8
	10	61	0.33	1.2
	20	34	0.25	1.6
	30	30	0.27	2.0
	40	23	0.25	2.4
	50	8	0.08	---
2,4-Difluoroestradiol	5	110	0.25	0.5
	10	101	0.33	0.7
	20	99	0.17	0.4
	30	95	0.25	0.6
	40	83	0.18	0.5
	50	45	0.17	0.8

[a]Average cloning efficiency for DMSO control (45%) taken as 100%.

The average of the transformation frequency (right hand column in Table V) minus the spontaneous background level (DMSO control) normalized to 10 µM concentration of estrogen ± s.e. was 2-fluoroestradiol, 4.74 ± 1.12; 4-fluoroestradiol, 0.81 ± 0.12; and 2,4-difluoroestradiol, 0.25 ± 0.10. Therefore, 2,4-difluoroestradiol was only marginally active in the neoplastic transformation of Balb/c 3T3 cells.

Since 2,4-difluoroestradiol is a biologically active estrogen with only weak transforming activity, we prepared the other 2,4-dihalogenated derivatives of estradiol in an effort to obtain a hormonally active derivative which was devoid of genotoxic activity. The results of the displacement curves for the binding of these derivatives are shown in Figure 9.

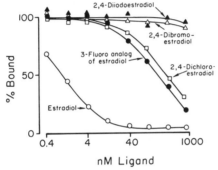

FIG. 9. Displacement curves for inhibition of [^{3}H]estradiol binding by unlabeled ligands using uterine cytosol from ovariectomized rats at 0°C.

The relative rates of catechol estrogen formation with the 2,4-dihalogenated derivatives using rat liver microsomes are shown in Figure 10.

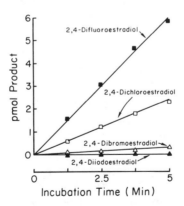

FIG. 10. Radioenzymatic assay for catechol estrogen formation using microsomes (104 µg protein) from male Sprague-Dawley rat liver.

HPLC analyses of the products from 2,4-dichloroestradiol demonstrated that dechlorination at C-2 had occurred to yield 2-hydroxy-4-chloroestradiol. Neither the 2,4-dibromo nor the 2,4-diiodo derivatives were converted at a significant rate to catechols (Table VI). However, the latter compounds showed less than 1% of the relative binding affinity of estradiol (Table VI).

TABLE VI. Summary of relative binding affinity (RBA) and rate of catechol estrogen formation with male rat liver microsomes.

Compound	% RBA[a] 0-4°C	Catechol Formed[b]
Estradiol	[100]	48.5 ± 1.6
2,4-Difluoroestradiol	90	11.3 ± 0.2
2,4-Dichloroestradiol	0.42	3.9 ± 0.1
2,4-Dibromoestradiol	< 0.1	0.2 ± 0.1
2,4-Diiodoestradiol	< 0.1	0.1 ± 0.1
3-Fluoro analog of estradiol	< 0.43	< 0.1

[a]Estradiol = 100%; calculated from data shown in FIG. 8.

[b]Calculated from data shown in FIG. 9 as pmol product/min/mg protein ± s.e.

DISCUSSION

The mode of action of estrogens in carcinogenesis is unknown; however, their failure to induce gene mutations in Salmonella/mammalian microsome mutagenicity assays has led to the presumption that they act as nongenotoxic tumor promoters [27], as cocarcinogens in estrogen-responsive tissues [28], or as epigenetic agents which induce aneuploidy and cell transformation due to interference with microtubule organization at mitosis [29,30]. The term "estrogen-induced genotoxicity" is used in this report to describe effects where some estrogens are either comutagenic in the presence of a genotoxic carcinogen (AAF), or induce the neoplastic transformation of heteroploid Balb/c 3T3 cells that are presumed to be preneoplastic [30]. These in vitro studies have been designed to determine

161

the role of estrogen metabolism in such genotoxic activity, versus the hormonal activity of the parent estrogen. Through this approach we might distinguish between promotional (hormonal) activity that influences cell growth and differentiation, and the role of metabolic activation (catechol formation) for nonmutagenic estrogens that mediate the carcinogenic process in vivo.

In the comutagenicity study, the arylamide AAF was selected because it is carcinogenic for the female rat mammary gland [31]. The formation of the DNA adduct, N-(deoxyguanosin-8-yl)-2-aminofluorene has been correlated with the induction of mutation by AAF in S. typhimurium [32]. The estrogen-enhanced mutagenicity of a low level of AAF (Table I) is selective; it depends on the structure of the estrogen rather than its hormonal activity. Moxestrol, the most potent estrogen in this series, is inactive as a comutagen with AAF, even though 2-hydroxymoxestrol is active in this respect (Figure 2). The 11β-methoxy group of moxestrol markedly reduces its metabolism to 2-hydroxymoxestrol in humans [33], in some experimental animals [34], and by some mammalian microsomes [14]. Estrogen 2-hydroxylase activity is present at a relatively high level in the hepatic microsomal activating system used in this study, and this activity appears to be a necessary requirement for the enhancement of mutagenicity of AAF and related mutagens by estrogen [11]. Thus, concentrations of 2.5 and 5 μM 2-hydroxyethinyl estradiol were more active as comutagens then equivalent concentrations of ethinyl estradiol (Figure 2). However, such concentrations of 2-hydroxymoxestrol were essentially inactive as comutagens, suggesting that further metabolism of a catechol estrogen to a semiquinone radical anion [18,35] may be required in this comutagenic process. The absence of a correlation between the relative rate of catechol formation and the enhancement of mutation by the active estrogens (Table 1) is consistent with such a mechanism, whereby catechol formation is an obligatory but not sufficient requirement for the comutagenicity of an estrogen. In the case of DES, we do not know if the catechol of DES or Z,Z-dienestrol, or both, are formed as major metabolites by the Aroclor-induced rat liver activating system.

The mechanism of the enhancement of mutagenicity by the active estrogens has not been established in detail. The hepatic mixed-function oxidase system used in this mutagenicity assay [9] is a complex mixture of flavoproteins and cytochromes, including those cytochrome P-450's responsible for catechol estrogen formation and N-hydroxylation and ring-hydroxylation of AAF. Evidence has been provided that ring hydroxylation at C-3, C-7, and C-9 of AAF was competitively inhibited by ethinyl estradiol and/or 2-hydroxyethinyl estradiol. [11] The comutagenicity of estrogens may therefore be due to a reduced detoxification of AAF (ring hydroxylation), with a concomitant increased activation (N-hydroxylation) of AAF. Since estrogen 2-hydroxylase activity represents the contribution from at least five of the cytochrome P-450 isoenzymes from rat liver [36,37], it is reasonable to assume that one or more of these isoenzymes will also catalyze ring-hydroxylation of AAF, which will be inhibited by estrogen substrates. The resulting alteration by estrogens of the relative balance between the detoxification and bioactivation of chemical carcinogens like AAF would therefore be expe   1 to depend on the interactions of the estrogen with specific P-   ı isoenzymes rather than with estrogen receptors.

The differences between the comutagenic ef ects of DES, estrone, estradiol and ethinyl estradiol versus estriol and moxestrol parallel the comparative ability of these estrogens to act as transforming agents of the A-31-1-13 subclone of Balb/c 3T3 cells [12]. Microsomes isolated from these cells bioactivate estradiol to both 2-hydroxy and 4-hydroxy catechols [12], but at a considerably reduced rate compared to liver and kidney microsomes (Tables IV and V). These catechols are more potent than estradiol as transforming agents [22]. Although the mechanism of neoplastic transformation of such preneoplastic cells has not been established for any carcinogen [30], their phenotypic alteration by some estrogens provides an in vitro model system for determining if the frequency of formation of Type III transformed foci following estrogen treatment is correlated with the hormonal activity of the estrogen.

The uterotrophic activity in immature rats of a mixture of the syn and anti forms of estrone methoxime was previously shown to be about 4% of that of estrone [38]. After purification of the minor syn component of this mixture, its relative binding affinity was found to be only 1-2% of that of estradiol (Table II). Using the catechol standards to correct for the yield of monomethyl ether products in the radiochemical assay, syn-estrone methoxime was an effective substrate for estrogen 2-/4-hydroxylase activity of the Balb/c 3T3 subclone. Therefore, this derivative, which was essentially inactive as a hormone, still retained both genotoxic activity and the ability to be bioactivated to a catechol.

The only 2,4-dihalogenated derivative of estradiol which had effective receptor binding was 2,4-difluoroestradiol (Table VI). This derivative had significant uterotrophic activity, but with Balb cell microsomes was a poor substrate for estrogen 2-/4-hydroxylase activity (Table IV), and was only marginally active as a transforming agent of Balb cells (Table V). Conversely, 2-fluoroestradiol was hormonally equipotent in vivo with 2,4-difluoroestradiol, and was both active as a transforming agent and as a

substrate for estrogen 2-/4-hydroxylase activity of Balb cells (Tables IV
and V). The genotoxic activity of 2- and 4-monofluoroestradiol would not be
expected to be the same here as was found by Liehr [23] in the Syrian
hamster kidney, since their relative rates of catechol formation in these
two systems are markedly different (Table IV). These differences in bioactivation are consistent with the 12/1 ratio of estrogen 2-/4-hydroxylase
activity found by Li et al. [39] using hamster kidney microsomes with
estradiol as substrate, versus the 1/1 ratio obtained with Balb cell microsomes [12]. The oxidative defluorination of the above fluoroestrogens,
analogous to the microsomal defluorination of 4-fluoroacetanilide [40] and
6-fluorobenzo(a)pyrene [41], emphasizes the requirement for metabolic
studies when the fluorine-probe methodology is used in studies of genotoxicity [42]. Until a biologically active estrogen is found which is not
genotoxic in vitro and in vivo, it is not possible to conclude from our
results with 2,4-difluoroestradiol that estrogen-induced genotoxicity does
not require receptor-mediated events.

SUMMARY

Diethylstilbestrol, ethinyl estradiol, estradiol, and estrone have
been shown to enhance the mutagenicity of a low level of a mammary
carcinogen, 2-acetylaminofluorene, in strain TA 98 of Salmonella
typhimurium in the presence of a rat liver microsomal activating system.
In studies thus far completed, the comutagenicity of these estrogens
requires their bioactivation to catechols. Since catechol estrogens
themselves had not yet been shown to be direct acting mutagens, we used the
neoplastic transformation of nontumorigenic Balb/c 3T3 cells as a more
sensitive test for estrogen-induced genotoxicity. While relative rates of
catechol estrogen formation, catalyzed by microsomes from these Balb cells,
usually paralleled the cellular transformation frequency induced by many
steroidal estrogens, the transformation frequency induced by an estrogen
could not be related to its relative binding affinity for uterine estrogen
receptors. An example of a genotoxic estrogen derivative with negligible
receptor binding is syn-estrone methoxime which is metabolized via catechol
formation. The hormonally active 2,4-difluoroestradiol is only a very weak
transforming agent, and is bioactivated to a small degree by Balb cell
microsomes through 2-defluorination. The dissociation between the genotoxicity of some estrogens and their hormonal activity indicates that
receptor-mediated actions need not be directly involved in the genesis of
estrogen related cancers.

164

ACKNOWLEDGEMENTS

This investigation was supported by grants CA 24629 and HD 13587
awarded respectively by the National Cancer Institute and National
Institute of Child Health and Human Development, DHHS (Bethesda, MD). The
authors are indebted to Mrs. Connie K. Durocher, Mr. Perry H. Moore, Jr.,
and Mr. Clifford Hurlburt for their excellent assistance in these studies.

REFERENCES

1. E. V. Jensen and E. R. DeSombre, Annu. Rev. Biochem. 41, 203-230
   (1972).
2. J. Gorski and F. Gannon, Annu. Rev. Physiol. 38, 425-450 (1976).
3. B. S. Katzenellenbogen, Annu. Rev. Physiol. 42, 17-35 (1980).
4. M. Ginsburg, B. D. Greenstein, N. J. MacLusky, I. D. Morris, and P. J.
   Thomas, Steroids 23, 773-792 (1974).
5. A. De Lean, P. J. Munson, and D. Rodbard, Am. J. Physiol. 235, E97-
   E102 (1978).
6. M. H. Teicher in: Biomedical Computing Information Center, Vanderbilt
   Medical Center, Nashville, TN, Program MED-64 (1983).
7. S. G. Korenman, Endocrinology 87, 1119-1123 (1970).
8. S. Franks, N. J. MacLusky, and F. Naftolin, J. Endocrinol. 94, 91-98
   (1982).
9. D. M. Maron and B. N. Ames, Mutat. Res. 113, 173-215 (1983).
10. T. Tsutsui, G. H. Degen, D. Schiffmann, A. Wong, H. Maizumi, J. A.
    McLachlan, and J. C. Barrett, Cancer Res. 44, 184-189 (1984).
11. R. H. Purdy and M. V. Marshall, Carcinogenesis 5, 1709-1715 (1984).
12. R. H. Purdy, J. W. Goldzieher, P. W. LeQuesne, S. Abdel-Baky, C. K.
    Durocher, P. H. Moore, Jr., and J. S. Rhim in: Catechol Estrogens, G.
    R. Merriam and M. B. Lipsett, eds. (Raven Press, New York 1983) pp.
    123-140.
13. M. M. Bradford, Anal. Biochem. 72, 248-254 (1976).
14. R. H. Purdy, P. H. Moore, Jr., M. C. Williams, J. W. Goldzieher, and
    S. M. Paul, FEBS Lett. 138, 40-44 (1982).
15. T. Kakunaga, K.-Y. Lo, J. Leavitt, and M. Ikenaga, Jerusalem Symp.
    Quantum Chem. Biochem. 13, 527-541 (1980).
16. T. Kakunaga, Int. J. Cancer 12, 463-473 (1973).
17. A. Sivak, M. C. Charest, L. Rudenko, D. M. Silveira, I. Simons, and A.
    M. Wood, Adv. Mod. Environ. Toxicol. 1, 133-180 (1980).
18. P. Ball and R. Knuppen, Acta Endocrinol. [Suppl.] 232, 1-127 (1980).
19. R. H. Purdy, L. L. Engel, and J. L. Oncley, J. Biol. Chem. 236, 1043-
    1050 (1961).
20. W. Zillig and G. C. Mueller, Fed. Proc. 15, 503-504 (1956).
21. D. F. Morrow and R. M. Hofer, J. Med. Chem. 9, 249-251 (1966).
22. R. H. Purdy, Prog. Cancer Res. Ther. 31, 401-415 (1984).
23. J. G. Liehr, Molec. Pharmacol. 23, 278-281 (1983).
24. J. G. Liehr, A. M. Ballatore, J. A. McLachlan, and D. A. Sirbasku,
    Cancer Res. 43, 2678-2682 (1983).
25. J. G. Liehr, Arch. Toxicol. 55, 119-122 (1984).
26. P. H. Jellinck, B. Norton, and J. Fishman, J. Steroid Biochem. 21,
    361-365 (1984).
27. A. C. Upton, D. B. Clayson, J. D. Jansen, H. S. Rosenkranz, and G. M.
    Williams, Mutat. Res. 133, 1-49 (1984).
28. M. B. Lipsett, Cancer 51, 2426-2429 (1983).
29. T. Tsutsui, H. Maizumi, J. A. McLachlan, and J. C. Barrett, Cancer
    Res. 43, 3814-3821 (1983).

30. J. C. Barrett, T. W. Hesterberg, and D. G. Thomassen, Pharm. Rev. 36, 53S–70S (1984).

31. R. C. Garner, and R. C. Garner. In: Chemical Carcinogens, C. E. Searle, ed. (American Chemical Society, Washington, D. C. (1976) pp. 366–461.

32. D. T. Beranek, G. L. White, R. H. Heflich, and F. A. Beland. Proc. Natl. Acad. Sci. USA, 79, 5175–5178 (1982).

33. J. Salmon, D. Coussediere, C. Cousty, and J. P. Raynaud, J. Steroid Biochem. 18, 565–573 (1983).

34. J. Salmon, D. Coussediere, C. Cousty, and J. P. Raynaud, J. Steroid Biochem. 19, 1223–1234 (1983).

35. S. D. Nelson, J. R. Mitchell, E. Dybing, and H. A. Sasame, Biochem. Biophys. Res. Commun. 70, 1157–1165 (1976).

36. D. E. Ryan, P. E. Thomas, L. M. Reik, and W. Levin, Xenobiotica 12, 727–744 (1982).

37. D. E. Ryan, S. Iida, A. W. Wood, P. E. Thomas, C. S. Lieber, and W. Levin, J. Biol. Chem. 259, 1239–1250 (1984).

38. J. Kärkkäinen, J. J. Ohisalo, J. Puranen, and T. Luukkainen. Contraception 12, 505–509 (1975).

39. S. A. Li, J. K. Klicka, and J. J. Li, Cancer Res. 45, 181–185 (1985).

40. J. W. Daly, G. Guroff, S. Udenfriend, and B. Witkop, Biochem. Pharmacol. 17, 31–36 (1968).

41. D. R. Buhler, F. Ünlü, D. R. Thakker, T. J. Slaga, A. H. Conney, A. W. Wood, R. L. Chang, W. Levin, and D. M. Jerina, Cancer Res., 43, 1541–1549 (1983).

42. M. K. Buening, W. Levin, A. W. Wood, R. L. Chang, I. Agranat, M. Rabinovitz, D. R. Buhler, H. D. Mah, O. Hernandez, R. B. Simpson, D. M. Jerina, A. H. Conney, E. C. Miller, and J. A. Miller, J. Natl. Cancer Inst., 71, 309–315 (1983).

DISCUSSION

KOLB–MEYERS: How did you identify the structure of the syn estrone methoxime? We have found that only one isomer was obtained in cases of estrone hydrazone and androstenedione 17-hydrazone, which we assigned the 17-anti configuration. The 17-syn hydrazones were not formed, as established from ^{13}C-NMR analysis. Examination of Dreiding models shows severe steric hindrance between NH$_2$ of the 17-syn hydrazones and the 12β-H (equitorial). Thus it appears that the syn estrone methoxime should suffer severe steric crowding since the methoxime group is comparable in size with the hydrazone group.

PURDY: The identification of syn estrone 17-methoxime was based on both ^{1}H and ^{13}C NMR spectra of this minor product of the reaction of estrone with methoxylamine hydrochloride and potassium acetate in methanol. These NMR spectra were clearly different from the ^{1}H and ^{13}C spectra of the major product, anti estrone 17-methoxime. As you indicate, steric hindrance is certainly present in the syn isomer, which was only obtained by HPLC in very low yield from the mother liquor after crystallization of the major product.

ABUL–HAJJ: In the metabolism of 2-fluoroestradiol, what happens to the 2-fluoro atom? Do you see an NIH shift of the 2-fluoro group?

PURDY: We assume that in the oxidative defluorination of 2-fluoroestradiol to 2-hydroxyestradiol the 2-fluoro group is eliminated as fluoride ion [analogous to the liver microsomal oxidation of 4-fluoroacetanilide to 4-hydroxyacetanilide, ref. 40]. No evidence was obtained for an NIH shift of the 2-fluoro group, since the major products of the reaction were

identified as the monomethyl ethers of 2-hydroxyestradiol by crystallization to constant specific activity.

KUPFER: How exhaustively did you search for the possible formation of
1-fluoro-2-hydroxyestradiol from 2-fluoroestradiol by an NIH shift? I
raise this question since it is possible that the above compound might not
interact with catechol-O-methyltransferase and hence will not be detected
by the radiometric method.

PURDY: The identified products of microsomal metabolism of 2-fluoro-
estradiol were the ^{3}H-labeled monomethyl ethers of 2-hydroxyestradiol and a
small amount of a product which was tentatively identified as 2-fluoro-
4-hydroxyestradiol 3-methyl ether by HPLC. It is certainly correct that
unless a catechol metabolite is a substrate for catechol-O-methyltransferase, it will not be detected as a product in this radioenzymatic
assay. Therefore, possible formation of 1-fluoro-2-hydroxyestradiol cannot
be ruled out until this catechol is available for use as a reference
standard in this assay.

STANCEL: Do you have any direct evidence for defluorination in vivo? Does
your Balb cell line have any high affinity estrogen binding sites?

PURDY: We have not studied the in vivo metabolism of 2-fluoroestradiol;
only its in vitro metabolism by a variety of mammalian liver microsomes
where the evidence has always supported its defluorination. The Balb/c 3T3
subclone does not have detectable high affinity estrogen receptors in the
cytosol.

ABUL-HAJJ: Since you propose that 2-hydroxylation is a prerequisite for
genotoxic activity, have you studied the activity of 2-methylestradiol?

PURDY: We have not studied the effects of 2-methylestradiol, since its
reported relative binding affinity to estrogen receptors is less than that
of estradiol. Our proposal is that estrogen 2-/4-hydroxylase activity is a
prerequisite for the genotoxicity of estrogens, which also includes the
formation of the 4-hydroxy catechols [e.g., the major catechol metabolite
of equilenin, ref. 14].

FORSBERG: You have demonstrated an effect by estrogenic compounds on cell
transformation in vitro. Are these transformed cells tumorigenic in vivo
and, if so, do the tumors kill the animals? Do you think that the effect
by your compounds could be related to activation of what we call an
oncogene?

PURDY: After treatment of Balb/c 3T3 cells with diethylstilbestrol,
estrone, estradiol and ethinylestradiol, cells from type III transformed
foci were further passaged and 5×10^6 cells inoculated subcutaneously in
NIH nude mice by Dr. Johng Rhim at the National Cancer Institute. All of
the cells which had been transformed by the above estrogens produced tumors
within 3 weeks in all animals, as opposed to the controls which were
nontumorigenic [see ref. 12]. The animals were killed after 5-6 weeks when
the tumors had grown to about 2 cm in diameter. These tumors were shown
histologically to be fibrosarcomas. We have no evidence that suggests that
the estrogen-induced transformation of these Balb cells is related to the
activation of an oncogene, although such preneoplastic cells can be
transformed by ras-like oncogenes [see ref. 30]. The subclone of these
Balb/c 3T3 cells used in our work was selected because it is particularly
sensitive to neoplastic transformation by polycyclic aromatic hydrocarbons
like 3-methylcholanthrene. Our working hypothesis is that the
bioactivation of estrogens is catalyzed by cytochrome P-450 activity in
these cells that similarly activates 3-methylcholanthrene.

MEYERS: As I understood you, your hormonal activities were based on receptor-binding activities, which you then correlated with tumor incidence. Since in vivo estrogenicity is not necessarily reflected (at least quantitatively) by binding affinities, isn't it dangerous to correlate tumor incidence data with binding-affinity data instead of with in vivo estrogenicity.....if true estrogenicity/carcinogenicity comparisons are desired?

PURDY: You are absolutely correct that any quantitative determination of both estrogenicity and carcinogenicity must ultimately be obtained using in vivo assay systems. Our efforts have first focused on the relative binding affinity (RBA) of various estrogen derivatives in order to obtain an index of markedly reduced RBA (estrone syn-methoxime) or retained RBA (2,4-difluoroestradiol) compared to estradiol. Then, in the cases of the fluoroestrogens and certain other compounds, we have extended the RBA measurements to a determination of uterotrophic activity in immature female rats [8]. As expected, these in vivo results were in qualitative but not quantitative agreement with RBA. In an analogous manner, the in vitro results of cell transformation need to be extended to animal studies such as the Syrian hamster model system that will be described in the subsequent report by Dr. Jonathan Li. Only through such in vivo studies can our short-term tests for the carcinogenic potential of an estrogen be translated into measurements of carcinogenicity in a tissue that responds to estrogen.

SOME BIOLOGICAL AND TOXICOLOGICAL STUDIES OF VARIOUS ESTROGEN MYCOTOXINS
AND PHYTOESTROGENS [1]

JONATHAN J. LI, SARA ANTONIA LI, JOHN K. KLICKA, AND JULIE A. HELLER

Medical Research Laboratories, V.A. Medical Center, and Department of Urolog-

ic Surgery, University of Minnesota Medical School, Minneapolis, MN 55417.

Our interest in natural and synthetic estrogens used therapeutically in

humans has now been extended to certain estrogen mycotoxins and phytoestro-

gens. They are characterized chemically into three classes, the resorcylic

acid lactones, coumestans, and isoflavones (Fig. 1). The estrogenic activity

of these plant and fungal products has been studied extensively [1-10]. Nu-

merous investigations have confirmed the binding of these compounds to estro-

gen receptors by competitive binding using tritiated estradiol in target

tissues of many species; the translocation of such ligand-receptor to the

nucleus; and their subsequent uterotropic and anabolic activities following

administration of these phytoestrogens and mycotoxins. Resorylic acid lac-

tones are produced by several species of _fusarium_ and are found as natural

contaminants in human food grains and animal feeds. Many different animals

are susceptible to toxicosis by these compounds, although swine are among

the most sensitive [11]. Fetal abnormalities have also been attributed to

estrogen mycotoxins [12,13], as well as squamous metaplasia and hyperplasia

[14]. Isoflavones, constituents of many forages and feed, are found in soya

beans. Coumestans are present in forages and legumes, such as alfalfa and

clover, at relatively low levels. While phytoestrogens do not presently have

any therapeutic or commercial use, the reduced estrogen mycotoxin derivatives

have shown to be effective in the treatment of postmenopausal syndrome [15]

and is widely employed as an implant for growth promotion in cattle [16].

Some of the metabolic biotransformations of these substances have been iden-

[1]
These studies were supported by Grant CA 22008 from the National Cancer
Institute, NIH, DHHS, and the General Medical Research Fund of the Veterans
Administration.

tified and their conjugation products isolated in tissues of various mammalian species [17-21], particularly the estrogen mycotoxins. Little is known,
however, about the details of the metabolism of these plant hormones in animals. The present investigation has been undertaken to study some of the
hormonal, metabolic, and carcinogenic properties of these natural non-steroidal compounds in the Syrian hamster, using methods well established in our
laboratory.

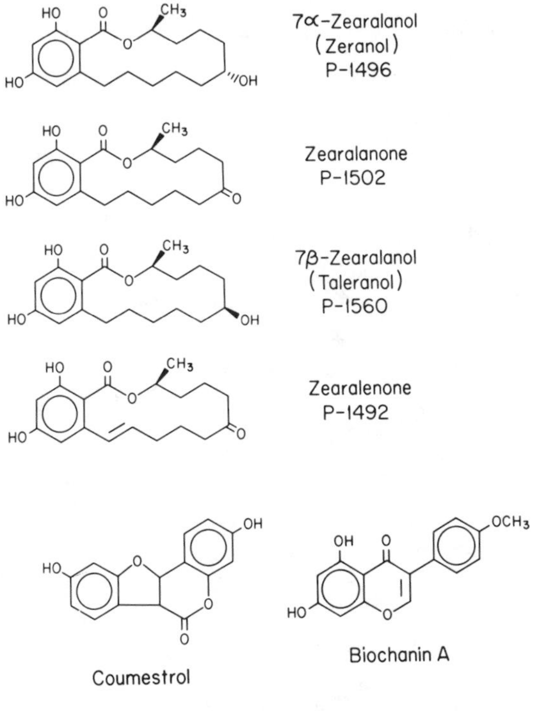

7α-Zearalanol
(Zeranol)
P-1496

Zearalanone
P-1502

7β-Zearalanol
(Taleranol)
P-1560

Zearalenone
P-1492

Coumestrol

Biochanin A

FIGURE 1. Structure of estrogen mycotoxins and phytoestrogens

Effect of Treatments on Body Weights

Male castrated Syrian golden hamsters were implanted with pellets of pure
phytoestrogens and mycotoxins. Body weights were monitored at one month intervals in the various treated groups (Fig. 2). To maintain similar daily ab-
sorptions, 20-mg pellets were implanted every 3-months in animals treated with
17β-estradiol, α-zearalanol, β-zearalanol, and zearalenone; two 30 mg. pel-

lets were implanted every two months in animals treated with zearalanone, coumesterol and biochanin A. The mean daily absorption was similar to 17β-estradiol in all treatment groups (241 ± 18 μg/day) except for coumesterol (60 ± 1 μg/day), despite additional exposure to coumesterol pellets. Both α-zearalanol and zearalenone exhibited a moderately suppressive effect on body weight following chronic exposure to these agents, which is similar to that observed following 17β-estradiol treatment. On the other hand, zearalanone and biochanin A treatments exhibited similar weight gains compared to un-treated chow-fed animals. Only continuous coumesterol administration showed slightly higher than normal weight gains, despite the lower absorption rate of this compound.

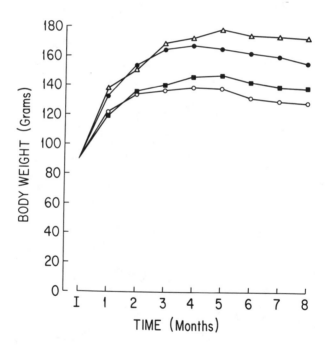

FIGURE 2. Effect of 17β-estradiol and various estrogen myco-toxins and phytoestrogens on body weight in castrated male Syrian golden hamsters. Initial body weights for all animals was 90 g. Control castrate without treatment (●), 7α-zeara-lanol (O), 17β-estradiol, zearalenone and 7β-zearalanol (■), zearalanone and biochanin A (●), coumestrol (△). Each point represents the mean body weight (grams) of 5 to 8 hamsters.

Competitive Binding to Estrogen Receptor

As previously reported [17,18], [³H]-17β-estradiol exhibited the characteristic binding profile for hamster renal carcinoma cytosol estrogen receptor. Of the estrogenic mycotoxins and phytoestrogens examined at lower competitive binding concentrations, 20 to 80-fold excess, only α-zearalanol showed
substantial binding affinity for this receptor (Fig. 3). However, all other
non-steroidal plant estrogens exhibited appreciable competitive binding at
100-fold excess for the 5nM radiolabeled estradiol. At 500-fold excess concentrations, all mycotoxins and phytoestrogens exhibited greater than 80%
competitive binding for the renal tumor cytosolic estrogen receptor (data
not shown).

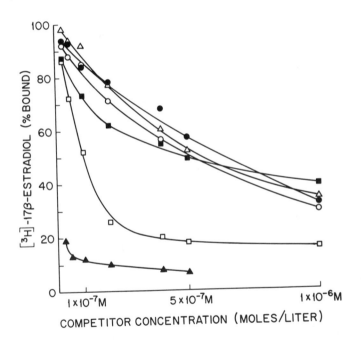

FIGURE 3. Competition of various estrogen mycotoxins and phytoestrogens for the binding of [³H]-17β-estradiol to the estrogen
receptor of the hamster renal carcinoma. Cytosols were incubated
with 5nM [³H]-estradiol alone or in combination with various
concentrations (1 to 200-fold excess) of non-labeled 17β-estra-
diol (▲), α-zearalanol (□), β-zearalanol (O), zearalenone
(●), zearalanone (△), and coumesterol (■). Each point
represents the mean of 5 to 7 individual determinations.

Induction of Progesterone Receptor and Serum Prolactin Elevation

We have previously reported an 8- to 13-fold increase in progesterone receptor in the untransformed hamster kidney after 3- to 4-months of either
17β-estradiol or diethylstilbestrol (DES) treatment, and a concomitant 6- to
8-fold elevation of serum prolactin levels [19-21], as determined by homologous radioimmunoassay [22]. The most potent estrogenic mycotoxin, α-zearalanol, produced a similar rise in the hamster renal progesterone receptor, as
well as a similar increment in serum prolactin as 17β-estradiol (Table 1).
Despite a 2.0- to 3.6-fold elevation in serum prolactin levels following either zearalanone or zearalenone treatment, the concentration of progesterone
receptor was not altered compared to untreated levels. Interestingly, phytoestrogen treatment produced similar changes in serum prolactin levels as
found with zearalenone, but somewhat greater stimulation of renal progesterone receptor concentrations than this estrogen mycotoxin intermediate.

Table 1. Induction of kidney progesterone receptor and elevation
of serum prolactin levels in castrated hamsters by various
estrogen mycotoxins and phytoestrogens

Treatment[a]	Progesterone Receptor Levels[b] (fmol/mg protein)	Serum Prolactin[b] (ng/ml)
Untreated control	4.1 ± 0.3	44 ± 3
17β-Estradiol	31.8 ± 1.8	226 ± 32
α-Zearalanol	29.8 ± 5.6	276 ± 65
β-Zearalanol	11.6 ± 4.0	202 ± 50
Zearalanone	5.1 ± 1.9	159 ± 28
Zearalenone	4.2 ± 0.9	90 ± 14
Biochanin A	8.9 ± 3.3	82 ± 10
Coumestrol	6.7 ± 2.0	69 ± 18

[a] Castrate males were treated for 3.5 months.

[b] Data represents the mean ± S.E. of four to ten separate determinations.

Relative Rates of Catechol Formation by Hamster Liver and Kidney Microsomal Estrogen Hydroxylase

Using a radioenzymatic assay [23,24], estrogen 2-/4-hydroxylase (ESH) was
assessed in liver and kidney microsomes of castrated hamsters with various

estrogen mycotoxins and phytoestrogens as substrates. These results are summarized in Table 2. In the liver, both estrone and 17β-estradiol, were equally effective substrates for this enzyme. When kidney microsomes were used,
estrone exhibited a 3.5-fold greater activity compared to 17β-estradiol. Of
the estrogen mycotoxins, zearalanone was as good a substrate for ESH as 17β-
estradiol in the liver and kidney, and zearalenone exhibited less activity in
both tissue microsomes. All the other estrogen mycotoxins were relatively
poor substrates for microsomal ESH when compared to 17β-estradiol. In contrast, both phytoestrogens, biochanin A and coumestrol, revealed substantial
activity as substrates for this enzyme.

Table 2. Microsomal estrogen hydroxylase activity and relative
catechol estrogen formation of various estrogen mycotoxins
and phytoestrogens in the hamster liver and kidney

Substrate[a]	Liver	Kidney
Estrone	9.6 ± 1.5[b]	5.2 ± 0.30[b]
17β-Estradiol	8.4 ± 0.8	1.5 ± 0.10
Zearalanone	6.3 ± 0.6	1.6 ± 0.30
Zearalenone	4.5 ± 0.8	0.4 ± 0.04
α-Zearalanol	3.1 ± 0.3	0.7 ± 0.10
β-Zearalanol	1.9 ± 0.3	0.4 ± 0.07
α-Zearalenol	1.3 ± 0.2	0.2 ± 0.01
β-Zearalenol	1.1 ± 0.03	0.2 ± 0.04
Biochanin A	12.0 ± 0.8	1.5 ± 0.06
Coumestrol	4.7 ± 1.3	1.2 ± 0.20

[a] Substrates (50 μM) were incubated with either hamster liver or
kidney microsomes (150 μg protein) for 10 min at 37°C. Estrogen hydroxylase activity is expressed in pmol/mg protein/min.

[b] Mean ± S.E. of at least four individual determinations.

Monomethyl Ether Product Formation from Estrogen Mycotoxins and Phytoestrogens

Following separation by HPLC, liver and kidney microsomal incubations
with either estrone or estradiol yielded characteristic monomethyl ethers of
the catechols, their retention times were identical to those of nonlabeled
authentic monomethyl ether standards obtained from 2- or 4-hydroxylation of

174

these substrates [25,26] as shown in Fig. 4. All estrogen mycotoxins exhibited essentially a single peak after HPLC (Waters Model 840 Data and Chromatography System) separation using isocratic followed by a linear gradient and
the radioactivity leaving the column was monitored with a flow detector using liquid scintillation counting (Flo-One Model IC, Radiomatic). HPLC retention times of monomethyl ether products of all compounds examined are summarized in Table 3. Although HPLC analyses of biochanin A did not yield good
resolution, apparently two catechol monomethyl ether peaks were observed after liver microsomal incubation and one peak of differing retention time in
the kidney. At the present time, the monomethyl ether product(s) of coumestrol could not be resolved, likely due to the very polar nature of the pro-
duct(s) formed.

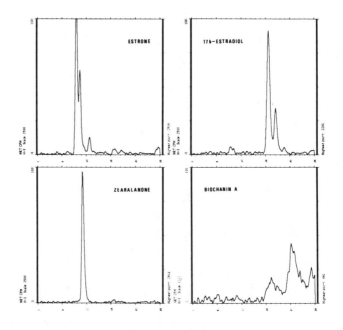

FIGURE 4. HPLC radiochromatograms of catechol monomethyl ether
products obtained from liver microsomal incubations using the
estrogen hydroxylase radioenzymatic assay.

The tritiated labeled catechol monomethyl ether product of zearalanone from liver microsomal incubations was identified by GC/MS analysis of the tri-methylsilylated (TMS) derivative of this product. A molecular ion of 494 mass units was obtained compared to a molecular ion of 464 units for the TMS derivative of the parent compound, zearalanone. This difference of 30 mass units indicates the addition of a methoxy group on the parent compound and is consistent with the microsomal hydroxylation of zearalanone to a catechol.

Table 3. HPLC retention times of monomethyl ether products from estrogen mycotoxins and phytoestrogens[a]

Substrate	Liver	Kidney
Estrone	8.8, 8.7, 10.7	8.0, 8.7, 10.7
17β-Estradiol	15.6, 17.1, 18.8	15.6, 17.1, 18.8
Zearalanone	9.3	9.3
Zearalenone	9.1	9.1
α-Zearalanol	9.3	9.3
β-Zearalanol	9.3	9.3
α-Zearalenol	9.3	9.3
β-Zearalenol	-	9.3
Biochanin A	20.3, 20.8	5.0
Coumestrol	-	-

[a] Catechol monomethyl ether products were obtained from microsomes using the estrogen hydroxylase radioenzymatic assay.

Hormonal Carcinogenicity of Various Estrogen Mycotoxins and Phytoestrogens

Of the estrogen mycotoxins and phytoestrogens studied, only α-zearalanol exhibited any carcinogenic activity in the hamster kidney of castrated male hamsters treated for 10-months. Compared to either 17β-estradiol or DES, however, the carcinogenic activity of α-zearalanol was particularly weak.

The present studies indicate that the natural non-steroidal estrogen mycotoxins and phytoestrogens have similar hormonal characteristics in the hamster as that of naturally occurring steroidal and synthetic stilbene estrogens. This was confirmed by the competitive binding of these compounds to the renal estrogen receptor, induction of progesterone receptor in the untransformed hamster kidney, and elevation of serum prolactin levels. Of the plant hormones that have currently been investigated, α- and β-zearalanol appeared to possess the most potent estrogenic activity in the hamster. Although the present observations are in general agreement with earlier studies regarding the estrogenicity of these compounds [1-4,6,10], the findings differ slightly from some reports in regard to the relative competitive binding of various estrogen mycotoxins to the estrogen receptor [5,7-9].

Numerous studies have demonstrated the bioconversion of either zearalanone to α- and β-zearalanol or zearalenone to α- and β-zearalenol in different mammalian tissues including liver, prostate, and erythrocytes [27-32]. Moreover, the conjugation of estrogen mycotoxins to glucuronic acid has been

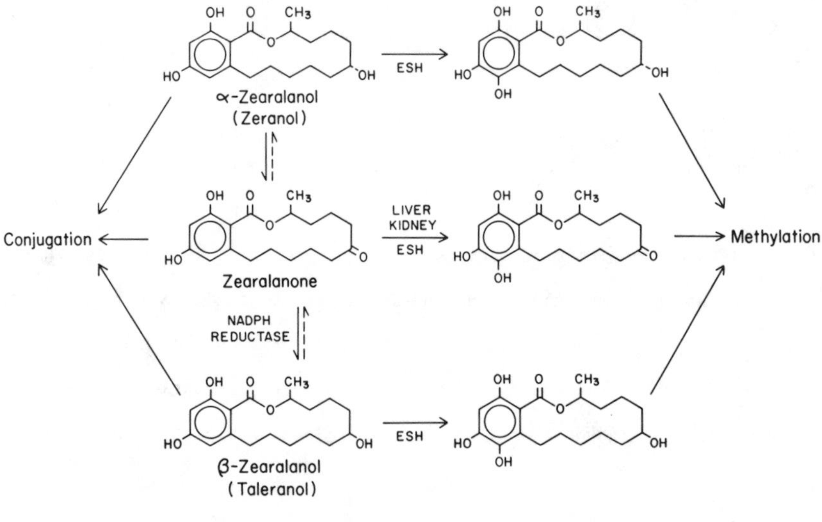

FIGURE 5. Metabolism of α-zearalanol to catechols

established [27,31,32]. However, little is currently known about the metabolism of phytoestrogens in animals. We now report a new pathway for the metabolism of estrogen mycotoxins and phytoestrogens to catechol intermediates (Fig. 5,6). Interestingly, there appears to be an inverse relationship between estrogenic activity and ability of a given estrogen mycotoxin to form catechols with hamster liver and kidney estrogen hydroxylase. Therefore, both α- and β-zearalanol, which possess appreciable estrogenic activity, exhibited relatively weak catechol forming activity. In contrast, both zearalanone and zearalenone were relatively good substrates for estrogen hydroxylase but demonstrated only poor estrogenic activity. Although both phytoestrogens studied showed substantial ability to form catechol metabolites, their estro-

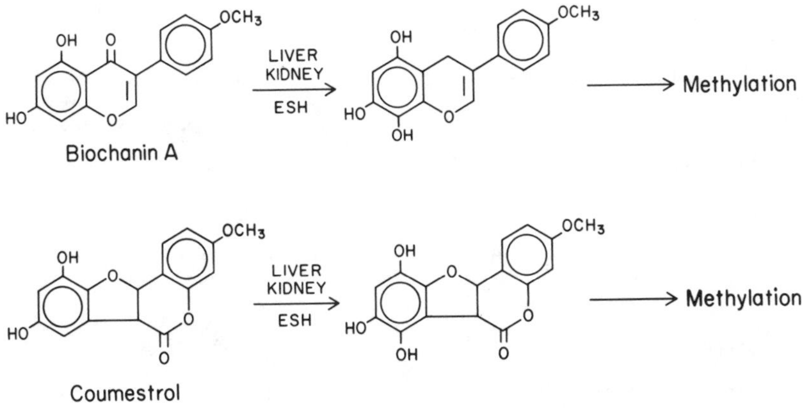

Biochanin A

Coumestrol

FIGURE 6. Metabolism of phytoestrogens to catechols

genic activity compared to either 17β-estradiol or DES was relatively weak. We have previously suggested that significant estrogenic activity and catechol intermediate formation may be pertinent for in-vivo cell-transformation in the hamster [25,33]. Therefore, it is not necessarily surprising that these plant hormones do not appear to exhibit appreciable carcinogenic activity in the hamster kidney. However, the ability of these compounds to metabolize to catechol intermediates could contribute importantly to the reproductive toxicities observed previously [12-14].

REFERENCES

1. Shutt, D.A., R.I. Cox. Steroid and phyto-oestrogen binding to sheep uterine receptors in vitro. J. Endocrinol. 52: 299-310, 1972.

2. Shemesh, M., H.R. Lindner, N. Ayalon. Affinity of rabbit uterine oestradiol receptor for phyto-oestrogens and its use in a competitive protein-binding radioassay for plasma coumestrol. J. Reprod. Fertil. 29: 1-9, 1972.

3. Boyd, P.A. and J.L. Wittliff. Mechanism of Fusarium mycotoxin action in mammary gland. J. Toxicol. Environ. Health 4: 1-8, 1978.

4. Martin, P.M., K.B. Horwitz, D.S. Ryan, and W.L. McGuire. Phytoestrogen interaction with estrogen receptors in human breast cancer cells. Endocrinology 103: 1860-1867, 1978.

5. Kiang, D.T., B.J. Kennedy, S.V. Pathre, and C.J. Mirocha. Binding characteristics of zearalenone analogs to estrogen receptors. Cancer Res. 38: 3611-3615, 1978.

6. Greenman, D.L., R.G. Mehta, J.L. Wittliff. Nuclear interaction of Fusarium mycotoxins with estradiol binding sites in the mouse uterus. J. Toxicol. Environ. Health 5: 593-598, 1979.

7. Katzenellenbogen, B.S., J.A. Katzenellenbogen, and D. Mordecai. Zearalenones: Characterization of the estrogenic potencies and receptor interactions of a series of fungal β-resorcylic acid lactones. Endocrinology 105: 33-40, 1979.

8. Verdeal, K., R.R. Brown, T. Richardson, D.S. Ryan. Affinity of phytoestrogens for estradiol-binding proteins and effect of coumestrol on growth of 7,12-dimethylbenz[a]anthracene-induced rat mammary tumors. J. Natl. Cancer Inst. 64: 285-290, 1980.

9. Powell-Jones, W.S. Raeford, and G.W. Lucier. Binding properties of zearalenone mycotoxins to hepatic estrogen receptors. Molec. Pharmacol. 20: 35-42, 1981.

10. Nelson, K., E.J. Pavlik, J.R. Van Nagell, Jr., M.B. Hanson, E.S. Donald-son, and R.C. Flanigan. Estrogenicity of coumestrol in the mouse: Fluorescence detection of interaction with estrogen receptors. Biochemistry 23: 2565-2572, 1984.

11. Stangroom, K.E. and T.K. Smith. Effect of whole and fractionated dietary alfalfa meal on zearalenone toxicosis and metabolism in rats and swine. Can. J. Physiol. Pharmacol. 62: 1219-1224, 1984.

12. Ruddick, J.A., P.M. Scott, and J. Harwig. Teratological evaluation of zearalenone administered orally to the rat. Bull. Environ. Contam. Toxicol. 15: 678-681, 1976.

13. Davis, G.J., J.A. McLachlan, and G.W. Lucier. Fetotoxicity and Teratogenicity of zearanol in mice. Toxicol. Appl. Pharmacol. 41: 138-139, 1977.

14. Rothenbacher, J., H.P. Wiggins, and J.J. Wilson. Pathological changes in endocrine glands and certain other tissues of lambs implanted with the synthetic growth promotant zearanol. Am. J. Vet. Res. 36: 1313-1318, 1975.

15. Utian, W.H. Comparative trial of P 1496, a new non-steroidal oestrogen analogue. Br. Med. J. 1: 579-581, 1973.

16. Baldwin, R.S., R.D. Williams, and M.K. Terry. Zeranol: A review of the metabolism, toxicology, and analytical methods for detection of tissue residues. Reg. Toxicol. Pharmacol. 3: 9-25, 1983.

17. Li, J.J., S.A. Li, and T.L. Cuthbertson. Nuclear retention of all steroid hormone receptor classes in the hamster renal carcinoma. Cancer Res. 39: 2647-2651, 1979.

18. Li, J.J., and S.A. Li. High yield of primary serially transplanted hamster renal carcinoma: Histologic and steroid receptor characteristics. Europ. J. Cancer 16: 1119-1126, 1980.

19. Li, S.A., and J.J. Li. Estrogen-induced progesterone receptor in the Syrian hamster kidney. I. Modulation by antiestrogens and androgens. Endo-

crinology, 103: 2119-2128, 1978.

20. Li, J.J., and S.A. Li. Estrogen-induced progesterone receptor in the Syrian hamster kidney. II. Modulation by synthetic progestins. Endocrinology, 108: 1751-1756, 1981.

21. Li, J.J., S.A. Li, J.K. Klicka, J.A. Parsons, and L.K.T. Lam. Relative carcinogenic activity of various synthetic and natural estrogens in the hamster kidney. Cancer Res. 43: 5200-5204, 1983.

22. Soares, M., P. Colosi, and F. Talamantes. Development of a homologous radioimmunoassay for secreted hamster prolactin. Proc. Soc. Exptl. Biol. Med. 172: 379-381, 1983.

23. Paul, S.M., J. Axelrod, and E. Diliberto, Jr. Catechol estrogen forming enzyme of the brain: Demonstration of a cytochrome P-450 monooxygenase. Endocrinology 101: 1604-1610, 1977.

24. Purdy, R.H., J.W. Goldzceher, P.W. LeQuesne, S. Abdel-Baky, C.K. Durocher, P.H. Moore, Jr., and J.S. Rhim. Active intermediates in carcinogenesis. In: G.L. Meeriam and M.B. Lipsett (eds.), Catechol Estrogens, pp. 123-140, New York, Raven Press, 1983.

25. Li, S.A., J.K. Klicka, and J.J. Li. Estrogen 2- and 4-hydroxylase activity, catechol estrogen formation, and implications for estrogen carcinogenesis in the hamster kidney. Cancer Res. 45: 181-185, 1985.

26. Li, J.J., R.H. Purdy, E.H. Appelman, J.K. Klicka, and S.A. Li. Catechol formation of fluoro- and bromo-substituted estradiols by hamster liver microsomes. Evidence for dehalogenation. Mol. Pharmacol. 27: 559-565, 1985.

27. Kiessling, K.H. and H. Pettersson. Metabolism of zearalenone in rat liver. Acta Pharmacol. et Toxicol. 43: 285-290, 1978.

28. Olsen, M., H. Pettersson, and K.H. Kiersling. Reduction of zearalenone to zearalenol in female rat liver by 3α-hydroxysteroid dehydrogenase. Acta Pharmacol. et Toxicol. 48: 157-161, 1981.

29. Ueno, Y., and F. Tashyro. α-Zearalenol, a major hepatic metabolite in rats of zearalenone, and estrogenic mycotoxin of Fusarium species. J.

Biochem. <u>89</u>: 563-571, 1981.

30. Thouvenot, D., R. Morfin, S. DiStefano, and D. Picart. Transformations of zearalenone and α-zearalanol by homogenates of human prostate glands. Eur. J. Biochem. <u>121</u>: 139-145, 1981.

31. Migadalof, B.H., H.A. Dugger, J.G. Heider, R.A. Coombs, and M.K. Terry. Biotransformation of zeranol: Disposition and metabolism in the female rat, rabbit, dog, monkey, and man. Xenobiotica, <u>13</u>: 209-221, 1983.

32. Chang, W.M., and J.K. Lin. Transformation of zearalenone and zearalenol by rat erythrocytes. Fd. Chem. Toxicol. <u>22</u>: 887-891, 1984.

33. Li, J.J. and S.A. Li. Estrogen-induced tumorigenesis in the Syrian hamster: Roles for hormonal and carcinogenic activities. Arch. Toxicol. <u>55</u>: 110-118, 1984.

ACKNOWLEDGEMENTS

We are grateful to Drs. Martin K. Terry and Bruce W. Martin, Animal Product Group, International Minerals and Chemical Corporation, Terre Haute, IN for generously providing the estrogen mycotoxins and for helpful discussions. We are also grateful to Dr. Jonathan A. Parsons for performing the hamster prolactin radioimmunoassays. We thank Cheron Carlson for expertly preparing this manuscript.

DISCUSSION

RAYNAUD: Did you incorporate phyto or fungal estrogens in the diet?

LI: This suggestion is well taken. I have been thinking of performing such studies using DES; surprisingly, such studies have not as yet been done. A comparison of carcinogenic activity following oral administration (in the diet) of DES with phytoestrogens and estrogenic myotoxins would be worthwhile.

COVEY: With regards to difficulty with HPLC separation of zealeranol, zearanol, zearalenone, zearalanone, and zearalenol, we have had success with reverse phase HPLC using 3 micron packing materials.

LI: I would be interested in the details of your separation of these estrogenic mycotoxins. However, our difficulty is the separation of the catechol monomethyl ether products of zearalanone, alpha- and beta-zearalanols and alpha- and beta-zearalenols, since they differ only by either a double-bond or a single hydrogen. We believe that separation can be achieved by modification of the gradient and/or solvent conditions.

MCLACHLAN: Did you do your tumorigenesis studies at equi-estrogenic doses of estradiol and zearanol?

LI: This is a pertinent question but difficult to resolve experimentally. First, one would have to agree on what constitutes estrogenic activity. It has been estimated that zearanol possesses 250-fold less activity in increasing rat uterine weight than estradiol. The other estrogenic mycotoxins are still less effective. It would, therefore, be most difficult to further increase appreciably the amount of estrogenic mycotoxin exposure to obtain equi-estrogenic potency. Reduction of the estradiol would not alter the data obtained with these natural nonsteroidal estrogens. Finally, we believe that estrogenicity is not the only property which contributes to the tumorigenic activity of this class of compounds.

NAFTOLIN: Your data showing a failure of carcinogenesis with these xenoestrogens is not convincing of their lack of tumorigenic activity. This is because of difficulties of absorption and the possibility that methylated compounds were formed which were inactive. Should you not check for biological activity to assure equivalent estrogenic doses and use other means of administration to avoid these problems? Would you be willing to accept these compounds as non-carcinogenic?

LI: I am personally against the addition of any unnecessary and non-essential additives either in meat producing animals or in processed foods. However, in regards to our hormone-inducing models in the kidney and liver of the hamster, the estrogenic mycotoxins appear to be appreciably less tumorigenic than most steroidal and stilbene estrogens tested.

SETCHELL: What was your rationale for using Biochanin A as a representative of the phyoestrogen? I would suggest that a better choice would have been daidzein or even equol because they may relate better to the in vivo situation. I should point out that in most animals, Biochanin A is degraded by gut bacteria into α-ethylphenol. This does not occur with the other phytoestrogens which are readily absorbed.

LI: Biochanin A was initially studied because of its relatively poor
binding affinity for the estrogen receptor in different species to
contrast the relatively high binding affinity of this receptor for
coumestrol. It appears evident from our present studies that demethylation occurs in vivo and in vitro to yield significant estrogenic responses
with Biochanin A and probable multiple catechol products. However, your
suggestion is well taken and we plan to extend these studies to other phytoestrogens as well.

Role of Metabolism in Determination of Hormonal Activity of Estrogens

ROLE OF METABOLISM IN DETERMINATION OF HORMONAL ACTIVITY OF ESTROGENS: INTRODUCTORY REMARKS

MANFRED METZLER
Institute of Pharmacology and Toxicology, University of Würzburg, Versbacher Strasse 9, D-8700 Würzburg, Fed. Rep. Germany

It is generally recognized that estrogens, both of endogenous and exogenous origin, are metabolized in the body basically in the same way as are other lipophilic compounds, i.e. by oxidation, reduction and conjugation, in order to increase their water-solubility and render them more readily excretable. As with other pharmacologically active compounds, the structural alterations of the molecule caused by its metabolism will most likely affect the biological activity. In the case of estrogens, basically four consequences of metabolism are conceivable: the metabolites may have

- decreased estrogenicity
- increased estrogenicity
- antiestrogenicity
- chemical reactivity.

Several of these effects of metabolism can be illustrated by the synthetic estrogen trans-diethylstilbestrol (E-DES). Thus, formation of the isomeric Z-DES or of Z,Z-dienestrol leads to products virtually devoid of estrogenicity (1,2), whereas the ortho-catechol and the olefinic epoxide of DES retain their estrogenic activity to a large extent (1,3). Finally, formation of a phenoxy radical and a para-quinoid product of DES stands as an example of chemically reactive metabolites, which may contribute to the long-term toxicity of this estrogen (4,5).

It is a well-established fact that the metabolism of a compound may vary between different species, strains, and sexes as well as between different tissues of the same organism. In the case of DES, pronounced species differences in the in vivo metabolism are known (6). More recent studies on the in vitro metabolism of DES with microsomes from the male and female rat and the hamster liver and kidney (7,8) and with different fetal mouse tissues in culture (9) have provided examples of the importance of tissue specific metabolism of estrogens.

These data emphasize the point that the metabolism of an estrogenic compound in a specific organ is an important determinant for the tissue dose of both hormonally and chemically active products and thus pertinent to understanding the hormonal and toxic effects of the estrogen on that organ.

The formation of a metabolite with a significantly higher estrogenicity as compared to the parent compound will naturally be unlikely for strong estrogens such as DES. However, compounds of weak or lacking hormonal activity may acquire such activity by metabolism. Examples for such proestrogens are methoxychlor and dimethylbenz(a)anthracene (DMBA). The metabolism of the widely used insecticide methoxychlor (2,2-bis(p-methoxyphenyl)-1,1,1-trichloroethane) involves demethylation to the bisphenolic compound, and it is assumed that this metabolite is responsible for binding to the estrogen receptor (10). Similarly, DMBA is metabolized to 3,9-dihydroxy-DMBA, the estrogenicity of which is approximately fifty times that of DMBA (11). Other examples of the generation of metabolites with enhanced hormonal activity are tamoxifen and zearanol, which will be discussed in detail in this morning's session.

In most cases, the estrogenicity of metabolites of pro-estrogens known to date is low to moderate. However, this should not lead us to underestimate this source of estrogenic compounds. There is an enormous number of organic compounds, both natural and man-made, already present in our environment, and this number is still increasing in industrialized countries. Many of these substances have aromatic structures, for which hydroxylation to phenolic products is the most general metabolic pathway. On the other hand, the phenolic ring structure appears to be a major prerequisite for high estrogenicity (12). Thus, it is not unreasonable to assume that among the many thousands of phenolic metabolites of environmental compounds there are certain ones which may have considerable hormonal activity. If exposure levels are sufficiently high, these environmental proestrogens must be expected to cause hormonal and toxic effects.

As the impact of estrogens on the development and health of animals and man becomes more and more obvious, there is an increasing need to develop strategies to at least detect and possibly avoid those proestrogens that are metabolically converted to strong estrogens. One obvious possibility would be a screening assay where microsomes are incubated with the test compound to account for metabolism. The mixture of parent compound and metabolites could then be assayed for estrogenicity in vivo or in vitro (13). It is conceivable that, in the future, such a test for estrogenicity will be added to the battery of assays presently required for mutagenicity, carcinogenicity, and teratogenicity clearance of compounds released into the environment in larger amounts.

REFERENCES

1. K.S. Korach, M. Metzler, and J.A. McLachlan, Proc. Nat. Acad. Sci. 75, 468-471 (1978).
2. G.H. Degen and J.A. McLachlan, Steroids 42, 253-265 (1983).
3. K.S. Korach, personal communication.
4. M. Metzler and J.A. McLachlan, Biochem. Biophys. Res. Comm. 85, 874-884 (1978).
5. M. Metzler in: Reviews in Biochemical Toxicology, Vol. 6, E. Hodgson, J.R. Bend, and R.M. Philpot, eds. (Elsevier Science Publishing Company Inc., New York 1984) pp. 191-220.
6. M. Metzler, CRC Crit. Rev. Biochem. 10, 171-212 (1981).
7. H. Haaf and M. Metzler, Carcinogenesis 6, 659-660 (1985).
8. H. Haaf and M. Metzler, Biochem. Pharmacol., in press (1985).

9. R. Maydl, R.R. Newbold, M. Metzler, and J.A. McLachlan, Endocrinology 113, 146-151 (1983).
10. J. Ousterhout, R.F. Struck, and J.A. Nelson, Biochem. Pharmacol. 30, 2869-2871 (1981).
11. S.L. Schneider, V. Alks, C.E. Morreal, D.K. Sinha, and T.L. Dao, J. Natl. Cancer Inst. 57, 1351-1355 (1976).
12. W.L. Duax and C.M. Weeks in: Estrogens in the Environment, J.A. McLachlan, ed. (Elsevier/North-Holland, New York 1980) pp. 11-32.
13. K.S. Korach in: Advances in Experimental Medicine and Biology, Vol. 138: Hormones and Cancer, W.W. Leavitt, ed. (Plenum Press, New York 1982) pp. 39-62.

190

IMPRINTING OF HEPATIC ESTROGEN ACTION

G. W. LUCIER, T. C. SLOOP, AND C. L. THOMPSON
The National Institute of Environmental Health Sciences, P.O. Box 12233,
Research Triangle Park, North Carolina 27709

ABSTRACT

Many aspects of liver biochemistry undergo sex
differentiation such that some enzymes are found in higher
concentrations in one sex compared to the other. These sex
differences are not expressed until puberty. In this paper,
we report our investigations on mechanisms of sex dimorphism
of a class of rat hepatic estrogen binding proteins which are
distinct from estrogen receptor. These sites are termed
higher capacity−lower affinity (HCLA) sites and are found
only in adult males. Imprinting of HCLA sites requires
neonatal exposure to androgen during a critical period
shortly after birth (approximately 9 days) and this effect is
pituitary dependent. HCLA sites possess an unusual binding
specificity and they appear to play a direct role in hepatic
androgen action. These sites function to prevent availability of steroidal estrogens for estrogen receptor
resulting in sex differences in hepatic estrogen responsiveness; females being more sensitive than males. HCLA sites do
not bind non-steroidal estrogens (diethylstilbestrol and
α-zearalanol) and no sex difference exists in hepatic
estrogen responsiveness for these compounds. Analysis of
sex-specific proteins by two-dimensional gel electrophoresis
provides compelling evidence that it is inappropriate to
construct a single unifying model to explain sex
differentiation of liver biochemistry.

INTRODUCTION

Many investigators have demonstrated that rat liver undergoes sex
differentiation such that some enzymes exhibit higher concentrations in
one sex than the other and several complete reviews are available on
this subject [1-3]. The approach used to investigate mechanisms of sex
differentiation of liver biochemistry has been based on the model
systems which were developed to explain sex dimorphism of behavioral
patterns [4-6]. According to these models, the hormonal milieu during a
well-defined developmental period, shortly after birth, plays a critical
role in imprinting for the expression of post-pubertal behavioral
changes. Most of these studies have been conducted in the rat and have
led to a generally-accepted explanation of the mechanism involved. The
critical components of the model are described below and these represent
the work of numerous researchers to whom the indicated references
provide a brief summary of credit [4-7].

It is thought that testosterone produced by the developing testes reaches target cells in the brain and is converted to 17β-estradiol (E_2) by aromatase enzymes which are found in high concentrations in discrete regions of the brain during the critical developmental period. E_2, formed in this way, binds to estrogen receptors which are also localized in these regions. Through a process, involving receptor-mediated events, specific nerve endings are programmed including some changes that are evident by histological analysis. The programmed nerve endings are thereby imprinted to become responsive to post-pubertal endocrine changes which causes expression of some male-specific behavioral parameters. The critical period for imprinting is the first week after birth and androgen deprivation during this time results in the expression of female behavioral patterns. Estrogen treatment during the critical period is not effective in imprinting male behavior because steroidal estrogens bind to α-fetoprotein in the blood and cerebrospinal fluid which prevents access of the estrogens to the target cells in the brain. However, non-steroidal estrogens, such as diethylstilbestrol (DES), do not bind well to α-fetoprotein and are capable of programming for post-pubertal expression of male behavioral characteristics in a manner similar to the effects of testosterone. Non-aromatizable androgens such as dihydrotesterone are not effective in imprinting sex differentiation of behavior because conversion of these compounds to estrogen is not possible.

Our investigations on the sex differentiation of liver have been designed to evaluate the similarities and/or differences in the above-described mechanisms for sex differences in behavior. In these studies we have focussed on sex differences of some drug-metabolizing enzymes as well as steroid binding proteins and protein synthesis profiles in isolated hepatocytes from endocrine-manipulated rats. In this paper we summarize and review our findings on the properties of a specific class of estrogen binding proteins which undergo sex differentiation.

SEX DIFFERENCES IN HEPATIC ESTROGEN BINDING SITES

Our lab as well as others have demonstrated that the liver contains estrogen receptor and is also a target organ for estrogens [8-12]. These studies have provided evidence that liver estrogen receptor possesses properties which have been assigned to receptor proteins in more classical estrogen target tissues such as uterus, vagina and brain.

These properties include high binding affinity, finite binding capacity and selectivity for estrogens. As with other target tissues, liver estrogen receptor can be localized in cytosol or nucleus depending on the procedures used to obtain subcellular fractions. The ligand-receptor complex is essential for retention of E_2 in the nucleus in cell free nuclear retention studies using purified liver nuclei. Further-more, E_2-receptor complexes, generated by incubating liver preparations with $^3H-E_2$, bind to DNA-cellulose and receptor deficient preparations do not exhibit DNA binding properties. Ontogeny studies on hepatic estrogen receptor have shown that receptor concentrations are low or non-detectable in prepubertal rats although substantial increases are evident immediately following puberty [12]. There is a good correlation between the ontogeny of estrogen responsiveness and concentrations of receptor in that administration of E_2 or DES to prepupertal rats produces no effect on hepatic synthesis of very low density lipoproteins whereas pronounced increases are seen in post-pubertal rats [13]. Similar results were obtained when ontogenetic differences in the hepatic production of renin substrate were examined [14]. No sex differences in receptor concentrations were observed [11,15] (Table I).

TABLE I. Ontogeny of total estrogen binding sites and estrogen receptor in rat liver cytosol[a]

| | | fmol/mg cytosol protein | | | |
| | | Age in days | | | |
		10	20	40	60
Total Binding	Males	103	234 ± 33	758 ± 344*	1895 ± 422*
	Females	107	267 ± 50	295 ± 68	331 ± 75
Receptor	Males	ND	1.2 ± 1.1	10.2 ± 2.8	11.3 ± 1.4
	Females	ND	0.5 ± 0.4	10.1 ± 2.3	9.5 ± 3.7

[a]To determine total binding sites, samples of cytosol were incubated (2 hr at 4°C with ^3H-estradiol (30 nM)). After subsequent treatment with dextran-coated charcoal, aliquots of supernatant were assessed for bound radioactivity. Receptor binding sites in partially-purified prepara-tions were determined by subtracting non-specific binding (binding in the presence of 100-fold excess of unlabelled ligand) from total binding. All Values are expressed as fmol/mg cytosol protein and repre-sent mean ± S.D., N = 5. Cytosolic protein concentrations were 8-10 mg per ml cytosol. ND indicates that values were not determined.

During the course of our investigations on hepatic receptor development we noticed that total $^3H-E_2$ binding was much greater in adult male rats than adult female rats although no sex differences in total binding were evident in immature animals (Table I).

TABLE II. Binding properties of estrogen receptor and HCLA sites from male liver.

	Estrogen Receptor		HCLA Sites	
	Property	Reference	Property	Reference
Binding affinity (K_d)	~ 0.2nM	[12]	20-40nM	[13]
Binding capacity (fmoles/mg cytosol protein)	~ 20	[12]	5000	[13]
Sedimentation on 5-20% sucrose density gradients	8-9S	[11]	4-5S	[11]
Localization in plasma	-	[11]	-	[11]
Binding to steroidal estrogens	+	[11]	+	[11,12]
Binding to non-steroidal estrogens (DES and α-zearalanol)	+	[11]	-	[12,19]
Binding to androgens (testosterone and dihydrotestosterone)	-	[12]	+	[11]
Binding to progestins and glucocorticoids	-	[12]	-	[12]
Involved in nuclear translocation/ retention of ^{3}H-E$_2$	+	[17]	+	[11]
Binding to DNA	+	[18]	-	[19]

Total binding sites in adult males have been shown to be comprised primarily of a class of sites distinct from estrogen receptor and we have termed them higher capacity-lower affinity (HCLA) sites [2]. We, as well as others, [9,11,15] have described the properties of HCLA sites and these properties are summarized in Table II. HCLA sites are not thought to be plasma contaminants because perfusion of adult male liver prior to preparation of subcellular fractions does not decrease the concentration of HCLA sites, no sex difference exists in plasma binding of ^{3}H-E$_2$ and cytosol from purified hepatocytes contain similar concentrations (fmol/mg cytosol protein) as cytosol from liver homogenates. HCLA sites are found in approximately 300-fold excess to hepatic estrogen receptor (~ 5000 fmoles/mg cytosol protein) and unlike receptors, their cytosolic localization appears not to be an artifact of biochemical fractionation procedures. Scatchard analysis of whole cytosol from male or female rats is demonstrated in Figure 1 and reveals that female cytosol exhibits receptor binding (Kd ~ 0.2 nM) and non-specific binding whereas cytosolic preparations from male liver contain at least two moderate affinity sites (K_d ~ 20 and 40 nM) and non-specific (non-saturable) sites. The moderate affinity sites are the

HCLA sites and can be removed by partial purification [11,13] which enables detection of estrogen receptor in male liver preparations. In fact, Scatchard analysis of E_2 binding in partially-purified male liver cytosol is indistinquishable from whole liver cytosol from females. Additional studies have demonstrated that HCLA sites are comprised of at least five different proteins [16]. Sucrose-density gradient analysis of liver estrogen binding proteins showed that HCLA sites sediment in the 4-5s region whereas estrogen receptor sediments in the 8-9s region [11].

The ability of various competitors to displace ^3H-E_2 from HCLA sites provides some interesting insights regarding the possible function of these sites. Steroidal estrogens such as unlabeled E_2 and estrone are effective competitors whereas non-steroidal estrogens such as DES and α-zearalanol do not displace ^3H-E_2 to any extent [11]. However, androgens such as dihydrotestosterone, testosterone, and 5α-androstane-3α,17β-diol are effective competitors [11]. Glucocorticoids and progestins, like non-steroidal estrogens, do not compete for HCLA sites. Other studies on the role of HCLA sites in steroid responsiveness have shown that they do not function to translocate/retain ^3H-E_2 in the nucleus nor does the ^3H-E_2-HCLA site complex bind to DNA [11,19] but these sites are involved in nuclear retention/binding of androgens. In fact, we have postulated that a portion of HCLA sites is the liver androgen receptor and that steroidal estrogens are antiandrogens in liver by virtue of binding to the androgen receptor [20].

In addition to evaluating the properties of HCLA sites, my laboratory has also evaluated modulation of the quantity of sites by various endocrine influences and our findings are summarized in Table III. Castration of adult male rats or ovariectomy of adult female rats had no effect on the concentrations of HCLA sites. However, castration of neonatal rats (day 2) prevented the post-pubertal expression of these sites [12]. Administration of testosterone propionate to neonatal castrates on days 2,6,9 and 13 of age was sufficient to imprint for expression of high concentrations of HCLA sites even though these animals had not been exposed to androgen for several weeks and the testosterone administered shortly after birth had long since been metabolized and excreted [21]. Therefore, it appears that sex differentiation of HCLA sites requires neonatal exposure to androgen during a critical period of early development and expression of these proteins is not dependent on continuous androgen exposure during adulthood. In order to more precisely ascertain the critical period for imprinting of HCLA sites a series of experiments were performed. First, male rats were castrated at day 2, day 6 or day 19 of age and HCLA sites quantified in these animals at 63 days of age. Results indicated that day 2 and day 6 castration prevented imprinting of HCLA sites whereas castration at day 19 had no effect on their post-pubertal expression [12]. Therefore, the critical period for neonatal androgen exposure is between day 6 and day 19 in rats. The second set of experiments involved castration of male rats at day 2 of age followed by a single administration of testosterone propionate at day 2,6,9,13,16 or 19 and the concentrations of HCLA sites were then quantified in each of the treatment groups at 63 days of age. These data revealed that androgen had virtually no effect on days 2,6,13,16 or 19 but imprinting did occur following androgen exposure at day 9 which demonstrates that the critical period for imprinting of HCLA sites is approximately 9 days of age in rats [21].

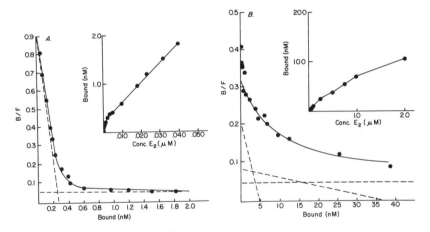

FIG. 1. Scatchard analysis of hepatic estrogen-binding proteins prepared from female or male cytosol. Cytosol (200 µl) prepared from female liver (A) was incubated (2 hr at 4°) with an equal volume of [³H]E₂ (0.1-3.0 nM). Cytosol (200 µl) prepared from male liver (B) was incubated 2 hr at 4°) with an equal volume of [³H]E₂ (0.1 - 6000 nM). Following the incubation, unbound ligand was removed by DCC treatment. Aliquots of the supernatant were assessed for bound radioactivity, and values obtained were plotted according to the method of Scatchard. The dashed lines were derived from a weighted nonlinear least-square analysis (analysis was performed on cytosol that was pooled from livers of at least three animals).

From the above experiments, it would seem possible that female rats could be imprinted to express HCLA sites. To test this hypothesis, female rats were administered testosterone propionate during the critical period and HCLA sites evaluated in the subsequent adult animals. Some of the rats were ovariectomized at 42 days of age. HCLA sites were detected in high concentrations in female rats receiving neonatal androgen provided that they were ovariectomized prior to sacrifice [21] (Table III). Since neonatal androgenized female rats, which were not ovariectomized, did not express HCLA sites it appears that estrogen blocks expression of the imprinting effect. In fact, administration of estrogen (E_2 or DES) represses synthesis of HCLA sites in adult males such that three days following estrogen exposure HCLA sites were not detected [22].

TABLE III. Influence of the endocrine environment on the expression of HCLA binding sites.

| Endocrine | Detection of high concentrations of HCLA sites[a] | | | |
| | Male | | Female | |
status	immature	mature	immature	mature
intact	–	+	–	–
castrate (day 1)	–	–	ND	ND
gonadectomized (day 21)	–	+	–	–
gonadectomized (day 42)	–	+	–	–
castrate (day 1) plus testosterone (day 2)	–	–	ND	ND
castrate (day 1) plus testosterone (day 9)	–	+	ND	ND
castrate (day 1) plus E_2 (day 9)	–	–	–	–
testosterone (day 9) ovariectomized (day 42)	ND	ND	ND	+
castrate (day 1) plus testosterone (days 23-30)	ND	–	ND	ND
castrate (day 1) plus dihydrotestosterone (day 9)	–	+	ND	ND
castrate (day 1 plus diethylstilbestrol (day 9)	–	–	ND	ND
castrate (day 1) plus α-zearalanol (day 9)	–	–	ND	ND
hypophysectomy (day 21)	ND	–	ND	–
hypophysectomy (day 42)	ND	–	ND	–
adrenalectomy (day 42)	ND	+	ND	–
thyroidectomy (day 42)	ND	+	ND	–

[a]HCLA sites measured in immature rats at day 28 and day 63 in mature rats. ND means experimental data not available.

According to the models for imprinting of behavioral sex differentiation, synthetic estrogens and aromatizable androgens are effective agents whereas steroidal estrogens and non-aromatizable androgens are not effective. To examine whether the same specificity exists for imprinting of HCLA sites, male rats were castrated immediately following birth and then administered testosterone propionate, dihydrotestosterone, E_2, DES or α-zearalanol during the critical neonatal period. Interestingly, testosterone propionate and dihydrotestosterone were equally effective in imprinting for HCLA sites but E_2, DES and α-zearalanol had no such effect [21]. These results demonstrate that imprinting of HCLA sites has a different mechanism than imprinting for male behavioral characteristics.

In order to further understand endocrine regulation of HCLA sites, adult rats were hypophysectomized, adrenalectomized or thyroidectomized. Adrenalectomy and thyroidectomy had no effect on expression of HCLA sites in either male or female rats but hypophysectomy abolished sex differences [23] indicating that the pituitary plays a dominant role in the regulation of hepatic sex differentiation. In fact, all known sex dimorphic patterns in rat liver are abolished by hypophysectomy [1-3]. Administration of growth hormone to hypophysectomized rats had no effect on expression of HCLA sites [23]. However, other investigators have reported that growth hormone feminized expression of some cytochrome P-450 dependent enzyme systems [24] as well as some steroid-metabolizing enzymes (25). The reason for this discrepancy is not clear but we feel that growth hormone may play an important role in the sex differentiation of some components of liver biochemistry but not others.

HCLA sites appear to play a direct role in promoting androgen action in liver but they do not seem to exert direct effects on estrogen action [3,11,13]. However, the presence of HCLA sites is correlated with resistance to hepatic estrogen responsiveness when using increased concentrations of very low density lipoproteins as the marker of responsiveness [13]. For example, four times as much E_2 is required to produce equivalent effects in males compared to ovariectomized females. The mechanism responsible for this sex difference is not entirely clear but several lines of evidence suggest a critical role for the HCLA sites: 1) In in vitro incubations much more ^3H-E_2 is required to saturate estrogen receptor preparations from male liver compared to female liver preparations although there are no apparent sex differences in the binding properties of estrogen receptor [11]; 2) Sex differences in receptor saturability are abolished if HCLA sites are removed by partial purification; 3) The presence of HCLA sites decreases nuclear translocation/retention of ligand-receptor complexes in cell free systems [11,13]; 4) Non-steroidal estrogens such as DES and α-zearalanol, which do not bind HCLA sites, produce similar hepatic responses in males and females [18].

SEX DIFFERENTIATION OF HEPATIC PROTEIN SYNTHESIS

This report has focussed on sex differentiation of hepatic estrogen binding proteins although numerous liver proteins are known to exhibit sex differences. However, it is important to refrain from generating a uniform mechanism of action for sex differentiation of liver based on only one group of proteins. For example, it appears that male specific components of the hepatic cytochrome P-450 dependent enzyme system and some steroid-metabolizing enzymes arise from similar but not identical mechanisms and each of these mechanisms is somewhat different than that for imprinting of steroid binding proteins [1-3,25-27]. In order to more fully evaluate the variety of mechanisms involved in the sex differentiation of liver biochemistry, we applied the technique of 2-dimensional gel electrophoresis of newly-synthesized proteins [28]. Our approach involved the preparation of isolated hepatocytes from endocrine manipulated rats and incubation of these parenchymal cells with ^{35}S-methionine and cysteine for periods of one to three hours. By using a short incubation period we were confident that we were evaluating protein synthesis arising from transcripts produced in vivo rather than in vitro. Following incubations, cells were lysed and protein-synthetic profiles examined on two-dimensional gels; SDS polyacrylamide in one direction and isoelectric focussing in the other. This approach allowed us to investigate protein synthetic profiles of approximately 500 different proteins. Some of the proteins were found only in male cells and others only in female cells whereas numerous proteins exhibited quantitative sex differences. Because this method involves a substantial amount of experimental error, we investigated endocrine regulation of only those proteins which exhibited qualitative sex differences and the properties of these proteins are summarized in Table IV and V.

These data demonstrate that some but not all female-specific proteins are expressed in neonatal male castrates. Moreover, expression of some but not all female-specific proteins found in male rats castrated neonatally is blocked by neonatal treatment of castrates with testosterone. If male rats receive androgen both during the critical period for imprinting and continuously during adult life none of the female-specific proteins are expressed in parenchymal cells. Expression of some but not all male-specific proteins is prevented by neonatal castration and some of these proteins are expressed in liver cells from rats receiving androgen only during the critical period. Expression of all the male-specific proteins requires androgen exposure during the critical period and continuous adult exposure.

TABLE IV. Molecular weight and isoelectric point values for proteins showing sex specific changes[a]

Female specific proteins			Male specific proteins		
Designation	MW	pI[b]	Designation	MW	pI
F1	55.4	5.77	M1	51.2	6.34
F2	47.8	7.03	M2	49.8	6.97
F3	43.8	6.66	M3	48.5	6.90
F4	36.5	7.23	M4	45.0	5.64
F5	35.3	6.06	M5	44.9	7.06
F6	32.4	7.12	M6	38.1	5.69
			M7	35.0	6.68
			M8	33.7	6.83

[a]Values quoted were from six separate determinations.
[b]MW, molecular weight; pI, isoelectric point.

TABLE V. Summary of sex-specific changes in hepatic cytosol protein profiles[a]

Female	Male	Male Neonatal Castrate[b]	Male Neonatal Castrate + Neonatal Testosterone
F1		F1	F1
F2			
F3		F3	
F4		F4	F4[c]
F5		F5	
F6		F6	
	M1		
	M2	M2	M2
	M3		M3
	M4	M4	M4
	M5		
	M6	M6	M6
	M7	M7	M7
	M8	M8	M8

[a]See Table IV for the molecular weight/isoelectric point values for these proteins. Castration on the day after birth; testosterone propionate (1.45 µmol) administered subcutaneously on day 9. Protein synthesis evaluated in parenchymal cells from 63 day old rats. F4 appears in the male castrate + testosterone but with diminished intensity compared to the male castrate or female.

For the above reasons, it is inappropriate to construct a single unifying mechanistic model to explain sex differentiation of liver biochemistry as it appears that there are numerous models with some overlapping components. Moreover, sex differentiation of liver biochemistry results from a different mechanism that controls sex differentiation of behavioral characteristics.

200

REFERENCES

1. H.D. Colby in: Advances in Sex Hormone Research, J.A. Thomas and R.L. Singhal, eds. (Urban Schuargenberg 1980) pp. 27-73.
2. G.W. Lucier, C.L. Thompson, T.C. Sloop, and R.C. Rumbaugh in: Sexual Differentiation, Basic and Clinical Aspects, M. Serio, M. Zanisi, M. Motta, and L. Martini, eds. (Raven Press 1984) pp. 207-223.
3. P. Skett and J.A. Gustafsson in: Reviews in Biochemical Toxicology, E. Hodgson, J. Bend and R. Philpot, eds. (Elsevier, Amsterdam 1979) pp. 27.
4. R.A. Gorski, J. H. Gordon, J.E. Shyryne, and A.M. Southam, Brain Res. 148, 333-346 (1978).
5. B.S. McEwen, Sci. Am. 235, 48-59 (1976).
6. P. Demoor and C. Denef, Endocrinology 82, 480-492 (1968).
7. F. Naftolin, K.J. Ryan, I.J. Davies, V.V. Reddy, F. Flores, Z. Petro, M. Kuhn, R.J. White, Y. Tokaoka and L. Wolin, Horm. Res. 31, 295-315 (1975).
8. R.F. Aten, R.B. Dickson, and A.J. Eisenfeld, Endocrinology 102, 433-442 (1978).
9. P.K. Eagon, S.E. Fisher, A.F. Inhoff, L.E. Porter, R.R. Stewart, D.H. Van Thiel, and R. Lester, Arch. Biochem. Biophys. 20, 486-499 (1980).
10. A.J. Eisenfeld, R. Aten, M. Weinberger, G. Hasselbacher, K. Halpern, and L. Krakoff, Science 191, 862-865 (1976).
11. W. Powell-Jones, C. Thompson, S.N. Nayfeh, and G.W. Lucier, J. Steroid Biochem. 13, 219-229 (1980).
12. W. Powell-Jones, C. Thompson, S. Raeford, and G.W. Lucier, Endocrinology 109, 628-636 (1981).
13. C. Thompson and G.W. Lucier, Mol. Pharmacol. 24, 69-76 (1983).
14. A.J. Eisenfeld, L.R. Krakoff and R.F. Aten, Biochem. Pharmacol. 26, 923 (1977).
15. R.B. Dickson, R.F. Aten, and A.J. Eisenfeld, Endocrinology 103, 1636 (1978).
16. C. Thompson, W. Powell-Jones and G.W. Lucier, Biochem. J. 194, 1-8 (1981).
17. W. Powell-Jones, S.N. Nayfeh, and G.W. Lucier, Biochem. Biophys. Res. Commun. 85, 167-173 (1978).
18. C. Mastri, P. Mistry, and G.W. Lucier, J. Steroid Biochem., in press.
19. C. Mastri and G. Lucier in: Endocrine Toxicology, J.A. Thomas, K.S. Korach, J.A. McLachlan, eds. (Raven Press 1985) pp. 335-355
20. R.C. Rumbaugh, Z. McCoy, and G.W. Lucier, J. Steroid Biochem. 21, 243-252 (1984).
21. T.C. Sloop, J.C. Clark, R.C. Rumbaugh, and G.W. Lucier, Endocrinology 112(5), pp. 1639-1646.
22. T.C. Sloop, G.W. Lucier, and R.C. Rumbaugh, Fed. Proc. 41(4), p. 1330 (1982).
23. G.W. Lucier, S.R. Slaughter, C. Thompson, C.A. Lamartiniere, and W. Powell-Jones, Biochem. Biophys. Res. Commun. 103, 872-879 (1981).
24. R.C. Rumbaugh and H.D. Colby, Endocrinology 107, 719-724 (1980).
25. A. Mode, G. Norstedt, P. Eneroth and P.A. Gustafsson, Endocrinology 113, 1250-1267 (1983).
26. H. Chao and L.W.K. Chung, Mol. Pharmacol. 21, 744-752 (1982).
27. L.W.K. Chung and H. Chao, J. Supramol. Structure 15, 193 (1980).
28. N.P. Illsley, C.A. Lamartiniere, and G.W. Lucier, J. Appl. Biochem. 1, 385-395 (1979).

DISCUSSION

KUPFER: The rat appears to be a "peculiar duck" with respect to the pronounced sexual dimorphism of hepatic mixed function oxidase (P-450). Has anyone determined whether, in other species in which the above sexual dimorphism is not evident or reversed, the high capacity, low affinity (HCLA) estrogen binding protein is present?

LUCIER: Other species also undergo hepatic sex differentiation, although the rat has certainly been the most studied animal model. Random-bred male mice also possess high concentrations of HCLA sites, and they also exhibit sexual dimorphism of some other aspects of liver biochemistry. Species such as hamster and guinea pig, which in general do not exhibit pronounced hepatic sex differences, do not possess HCLA sites. So, it appears that in species where hepatic sex differences are readily apparent, HCLA sites are present, whereas in other species HCLA sites are not present.

NAFTOLIN: Is this 4 S material an enzyme?

LUCIER: It is possible that HCLA sites have enzymatic activity, but this is doubtful because the radioactive 17β-estradiol or androgen used in our binding studies is recovered as unmetabolized ligand when the ligand-receptor complex is extracted with organic solvents. However, our studies have shown that HCLA sites are comprised of at least five different proteins. At least one of these appears to be the hepatic androgen receptor as judged by nuclear retention studies, DNA binding studies, competition studies, and a positive correlation between the presence of binding protein and liver responsiveness to androgen.

NAFTOLIN: Is the factor controlling this material growth hormone?

LUCIER: Growth hormone does not appear to regulate expression of HCLA sites, although studies by Gustafsson indicate that growth hormone may be the feminizing factor for at least two steroid-metabolizing enzymes that undergo liver sex differentiation. Our studies have shown that hypophysectomy abolishes sex differences of HCLA sites like it does to other liver components that exhibit sex differences. However, administration of growth hormone to hypophysectomized rats does not restore sex differences in HCLA sites, nor does growth hormone have an effect on these sites in intact male or female rats. These results, taken together with Gustafsson's data, demonstrate that there is not a single unifying mechanism of action to explain all aspects of liver sexual dimorphism.

RAYNAUD: Have you tried to add an antiandrogen to reverse the effect of androgen and demonstrate that the response is androgen mediated?

LUCIER: No we have not, but this would be an interesting thing to do. We would have to be sure that the compound used possessed only antagonistic actions in the brain cells that are important to the imprinting of liver biochemistry. Otherwise, the results would be meaningless.

RAYNAUD: Moxestrol does not bind to α-fetoprotein. One has to take into account that there is a larger amount of α-fetoprotein at birth in the rat and that the affinity constant is not negligible in respect to estrogen receptor. The situation is also complicated by the fact that the half-life of α-fetoprotein is six days, and the distribution between α-fetoprotein and receptor will be extremely time-dependent.

202

LUCIER: Moxestrol would be an interesting agent to use in studies involving sex differentiation of behavior where conversion of androgens to estrogens in brain is critical to the mechanism of action. However, estrogens are not involved in sex differentiation of HCLA sites as demonstrated by our results that non-steroidal estrogens (DES and α-zearalanol) which do not bind α-fetoprotein also do not imprint for sex differentiation of HCLA sites. Moreover, non-aromatizable androgens, like dihydrotestosterone, do imprint HCLA sites. For these reasons, we are not concerned about influences of α-fetoprotein in our studies.

SONNENSCHEIN: I wonder whether the role of AFP in this imprinting process is adequately established when evidence has been presented showing that AFP enters cells in the rat hypothalamus during this perinatal period.

LUCIER: As stated in the answer to the previous question, α-fetoprotein does not influence imprinting of HCLA sites, although it does exert a profound influence on the imprinting of behavioral patterns. If α-fetoprotein-estrogen complexes do enter the cells of the developing brain and the estrogen is available for binding to its receptor, then 17β-estradiol should imprint for behavioral sex differentiation. The fact that 17β-estradiol is not an effective imprinter of behavior indicates that transport of α-fetoprotein into brain cells is probably not important to the imprinting process.

ESTROGEN PRODUCTION AND METABOLISM IN RELATION TO CANCER

PENTTI K. SIITERI PH.D., JAMES MURAI, PH.D., AND NIKLAS SIMBERG, M.D.
Department of Obstetrics/Gynecology and Reproductive Sciences,
University of California at San Francisco, San Francisco, CA 94143

INTRODUCTION

The role that estrogens may play in the development of human reproductive tract cancers remains to be defined. The multitude of endocrine studies aimed at finding specific abnormalities in urinary excretion, plasma levels or production rates of estrogens, or other hormones, in women either at risk or with cancer of the endometrium or breast generally have been unrewarding [For reviews see 1-3]. Although the association between obesity and endometrial cancer appears to be explained by both increased peripheral estrogen synthesis from adrenal precursors [4,5] and increased availability of plasma estradiol [6,7], other factors, such as the level of exposure to carcinogens must be equally important since most obese postmenopausal women do not develop endometrial cancer. The relationship between endogenous estrogens and breast cancer is even less clear. Even when many plasma and urinary hormones were examined in familial breast cancer patients, only subtle differences in conjugation of urinary estrogens between patients and controls were found [8]. These and many other negative studies can be interpreted in several ways. First, it is possible that estrogens have no direct role in human breast cancer. This seems highly unlikely given the 100 fold difference in breast cancer incidence between the sexes. However, the alternative interpretation of the sex difference is that men are protected from breast cancer. Testosterone, or one of its metabolites, clearly antagonize the effects of estrogen on the male breast as shown in studies of gynecomastia [4,9]. Adrenal androgens may also be important in this context [10] and indeed the early studies of Bulbrook and colleagues suggested that production of dehydroepiandrosterone sulfate (DHEAS) is subnormal in women at risk for developing breast cancer [11]. Poortman, Thijssen and their colleagues subsequently proposed that adrenal androgens such as androst-5-ene-3β,17β-diol (ADIOL) which is largely derived from DHEAS may antagonize estrogen action in normal or cancer cells [12]. Other investigators have suggested the possibility that ADIOL may act as an estrogen agonist via the estrogen receptor [13]. However, the fact that postmenopausal women and men have similar estrogen production

rates and plasma estrone (E1) and estradiol (E2) levels clearly
suggests that the antiestrogenic properties of androgens are of
paramount importance. As suggested by many authors, differences in
androgens or other natural antiestogens such as progesterone [14],
rather than estrogens, may ultimately prove to be of vital importance
in determining cancer susceptibility.

Another possible reason for the failure to detect hormonal
abnormalities in cancer patients is that plasma and urinary hormone
levels do not reflect the hormonal milieu of the breast itself. There
is considerable evidence in support of this view. A number of reports
have shown that the hormone content of breast cyst fluid [3] or fluid
aspirated from the breast nipple [15,16] is extremely high relative to
the blood circulation. Milk and breast fluid contains many normal
constituents derived from blood or formed during turnover of breast
cells as well as foreign substances such as nicotine in cigarette
smokers [17]. Studies by Petrakis and his colleagues [18,19] showing
high levels of cholesterol and its epoxides which are known carcinogens
in breast nipple fluid suggest that further study of this material may
help elucidate the local hormonal environment that promotes breast
disease.

Unfortunately, little is known concerning the mechanism(s) by
which substances accumulate in the breast. The simplest explanation is
that they arise from normal transcapillary passage of plasma
constituents through the alveoli into the ductal system where to a
greater or lesser extent they are trapped when resorption via lymphatic
and venous systems is incomplete in the nonfunctioning breast. The
idea of breast "stagnation" as a cause of breast cancer arose in
ancient times and has received both clinical and experimental support
from time to time. For example, breast cancer incidence is increased
unilaterally in mice when egress from these breasts is prevented by
nipple cauterization [20]. Although this notion is intuitively obvious
and acceptable, experimental proof of its importance in development of
human breast disease is not easily obtainable. Nevertheless, it could
help explain several facets of the breast cancer puzzle. For example,
breast cancer is extremely rare in lower primates who like most other
mammalian species do not achieve full breast development until their
first pregnancy. Does pubertal breast enlargement in women long before
they become pregnant increase exposure of breast ductal cells to cancer
causing agents? If so, the protective effect of early pregnancy may be
explained simply by full maturation of the ductal system which

facilitates removal of hormones and noxious agents not only during
lactation but throughout a woman's reproductive life. In contrast to
earlier epidemiologic studies, a recent report which carefully examined
lactational performance strongly suggests that breast feeding protects
premenopausal women against breast cancer [21]. The observation by
Petrakis et al [22] that Chinese boat women who nurse their offspring
from only one breast have a 4 fold higher incidence of cancer in the
nonsuckled breast is in accord with this view. Furthermore,
geographical variations in breast cancer rates may be explained at
least in part by social and other factors which influence turnover of
the breast fluids. The high incidence of breast cancer in Western
women relative to African women who are either pregnant or breast
feeding throughout their fertile years may reflect both greater
exposure to environmental carcinogens and their retention in the
breasts of modern women with low fecundity. Do similar considerations
apply to the nonpregnant state? The breasts are properly considered as
excretory organs even in the nonlactating state but the significance of
this function is unclear. The amount of fluid obtainable by applying
slight negative pressure to the nipples of nonlactating women varies
widely [17]. Does this mean that some women can relieve stagnation by
voiding their breasts of noxious agents by excretion as well as
resorption? What are the anatomical and hormonal factors which
regulate this process? These are only a few of the questions that
arise in light of recent analyses demonstrating the richness and
complexity of the hormonal milieu within the breasts.

Transport of Estrogens

Endocrinologists generally believe that only the free (protein
unbound) fraction of steroid and thyroid hormones in plasma are able to
enter target cells and exert biological effects. According to this
view the specific high affinity binding proteins in blood such as
corticosteroid binding globulin (CBG), sex hormone binding globulin
(SHBG) and thyroxine binding globulin (TBG) function only to regulate
the plasma free concentrations of the hormones which they bind. We
became interested in reevaluating this question when we found that the
concentration of SHBG was severely depressed in obese postmenopausal
women [6, 7]. These results suggested that the reduced binding
capacity of SHBG would increase the percentage of free estradiol in

plasma as had been noted for testosterone in hyperandrogenic states by
many authors. Despite the elegant studies of Anderson [23], however,
little attention had been given to binding of estradiol in plasma.
Clear evidence was presented for reciprocal variations in free
estradiol and SHBG levels [24], whereas others concluded that estradiol
binding to SHBG was insignificant under physiologic conditions [25].
In view of these controversial results we developed a new approach to
the measurement of free steroids in plasma that could yield
physiologically relevant information. The procedure that evolved,
isodialysis, combines the principles of dialysis, ultrafiltration and
double isotope methodology [26]. This method permits the rapid
determination of the percentage of free steroid in many small samples
(0.2 ml) of whole plasma at $37^{\circ}C$. Using this method we obtained
unequivocal evidence for binding of estradiol to SHBG and demonstrated
that the percentage of free E2 is inversely related to the plasma SHBG
concentrations [27]. When postmenopausal women with and without
endometrial cancer were studied the expected increase in percentage of
free E2 in obese subjects with low SHBG binding capacity was observed
in both groups [6,7]. Thus, the effects of increased estrogen
production in obese women appears to be augmented by increased
availability of plasma estrogens to target tissues. The failure to
find differences between women with and without endometrial cancer was
not surprising since estrogens are generally considered to be promoters
of cancer rather than carcinogens themselves. However, as stated
earlier women with cancer may have experienced greater exposure to
carcinogens or lacked adequate amounts of some natural estrogen
antagonist. We also carried out studies of E2 binding in plasma of
women with breast cancer and the influence of obesity was evident
particularly in postmenopausal women since elevated free estradiol
levels were observed [28]. In addition, there appeared to be a small
number of patients who had elevated free E2 levels despite normal
plasma SHBG [29]. These intriguing results suggested that other
mechanisms such as competing ligands or an abnormal SHBG binding site
might chronically elevate free estradiol levels in some women.
Subsequent work by others has been controversial with both supportive
[30] and negative findings [31] reported. An intriguing possibility
was raised by Bulbrook and associates who found a difference in binding
of E2 to albumin such that Japanese women have a greater fraction of
total E2 bound to SHBG than British women [32].

More recently we have been engaged in a large scale study of
plasma and breast fluid estrogens in women with benign or malignant
breast disease and appropriate controls. Preliminary analysis of
results obtained for Caucasian women only has yielded the expected
inverse relationships between plasma SHBG binding capacity and body
weight and also percentage of free E2 in both pre- and postmenopausal
women in all three catagories. Table I shows the values obtained for

Table I.

	Premenopausal		Postmenopausal	
	Control	Cancer	Control	Cancer
E2 (pg/ml)	117 ± 85* (306)	134 ± 84 (52)	21 ± 23 (54)	17 ± 14 (45)
E1 (pg/ml)	84 ± 45 (305)	103 ± 66 (51)	38 ± 25 (54)	38 ± 23 (45)
% FE2	1.65 ± .39 (305)	1.49 ± .32 (52)	1.68 ± .43 (55)	1.68 ± .37 (45)
SHBG (nM)	47 ± 21 (305)	57 ± 31 (52)	46 ± 23 (55)	46 ± 22 (45)

*Mean ± S.D. (n)

plasma E1, E2, SHBG and percentage free E2 in cancer patients and
controls. Women who were pregnant or had their last menstrual period
less than one year from the time of blood sampling have been excluded
as were women receiving birth control preparations or thyroid
medications. As seen, no significant differences in estrogen
concentrations, SHBG or percentage of free E2 was observed in
postmenopausal women. The lower percentage of free E2 (1.49%) in
premenopausal cancer patients is explained by the significantly higher
SHBG levels (57 ± 31 vs 47 ± 21). The difference in SHBG levels may be
due to differences in estrogen and/or androgen levels or other factors
since no significant difference in mean body weights was observed
(control = 131 ± 22 vs. cancer = 131 ± 27 lbs).

In examining the various possibilities that could explain our
current failure to find higher mean percent free E2 in cancer patients
we considered the effects of long term storage of serum on values of
percentage of free E2. Isodialysis assays for percent free E2 were

repeated on a limited number of samples after storage for a period of 3-4 years. The results shown in Table II indicate that the values for percentage free E2 increased upon storage for both control and cancer

Table II. The effect of storage on serum % free E2.

	First Assay 3.1 ± 1.2 mos[+]	Second Assay 39 ± 3.8 mos
Controls (n = 14)	1.67 ± .41*	1.79 ± .42
Cancers (n = 14)	1.53 ± .27	1.83 ± .36**

* Mean ± S.D.
** Differs significantly from first assay by the Wilcoxon signed rank test for paired observations (p < .01)
[+] Mean time of storage from serum blood sampling

sera although only the change in the cancer group was statistically significant when analyzed by the Wilcoxon signed rank test for paired observations. While these results can still be interpreted to mean that some inherent difference exists in the SHBG of some patients we cannot conclude at the present that breast cancer patients exhibit increased availability of plasma E2 beyond that amount which is predicted from the plasma SHBG binding capacity. Possible differences in affinity for albumin and distribution of E2 in serum of cancer patients were also sought by the methods we previously described [27] but these results were also negative.

Steroids in Breast Fluids

The ready availability of fluids from breast cysts has led to numerous investigations of its contents including the steroid hormones. The most extensive analysis of steroids is that of Bradlow et al [32] who analyzed samples from more than 1000 subjects. These workers found that the concentrations of circulating hormones including cortisol, progesterone, testosterone, estrone and estradiol were similar to those found in plasma. In marked contrast, the sulfates of the C-19 17-ketosteroids, androsterone (A) and dehydroepiandrosterone (DHEA) were present at levels 100 to 1000 fold greater than those found in plasma. Dihydrotestosterone (DHT) concentrations also were elevated in cyst fluid about five fold over plasma. Dramatically higher levels of estrone and estradiol sulfates were also found in cyst fluid. To investigate the origin of steroids in cyst fluid these workers administered labeled steroids intravenously and found significant uptake in cyst fluid only of DHEA sulfate. Since limited uptake of labeled water or antipyrine was observed these authors concluded that an active process is involved in uptake of DHEAS and that synthesis of other steroid sulfates occurs within breast tissues. Similarly, Raju et al [33] could not account for the high levels of estriol-3-sulfate (E3-S) in cyst fluid by accumulation from blood.

High levels of DHEAS [16], E2 and prolactin [15] have also been found in nipple secretions. In our epidemiologic-endocrine study of breast cancer we also have measured levels of unconjugated E1 and E2 in breast fluids obtained from patients and controls as previously described [17-19]. Samples were stored at $-70^{o}C$ prior to radioimmunoassay using highly specific antisera for E1 and E2 as reported previously [28]. A preliminary analysis of the results for caucasian women is shown in Table III. Excluded from consideration are subjects who were currently taking hormonal birth control or estrogen

TABLE III. BREAST FLUID ESTROGENS (ng/ml)

Age (n)	E1 (SD)	E2 (SD)
	Control	
20-29 (15)	1.9 (1.6)	1.7 (1.3)
30-39 (40)	2.4 (3.9)	1.0 (1.2)
40-49 (17)	3.2 (4.8)	1.6 (1.5)
50-59 (7)	1.5 (1.3)	0.9 (0.8)
	Benign Disease	
20-29 (10)	2.9 (2.0)	2.2 (1.4)
30-39 (54)	2.5 (2.9)	1.3 (1.1)
40-49 (33)	2.6 (2.2)	1.5 (1.2)
50-59 (3)	1.6 (1.0)	0.9 (0.7)
	Breast Disease	
30-39 (5)	1.6 (1.4)	0.9 (0.7)
40-49 (9)	2.3 (1.4)	1.2 (0.5)

replacement preparations and those who were either pregnant or lactating. First it is apparent that the mean values for both E1 and E2 are in the ng/ml range as compared to serum values which range from

20 to 400 pg/ml. The breast fluid concentrations are highly variable
as evidenced by the large standard deviations. Although the values for
both estrogens tend to be higher in young women (20-40) with benign
breast disease than in controls this difference is not significant
because of the large variability. Unfortunately, too few values are
yet available for breast cancer patients to draw meaningful
conclusions. The ratio of breast fluid to serum estrogen
concentrations also was highly variable (<1 to >200). Nevertheless
significant but weak correlations were found for the breast fluid/serum
ratios of E1 (r = 0.189, p = .05) and E2 (r = 0.39, p = <.001) with age
in control but not diseased women. These results suggest that the
retention (or synthesis) of estrogens within the breast increases with
age. Interestingly, the breast fluid/serum ratio of E2 in pregnant
women was uniformly less than one despite the higher plasma levels
(Fig. 1). These results suggest that the turnover of breast estrogens

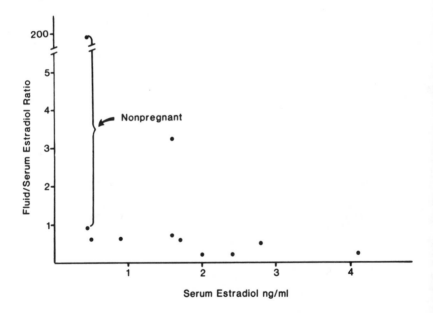

Figure 1 Ratio of breast fluid/serum estradiol concentrations are
plotted against serum estradiol values for 10 pregnant women. Note
that the ratio is less than one for all but one subject whereas the
ratio varies from 1 to 200 for nonpregnant women.

is more rapid during pregnancy perhaps due to the stimulation of ductal growth and increased blood flow caused by the elevated levels of estrogen and progesterone.

Low level ($r = .15-.2$) but significant correlations were also found between the percentage of free E2 in serum and E1 and E2 concentrations in breast fluid suggesting that at least a portion of the estrogens found in breast fluids may have arisen by diffusion from blood. Obviously further study is needed to substantiate this or any other mechanism for estrogen accumulation. In any event it would appear that both E1 and E2 are present in both normal and diseased breast nipple aspirates at levels which exceed the plasma concentrations by 10-100 fold. The difference in protein unbound E2 levels may be even larger since unlike serum, breast fluid contains low levels of proteins including SHBG [27]. In contrast to the above results Bradlow et al [32] found E1 and E2 levels in cyst fluid to be lower than plasma levels although both E1 and E2 sulfates were present in concentrations many fold higher. It is possible that cyst fluid is a more stagnant pool in which estrogens are extensively sulfurylated. Since conjugated steroids are thought to be biologically inactive, sulfurylation of steroids may provide local protection as is the case in human fetal tissues [34].

These results raise important questions concerning not only the source but also the potential effects of high local estrogen levels on ductal epithelial cells within the breast. Clearly, responsive cells would be expected to be maximally stimulated unless the estrogens are inhibited by antagonists. Viewed in this context, there is a great need to identify and elucidate the mechanisms of action of potential or unknown naturally occuring estrogen antagonists [35]. The breasts undergo cyclical changes in response to ovarian estrogens and progesterone although the histological changes are poorly characterized. Localized hormonal effects are evident even in teenage girls who may experience changes in "lumpiness" during their menstrual cycles. The large variety of focal cellular changes varying from the normal presence of microcysts to gross cysts, intraductal papillomas and other epithelial proliferations indicates that local conditions vary throughout the mass of breast tissue under normal circumstances. Clearly the high levels of E1 and E2 in breast fluids not only could result in local proliferation of cells but they also may give rise to carcinogens. Although little evidence is presently available for catechol estrogen synthesis in the breast, this pathway to carcinogenic metabolites demonstrated by the studies by McLachlan and others [36] may be extremely important when local E1 and E2 concentrations are elevated.

In addition to transport from blood into breast tissue synthesis from blood-borne steroidal precursors may contribute to the high levels of free E1 and E2 found in breast fluid. Aromatization of androgens and release of E1 from estrone sulfate, the major estrogen in human plasma, have been considered. Many investigators have examined normal and tumorous breast tissue and cells for the presence of the aromatase enzyme [37-41]. Most of these reports are difficult to interpret either because of uncertain identification of estrogenic products formed from precursors, such as labelled androstenedione, or the failure to provide data which convincingly demonstrate enzymatic activity. In our own studies we have found very few breast tumors in which aromatase activity was clearly present using the tritium release assay [42]. Few studies have addressed the question of whether the aromatase enzyme is present in normal breast epithelial or adipose cells. Thus it is not yet known whether both stromal and adipose cells of breast contain the aromatase enzyme as shown by Simpson and his colleagues for abdominal fat [43]. Controversy also exists concerning the ability of tumor cell lines to synthesize estrogens. The careful studies of McIndoe indicate that estrogen derived from androgen can interact with the estrogen receptor of MCF-7 human breast tumor cells [44]. However, others have concluded that aromatase activity is not important in breast tumors since no correlation was found with progesterone receptor levels [45].

Estrone sulfate (E1S) is the most abundant estrogen in the blood of humans and the possibility that it is a precursor of E1 and E2 within breast tissues has been considered by several investigators [46-50]. However, steroid sulfokinase activity has also been demonstrated in breast tissue [51]. The interconversion of E1 and E2 by estradiol 17 β-dehydrogenase (17β-HSD) occurs in many tissues including the breast. Thus the potential exists to form the more active E2 from E1 and E1S. Nevertheless, it is difficult to assess the physiologic importance of plasma-borne steroids as a source of active estrogens within the breast from these in vitro studies.

Mechanism of Estrogen Action

It is becoming increasingly evident that the central dogma of receptor mediated steroid action established over the past 25 years has many flaws. This is nowhere more apparent than the present controversy concerning the manner by which estrogens stimulate target cell proliferation. Virtually every conceivable mechanism including direct receptor mediated effects, production of local autocrine or distant paracrine growth factors, and estrogen mediated relief of growth inhibition by serum factors has some experimental support. Furthermore, we still do not fully understand how estrogen antagonists including the many synthetic antiestrogenic compounds or progestational, androgenic and glucocorticoid hormones act. In contrast it seems to be generally agreed that some effects of estrogens such as stimulation of progesterone receptor synthesis are exerted through binding to the estrogen receptor (ER) and interaction of the complex with specific genes in the nucleus of target cells. However, even the mechanism by which ER interacts with the genome has come into question recently. Our early observations on the kinetics of accumulation of 4S and 5S ER in uterine cell nuclei [52,53] strongly suggested the possibility that the receptor is present in the nucleus rather than being translocated from the cytoplasm as proposed by Jensen, Gorski and others in the "two step" mechanism. Recent studies using antibodies to ER [54] and cell enucleation techniques [55] appear to provide convincing evidence that the native estrogen receptor resides in the nucleus of target cells. Furthermore, recent studies have shown that the 4S→5S transformation of ER takes place in the nucleus of MCF-7 human tumor cells also [56].

Our recent studies of estrogen availability in blood of hyper- and hypo-estrogenic postmenopausal women showed that the plasma free E2 levels were extremely low (10^{-12} M) and that the mean difference in obese and thin women was less than 3 fold [7]. These results raised several important questions regarding the ability of the estrogen receptor to discriminate between these low levels of E2. As a consequence we reexamined the binding of E2 to the rat uterine estrogen receptor (ER) under physiologic conditions using a slight modification of the isodialysis method in which free rather than bound ligand concentrations are measured [26]. This approach eliminates erroneously low estimates of receptor binding affinity which arise with commonly employed methods due to binding of ligand to nonreceptor components in crude preparations at equilibrium [57]. In summary, these results have demonstrated that 1) the binding affinity of E2 for ER ($K_D \approx$ 1-3 x 10^{-11} M) is considerably higher even at $37^{\circ}C$ than previously estimated when free E2 concentrations are calculated rather than measured. 2)

When receptor preparations are warmed in the absence of reducing agents such as DTT the K_D slowly increases to values around 1 nM giving the appearance of Type II binding sites. 3) In agreement with the reports of Notides [58,59] positive cooperativity of binding is observed which can be blocked by compounds such as estriol. The consequence of these findings [60] is that levels of E2 consistent with the free and albumin fractions found in plasma of obese postmenopausal women can be effective in vivo since the value of K_D falls in this range. Furthermore, as illustrated in Fig. 2, positive cooperativity of

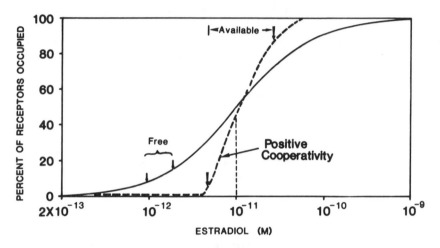

Figure 2 Theoretical saturation plot (solid line) for estradiol binding to the estrogen receptor with a K_D of 2×10^{-11}. Dashed line shows the effect of positive cooperativity obtained with rat uterine cytosol when binding was studied by measuring free estradiol over a broad range as described (57). Available refers to the range of free and albumin bound estradiol observed in postmenopausal women (7).

binding dramatically reduces the range of E2 required to saturate the receptor which offers an explanation for the small difference in E2 concentrations between hypo- and hyperestrogenic women. These results further suggest that inhibition of positive cooperativity may be an important mechanism by which estrogen action can be antagonized. Further studies are in progress to define the range of compounds which have the ability to block cooperative binding of E2. It should be noted that the elegant studies of Jordan and his colleagues indicate that antiestrogens such as Tamoxifen may act by blocking a

conformational change in the ER required to convert it to the
biologically active form [60]. The presence of endogenous steroids
which act similarly in breast fluids may be of vital importance to our
understanding of the role of estrogens in breast cancer.

Concluding Remarks

It would appear that estrogens are necessary but not sufficient to cause cancer of reproductive tract tissues in humans. This follows from the fact that only a fraction of obese postmenopausal women or those who consume exogenous estrogens develop endometrial cancer. It is unlikely that specific abnormalities in estrogen production, plasma levels or metabolism are associated with reproductive tract cancers. The increased estrogenicity observed in obese postmenopausal women can be accounted for by 1) increased peripheral production of E1 from androstenedione 2) increased tissue transport of E2 owing to reduced SHBG and 3) the absence of the antagonistic actions of progesterone or perhaps other steroids such as adrenal androgens. The decline in adrenal androgen secretion with age may explain the continuing rise in endometrial cancer despite the relatively low estrogen levels. The apparent increase in target tissue sensitivity may be brought about by withdrawal of an antagonist related to DHEAS. However, differences in metabolism of estrogens may also be important. Fishman and coworkers [62] have proposed that factors which favor 16 α-hydroxylation over 2-hydroxylation of estradiol may promote cancer formation because estriol is a relatively more potent agonist as compared to the catechol estrogens such as 2-hydroxy-E2. This view is difficult to reconcile with the extremely low circulating levels of E3, and its precursor 16α -hydroxy estrone, and the low potency of both of these compounds relative to E2. Even if one proposes that local formation of metabolites within target tissues may be important, the prevention of cooperative binding to ER of E2 by E3 is consistent with antiestrogenic rather than estrogenic properties of the latter.

The situation is even more complex in breast cancer since it appears that the local hormonal environment of the breast may be modified by factors other than the availability of hormones from blood. These include local synthesis of both agonists and antagonists as well as the poorly understood dynamics of turnover within the breast ductal system. The studies of Petrakis demonstrating the presence of both endogenous and exgenous substances in breast fluid suggest that environmental estrogens (or antagonists) may also accumulate in the breast. Unfortunately, no information is yet available concerning this important aspect of breast disease. The hormonal milieu of the normal breast in young women likely reflects the changes in ovarian secretion of estrogens and progesterone but in the absence of full maturation associated with pregnancy and lactation the ability of the breast to

clear itself of hormones and other substances may not develop fully or
may become impaired. The local hormonal milieu in the nulliparous
woman may lead to foci of atypical cellular growth, cyst formation and
in some cases neoplasia. If this scenario is correct then it is clear
that inhibition and/or reversal of such changes becomes of paramount
importance. The problem must be examined not from the perspective of
plasma hormone levels but rather from the breast itself. A step in
this direction has already been taken by Mauvais-Jarvais and colleagues
who advocate topical progestin administration for treatment of benign
breast disease [63].

REFERENCES

1. J.A. Nisker, and P.K. Siiteri in: Clinical Obstetrics and
    Gynecology R.J. Worley, ed. (Harper and Rower, Hagerstown
    1981) pp. 301-322.
2. M.C. Pike, P.K. Siiteri and C.W. Welsh eds. Banbury Report 8:
    Hormones and Breast Cancer, (Cold Spring Harbor, N.Y 1981)
3. A. Angeli, H.L. Bradlow, and L. Dogliotti eds. Endocrinology
    of Cystic Breast Disease, (Raven Press, N.Y. 1983)
4. J.D. Wilson, and P.K. Siiteri, Proc. of the 4th Int. Congress of
    Endocrinology, Excerpta Medica Foundation, Int. Congress
    Series 273, 1051-1056 (1973).
5. P.C. MacDonald, C.D. Edman, D.L. Hemsell, J.C. Porter, and
    P.K. Siiteri, Am. J. Obstet. Gynecol. 130, 448-455 (1978).
6. R.J. Davidson, J.C. Gambone, L.D. Lagasse, T.W. Castaldo, G.L.
    Hammond, P.K. Siiteri, and H.L. Judd, J. Clin. Endo. Metab.
    52, 404-408 (1981).
7. L.R. Laufer, R.J. Davidson, R.D. Ross, L.D. Lagasse, P.K. Siiteri,
    and H.L. Judd, Am. J. Obstet. Gynecol. 145, 585-590 (1983).
8. J. Fishman, H.L. Bradlow, D.K. Fukushima, J. O'Connor, R.S.
    Rosenfeld, F.J. Graepel, R. Elston, and H. Lynch, Cancer Res.
    43, 1884-1890 (1983)
9. J.D. Wilson, J. Aiman, and P.C. MacDonald, Adv. Intern.
    Med. 29, 1-32 (1980).
10. D.C. Moore, L. V. Schlaepfer, L. Paunier, and P.C. Sizonenko
    J. Clin. Endo. Meta. 58, 492-499 (1984).
11. R.D. Bulbrook, J.L. Hayward, and C.C. Spicer, Lancet ii,
    395-398 (1971).
12. A. A. J. van Landeghem, J. Poortman, M. Nabuurs, and J.H.H.
    Thijssen, Cancer Res. 45, 2907-2912 (1985).
13. J.B. Adams in: Commentaries on Research in Breast Disease
    Volume 3, R.D. Bulbrook, D.J. Taylor eds. (Alan R. Liss, Inc.,
    N.Y. 1983) pp. 131-161.
14. R. Grattarola, Cancer 17, 1119-1122 (1964).
15. E.L. Wynder, and P. Hill, Lancet ii 840-842 (1977).
16. W.R. Miller, V. Huneniuk, and R.W. Kelly, J. Ster. Biochem.
    13, 145-151 (1980).
17. N.L. Petrakis, L.D. Gruenke, T.C. Beelen, J.C. Craig, and N.
    Castagnoli, Science 119, 303-305 (1978).
18. N. L. Petrakis, L.D. Gruenke, and J. C. Craig, Cancer Res. 41,
    2563-2565 (1981).

218

19. N.L. Petrakis, M.E. Dupuy, R.E. Lee, M.L. Lyon, C.A. Maack, L.D. Gruenke, and J.C. Craig in: Banbury Report 13, Indicators of Genotoxic Exposure (Cold Spring Harbor Laboratory, N.Y. 1982) pp. 67-82.
20. F. E. Adair, H.J. Bagg, Internat. Clinics (thirtyfifth series), 4, 19-27 (1925).
21. T. Byers, S. Graham, T. Rzepka, and J. Marshall, Am. J. Epidem. 121, 664-674 (1985).
22. R. Ing, J.H.C. Ho, N.L. Petrakis, Lancet ii, 124-127 (1977).
22a. R. Ing, J.H.C. Ho, N.L. Petrakis, Lancet ii, 655-657 (1977).
23. D.C. Anderson, Clin. Endo. 3, 69-96 (1974).
24. C.H. Wu, T. Motonashi, H.A. Abel-Rahman, G.L. Flickinger, and G. Mikhail, J. Clin. Endo. Metab. 43, 436-445 (1976).
25. R. A. Vigersky, S. Kong, M. Sauer, M.B. Lipsett, and D.L. Loriaux, J. Clin. Endo. Metab. 49, 899-904 (1979).
26. G.L. Hammond, J.A. Nisker, L.A. Jones, and P.K. Siiteri, J. Biol. Chem. 255, 5023-5026 (1980).
27. P.K. Siiteri, J.T. Murai, G.L. Hammond, J.A. Nisker, W.J. Raymoure, and R.W. Kuhn Rec. Prog. Hormone Res. 38, 457-510 (1982).
28. J.W. Moore, G.M.G. Clark, R.D. Bulbrook, R.D. Hayward, J.T. Murai, G.L. Hammond, and P.K. Siiteri, Intl. J. Cancer 29, 17-21 (1982).
29. P.K. Siiteri, G.L. Hammond, and J.A. Nisker in Banbury Report 8: Hormones and Breast Cancer M.C. Pike, P.K. Siiteri, and C.W. Welsh eds. (Cold Spring Harbor, N.Y. 1981) pp. 87-106.
30. M.J. Reed, R.W. Cheng, C.T. Noel, H.A.F. Dudley, and V.H.T. James, Cancer Res. 43, 3940-3943 (1983).
31. P.F. Bruning, J.M.G. Bonfrer, and A.A. M. Hart, Br. J. Cancer 51, 479-484 (1985).
32. J.W. Moore, G.M.G. Clark, O. Takatani, Y. Wakabayashi, J.L. Hayward, and R.D. Bulbrook, J. Clin. Invest. 71, 749-754 (1983).
33. U. Raju, M. Ganguly, and M. Levitz, J. Clin. Endo. Meta. 53, 847-851 (1972).
34. P.K. Siiteri, and P.C. MacDonald, J. Clin. Endo. Meta. 26, 751-761 (1966).
35. B.M. Markaverich, R.R. Roberts, M.A. Alejandro, and J.H. Clark, Cancer Res. 44, 1515-1519 (1984).
36. J.A. McLachlan, A. Wong, G.H. Degen, and J.C. Barrett, Cancer Res. 42, 3040-3045 (1982).
37. Y. J. Abul-Hajj, Steroids 26, 488-500 (1975).
38. J.B. Adams, and K. Li, Br. J. Cancer 31, 429-433 (1975).
39. K. Li, D.P. Chandra, T. Foo, J.B. Adams, and C. McDonald, Steroids 28, 561-574 (1976).
40. W.R. Miller, and A.P.M. Forrest, Lancet 2, 86-88 (1974).
41. P.K. Siiteri, and M. Serron-Ferre in: The Endocrine Function of the Human Adrenal Cortex, V.H.T. James, M. Serio, G. Giusti, and L. Martini eds. (Academic Press, Inc., N.Y. 1978) pp. 251-264.
42. P.K. Siiteri, Cancer Res. (supplement) 42, 3269s-3273s (1982).
43. E.V. Simpson, W. H. Cleland, and C.R. Mendelson, J. Steroid Biochem. 19, 707-713 (1983).
44. J.H. MacIndoe, G.R. Woods, L.A. Etre, and D.F. Covey, Cancer Res. (supplement) 42, 3378s-3381s (1982).
45. N. Tilson-Mallett, S.J. Santner, P.D. Feil, and R.J. Santen, J. Clin. Endo. Metab. 57, 1125-1128 (1983).

46. T.L. Dao, C. Hayes, and P.R. Libby, Proc. Soc. Exp. Biol. Med. 146, 381-384 (1974).
47. J. Koudstaal, Eur. J. Cancer 11, 809-813 (1975).
48. N. Wilking, K. Carlstrom, S.A. Gustafsson, H. Skoldefors, and O. Tollbone, Eur. J. Cancer 16, 1339-1344 (1980).
49. F. Vignon, M. Terqui, B. Westley, D. Derocq, and H. Rochefort, Endocrin. 106, 1079-1086 (1980).
50. O. Prost, M.O. Turrel, N. Dahan, C. Craveur, and G.L. Adessi, Cancer Res. 44, 661-664 (1984).
51. J.B. Adams, D.P. Chandra, Cancer Res. 37, 278-284 (1977).
52. P.K. Siiteri, B.E. Schwarz, I. Moriyama, R. Ashby, D. Linkie, and P.C. MacDonald, Adv. Exp. Med. Biol. 36, 97-112 (1973).
53. D.M. Linkie, and P.K. Siiteri, J. Steroid Biochem. 9, 1071-1078 (1978).
54. W.J. King, and G.L. Greene, Nature 307, 745-747 (1984).
55. W.V. Welshons, M.E. Lieberman, and J. Gorski, Nature 307, 747-749 (1984).
56. A. Kasid, J.S. Strobl, K. Huff, G.L. Greene, and M.E. Lippman, Science 225, 1162-1166 (1984).
57. P.K. Siiteri, Science 223, 191-193 (1984).
58. A.C. Notides, N. Lerner, and D.E. Hamilton, Proc. Natl. Acad. Sci. USA 78, 4926-4930 (1981).
59. S. Sasson, and A. Notides, J. Biol. Chem. 258, 8118-8122 (1983).
60. M.A. Thompson, J.T. Murai, and P.K. Siiteri, submitted to J. Biol. Chem. (1985).
61. V.C. Jordan, Pharm. Rev. 36, 245-276 (1984).
62. J. Schneider, D. Kinne, A. Fracchia, V. Pierce, K.E. Anderson, H. L. Bradlow, and J. Fishman, Proc. Natl. Acad. Sci. 79, 3047-3051 (1982).
63. F. Kuttenn, S. Fournier, R. Sitruk-Ware, P. Martin, and P. Mauvais-Jarvis in: Endocrinology of Cystic Breast Disease A. Angeli, H.L. Bradlow, L. Dogliotti eds. (Raven Press, N.Y. 1983) pp. 231-252.

220

DISCUSSION

PASQUALINI: Do you have any quantitative data on the concentration levels of estrogen sulfates in the breast fluids in normal and cancer patients?

SIITERI: Preliminary results with a small number of samples have revealed very high levels of estrone sulfate, but differences have not been detected thus far.

STANCEL: Have you measured the K_D of the nuclear form of the estrogen receptor via isodialysis?

SIITERI: Not yet.

STANCEL: What oncogene were you referring to in your last slide?

SIITERI: I have no specific information at this point in time.

STANCEL: One possibility to explain why breast tissue doesn't continuously grow in response to the high local estrogen may be the high level of estrogen per se. You may not need to postulate an antagonist, since in some systems high estrogens can "block" cell division.

SIITERI: That is true, but the distinction between a cytostatic and cytotoxic effect at high estrogen levels is difficult to make.

SETCHELL: The high levels of cholesterol in breast fluid of postmenopausal women is interesting. Have studies of the lipoproteins been carried out and, if so, how do they differ? Would you care to speculate as to the reason for this difference--is it a direct effect of estrogen?

SIITERI: I do not know of any studies on lipoproteins in breast fluids.

KUPFER: In collaboration with Dr. Chris Longcope (Worcestor), we determined the K_D for ^{3}H-estradiol in cytosol from numerous human breast tumors, using dextran coated charcoal (DCC) and Scatchard plot analysis. We often obtained a K_D of 10^{-11} M. This points out that the use of DCC does not always yield a high K_D and, hence, under appropriate conditions provides the proper measurements.

SIITERI: Quite true. As I pointed out, the degree of error in calculated free ligand values is variable depending upon the composition of the cytosol. In some cases, it may be negligible.

RAYNAUD: If you measure rate of association and dissociation and calculate the association equilibrium constant from the ratio of the two rates, you obtain values which are similar with those you have shown with your ultrafiltration dialysis system.

SIITERI: Thank you. We are aware of this fact and feel that this helps to substantiate our values as being correct.

PROLACTIN SYNTHESIS BY CULTURED RAT PITUITARY CELLS: AN ASSAY TO STUDY
ESTROGENS, ANTIESTROGENS AND THEIR METABOLITES IN VITRO

V. CRAIG JORDAN, R. KOCH AND R.R. BAIN
Department of Human Oncology, Wisconsin Clinical Cancer Center,
University of Wisconsin, Madison, WI 53792

ABSTRACT

Since non-steroidal antiestrogens are extensively metabolized in
vivo it has been difficult to dissect the role of individual metabolites
in the overall pharmacology of the drugs. A primary route of metabolism
is the formation of hydroxylated metabolites with a high binding affinity
for the estrogen receptor and, as a result, an increased antiestrogenic
potency. An assay system utilizing estrogen-stimulated prolactin synthesis by primary cultures of immature rat pituitary cells, has been developed to study the structure-activity relationship of compounds in vitro.
The assay has been used to describe the structural requirements for compounds to stimulate or to inhibit prolactin synthesis. A drug-receptor
map of the estrogen receptor is proposed to predict the pharmacology of
binding ligands. Recently the phytoestrogens have attracted attention as
potential environmental agents which may produce infertility problems or
promote the growth of breast cancer. Only small quantities of the phytoestrogens are available as pure compounds and the prolactin synthesis
assay is ideal to classify their pharmacology. Equol is known to be a
metabolite of the phytoestrogens formononetin and diadzein. Equol is
more potent than formononetin but is less potent than coumestrol, which
is the most potent of the phytoestrogens. In the future, the prolactin
synthesis assay can be used to evaluate the pharmacology of a broad range
of environmental agents with potential estrogenic activity.

INTRODUCTION

The last 50 years has seen an exponential rise in the published
reports about estrogen action. This chapter traces the development of
potent estrogenic and antiestrogenic compounds by the study of their
structure-activity relationships. Studies of structure-activity relationships in vivo using Allen-Doisy or 3-day uterine weight tests can
provide much valuable information, but the assays suffer from the complex
problems of pharmacokinetics and metabolic transformation. Studies in
vitro using primary cultures of rat pituitary cells to assay the ability
of a compound to induce prolactin synthesis respectively, can provide
essential information about the structural requirements for a compound to

produce estrogenic and antiestrogenic effects. Nevertheless, it should
be pointed out that studies in vivo are required to determine whether a
compound is metabolically activated to an estrogen. Estrogen receptor
binding models will be presented to describe the changes in a molecule
that will predict high affinity for the ligand and agonist, partial
agonist and antagonist properties of the ligand-receptor complex. Most
phytoestrogens conform to the predictions of the estrogen receptor
binding model.

THE METABOLISM OF TAMOXIFEN IN DIFFERENT SPECIES

Fromson and coworkers [1,2] were the first to describe the metabolism of tamoxifen in laboratory animals and women. Initially a range of
metabolites (A-F) were characterized in laboratory animals by the isolation of radiolabelled metabolites of ^{14}C-labeled tamoxifen using thin
layer chromatography. R_f's were compared with synthetic standards and
the structure of some metabolites was confirmed by gas chromatography/
mass spectrometry. Initially, metabolite B (4-hydroxytamoxifen) was
believed to be the major metabolite in man [2], however, there is now
adequate evidence to prove that N-desmethyltamoxifen (known also as
metabolite X) is the major metabolite [3]. The pharmacology of the
different metabolites of tamoxifen has been reviewed [4]. We recently
described [5] an HPLC method to determine tamoxifen and its metabolites
in biological fluids and have used this to identify primary metabolites
in different species. Representative chromatograms for patients undergoing tamoxifen therapy are shown in Fig. 1.

Tamoxifen exhibits different actions in different species and it is
possible that differential metabolism is responsible for increased estrogenicity. Tamoxifen is fully estrogenic in the mouse [6-8], completely
antiestrogenic in the chicken [9] and frog (A.C. Tate and D. Schonberg,
personal communication) and exhibits estrogenic and antiestrogenic
actions in the rat [6-8] and human [10]. However, no dramatic metabolic
changes have been observed in chickens, mice and rats [11] using radio-
isotopes; 4-hydroxytamoxifen is the principal metabolite. Similarly,
HPLC analysis demonstrates the proportion of metabolites in different
species (Table 1). It seems that a strong case cannot be made at
present, to support the hypothesis that the conversion of tamoxifen to
estrogenic metabolites is responsible for species differences. Nevertheless, it must be conceded that potent unidentified metabolites might
be responsible for the effects.

METABOLISM IN HUMANS

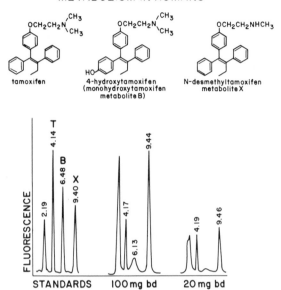

Fig. 1. The identification of metabolites of tamoxifen in human serum. Triphenylethylenes are separated from extracted serum by HPLC [5] and quantitated by post-column fluorescence activation. The triphenylethylenes are converted to phenanthrenes by on line UV lamps.

To investigate the contribution of metabolic activation in the actions of antiestrogens in vivo we have evaluated the estrogenic and antiestrogenic properties of a series of structural derivatives of tamoxifen (Fig. 2). It is interesting to note that the introduction of a methoxy group into tamoxifen did not significantly alter the partial estrogenic and antiestrogenic properties in the 3 day immature rat uterine weight test (Fig. 3). If methoxy derivatives of non-steroidal antiestrogens are demethylated prior to exerting their biological effects [12], then hydroxylation of tamoxifen in vivo to form 4-hydroxytamoxifen may make a significant contribution to the pharmacology of the drug. Certainly 4-hydroxytamoxifen has a high binding affinity for the estrogen receptor [13]. Nevertheless, the finding that compounds that cannot undergo metabolic p-hydroxylation (p fluoro, chloro, methyl) are also antiestrogenic in vivo [14] (Fig. 3) demonstrates that these substituted triphenylethylenes have inherent antiestrogenic properties. Thus it

TABLE 1. The relative abundance of various metabolites of tamoxifen, determined by HPLC [5], during the administration of the drug to different species.

Species	Metabolite	
	4-OH Tamoxifen	N-Des CH$_3$ Tamoxifen
Xenopus	++++	---
Chicken	+++	---
Mouse	+	---
Rat	+	+
Human	+	+++

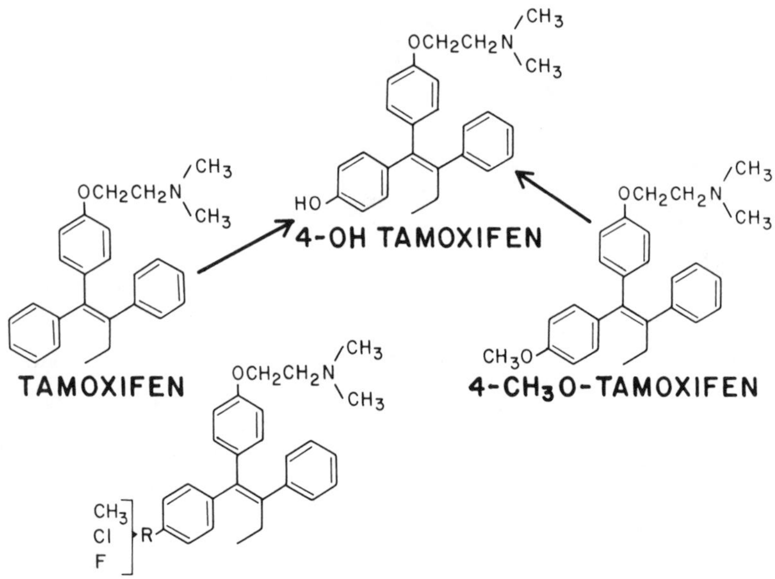

Fig. 2. The possible conversion of triphenylethylenes to 4-OH tamoxifen. There is either para hydroxylation or demethylation. The substituted compounds (para methyl, chloro and fluoro) were synthesized to determine the role of para hydroxylation in the pharmacology of tamoxifen.

appears to be an advantage, but not a requirement, for antiestrogens to undergo metabolic activation.

To dissect the contribution of different metabolites in the overall pharmacology of tamoxifen we have developed an assay system in vitro to determine structure activity relationships.

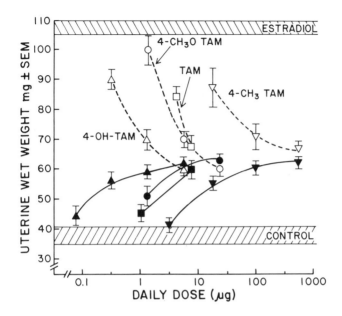

Fig. 3. The estrogenic and antiestrogenic activity of triphenylethylenes in the 3 day immature rat uterine wet weight test. Compounds (tamoxifen, TAM; 4-methoxytamoxifen, 4-CH$_3$O TAM; 4-hydroxytamoxifen, 4-OH TAM; 4-methyltamoxifen, 4-CH$_3$ TAM) or estradiol (0.16 µg) were administered daily for 3 days and the uterine weights determined on day 4. Compounds were either administered alone (solid lines) or with etradiol (broken lines).

REGULATION OF PROLACTIN SYNTHESIS IN VITRO--AN ASSAY TO STUDY STRUCTURE ACTIVITY RELATIONSHIPS

Primary cultures of rat pituitary cells respond to physiological concentrations of estradiol by a specific increase in prolactin synthesis [15]. This model system for estrogen action (illustrated in Fig. 4) has been validated for the study of structure-activity relationship within groups of nonsteroidal estrogens and antiestrogens. The antiestrogens, tamoxifen and 4-hydroxytamoxifen, competitively and reversibly inhibit estradiol-stimulated prolactin synthesis [16]. Their potencies are consistent with their relative binding affinities for the estrogen receptor; 4-hydroxytamoxifen is 30 times more potent than tamoxifen. To avoid the possibility that tamoxifen is metabolically activated to 4-hydroxy-

226

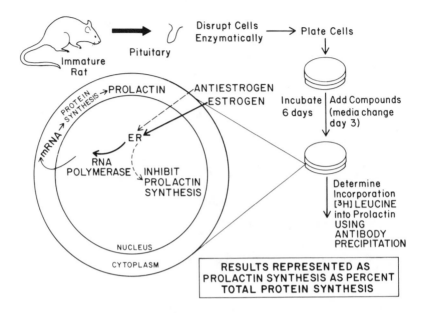

Fig. 4. A diagramatic representation of the method involved to study the modulation of prolactin synthesis in primary cultures of rat pituitary cells by estrogens and antiestrogens [16].

tamoxifen in vitro, the para substituted derivatives of tamoxifen (4-methyl, chloro and fluoro) that are unlikely to be metabolized to 4-hydroxytamoxifen [14,16] have been tested. The substitution does not affect the binding of the compounds to the estrogen receptor [14,16] and the derivatives of tamoxifen inhibit estradiol-stimulated prolactin synthesis consistent with their relative binding affinities for the receptor (Fig. 5).

STRUCTURE-ACTIVITY RELATIONSHIPS

A hypothetical model of the ligand interaction with the estrogen receptor binding site has been developed to describe the structural features necessary to initiate or to inhibit prolactin synthesis in vitro.

A correctly placed alkyl-aminoethoxyside chain is important to prevent the initiation of prolactin synthesis via the estrogen receptor [17]. We have focused upon this area of interaction at the ligand binding site and found that the compounds related to bisphenol (4-hydroxytamoxifen without the alkylaminoethylside chain) are particularly

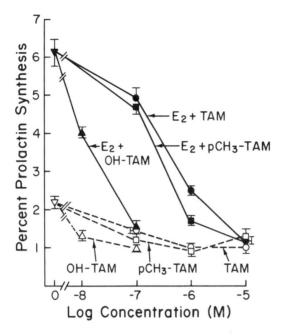

Fig. 5. Comparison of the effects of 4-OH tamoxifen, 4 CH_3 tamoxifen and tamoxifen on prolactin synthesis. Pituitary cells ($2x10^5$/dish) were cultured for 6 days in DMEM + serum containing the following additions: 0.1% ethanol (V), 1 nM estradiol (▼), the indicated concentration of compounds with (solid lines) or without (broken lines) estradiol. Prolactin synthesis is expressed as a fraction of total protein synthesis. Values are means ± S.E. for three cultures per point.

interesting as they are all partial agonists in vitro [18,19]. Belleau's macromolecular perturbation theory [20], which was originally proposed to explain agonist, partial agonist and antagonist activity of drugs at the muscarinic cholinergic receptor, may be used to explain partial agonists in terms of the estrogen receptor model. According to Belleau's hypothesis, antagonists bind to the receptor and produce a non-specific conformation perturbation (NSCP) and the complex has zero intrinsic activity. An agonist, on the other hand, binds to the receptor and induces a specific conformational perturbation (SCP). Between these extremes, a partial agonist binds to the receptor and produces an equilibrium mix of agonist and antagonist receptor complexes. Applying these definitions to the estrogen receptor (Fig. 6), estradiol binds with high affinity to the resting receptor and induces a SCP which results in the ligand being locked into the binding site. 4-Hydroxytamoxifen

228

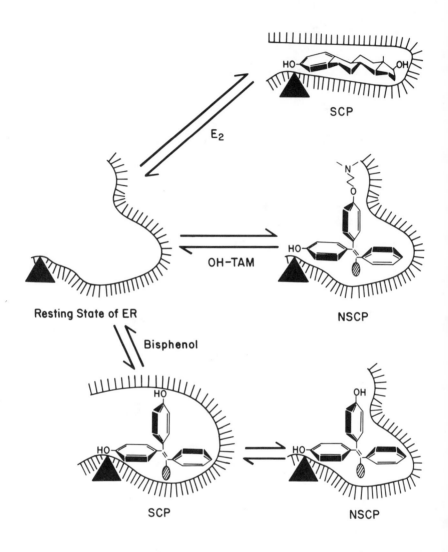

Fig. 6. Adaptation of Belleau's macromolecular perturbation theory to describe the interaction of agonists, antagonists and partial agonists with the estrogen receptor (ER). The phenol group of the ligand interacts with phenolic site on the ER (Δ) and produces a high-affinity interaction if the geometry of the ligand is correct. Estradiol (E_2) an agonist, induces a specific conformational perturbation (SCP), whereas 4-hydroxytamoxifen (OH-TAM) an antagonist, only induces a nonspecific conformational perturbation (NSCP). Bisphenol, a partial agonist, produces a mixture of SCP and NSCP in the ER.

(antagonist) wedges into the resting receptor and only produces a NSCP. Bisphenol (partial agonist) interacts at the ligand binding site, but while some of the receptors can be induced to lock the ligand into the protein, other ligand interactions are only able to induce a NSCP in the complex.

An adequate assay system is now established and validated to dissect the structural constraints of a ligand to modulate estrogen-dependent events via the estrogen receptor. Nonsteroidal compounds can now be classified experimentally into agonists and antagonists and partial agonists based upon their structures. We have used the assay to study the biological activity of several phytoestrogens.

PHYTOESTROGENS

Plants [21] contain estrogens that are suspected of contributing to infertility problems in farm animals. There is also the possibility that phytoestrogens in the diet can contribute to the growth of hormone-dependent breast tumors in post-menopausal patients [22]. Other than the potentially harmful effects of estrogens, they are apparently important to improve the quality of meat. Grazing animals in areas that are rich in phytoestrogens could provide economic advantages.

There are three major chemical types of phytoestrogens in plants: coumestans, flavones and isoflavones. Coumesterol is the most potent of the estrogens in forage crops [23] and, consistent with this observation, has a higher binding affinity for the estrogen receptor than genistein [24,25]. In contrast, the flavones are very weak estrogens. The methoxyflavone, tricin, is a constituent of alfalfa [26] but is very weakly estrogenic in the mouse. The isoflavone derivatives have attracted much attention as estrogenic compounds in clover. The early studies of the structure-activity relationships have been reviewed by Bradbury and White [27]. Genistein is the most active estrogen in this group with the highest binding affinity (RBA 0.9) for the estrogen receptor [25]. The methoxy derivative, Biochanin A, does not bind to the estrogen receptor but is estrogenic in vivo [25,28]. Similarly, diadzein (Fig. 7) has a higher binding affinity for the estrogen receptor than the methoxy derivative, formononetin (Fig. 7). Both compounds are weak estrogens in vivo [25,28].

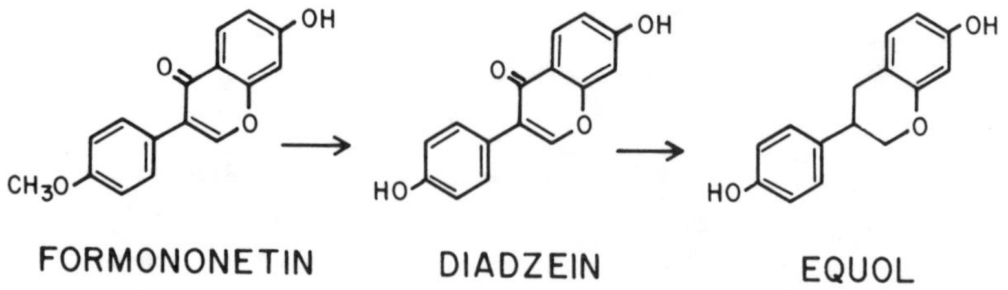

FORMONONETIN   DIADZEIN   EQUOL

Fig. 7. The metabolic activation of formononetin to equol described in sheep [29].

The metabolism of formononetin and Biochanin A by micro-organisms in the sheep rumen has been described [29]; however, diadzen is further reduced to equol (Fig. 7). Currently there is much interest in the detection of phytoestrogens in human urine because of the possibility that changes in diet might cause the activation of hormone-dependent breast cancer. Several studies have reported phytoestrogens in the urine [30,31]; however, the recent reports by Setchell and coworkers [32,33] are particularly interesting because they document that certain individuals have the ability to produce equol from soya products. Clearly this will be a significant area of research in the future.

The structure of formononetin and the conversion to diadzein is reminiscent of the metabolic activation of mestranol to ethinyl estradiol [34,35] (Fig. 8). We have tested these steroids in the pituitary prolactin assay in vitro (Fig. 9). Both compounds are fully estrogenic but consistent with the lower relative binding affinity of mestranol for the estrogen receptor, the estrogenic potency is about 1% of ethinyl estradiol's. Similarly, diadzein is a more potent estrogen in the prolactin synthesis assay than formononetin (data not shown) and has equivalent activity to equol (Fig. 10). Coumestrol is the most potent of the phytoestrogens that we have tested (Fig. 10).

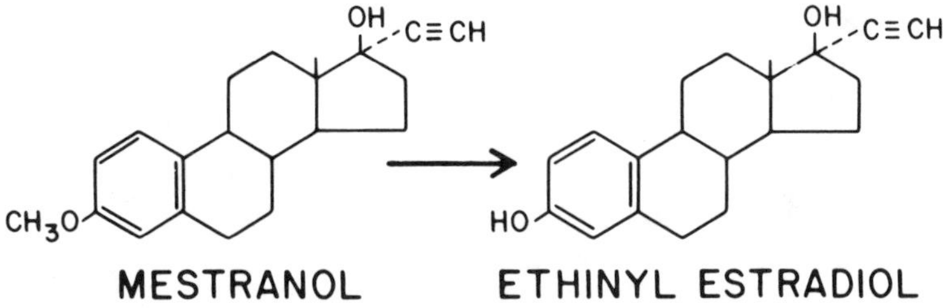

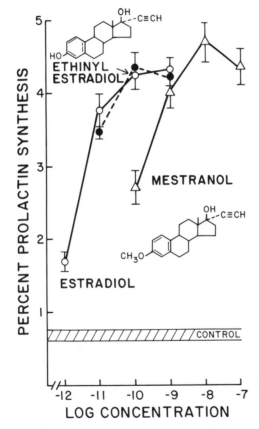

MESTRANOL   ETHINYL ESTRADIOL

Fig. 8. The metabolic activation of mestranol to ethinylestradiol [34,35].

Fig. 9. The relative estrogenic potencies of ethinyl estradiol, estradiol and mestranol using the prolactin synthesis assay in primary cultures of immature rat pituitary cells.

232

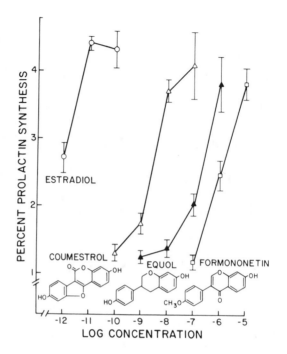

Fig. 10. The relative estrogenic potencies of estradiol, coumestrol, equol and formononetin using the prolactin synthesis assay in primary cultures of immature rat pituitary cells.

Recently, a novel compound, enterolactone (HPMF), has been isolated from human urine [36,37] (Fig. 11). No biological properties or function have been ascribed for enterolactone, but it appears to be a product of

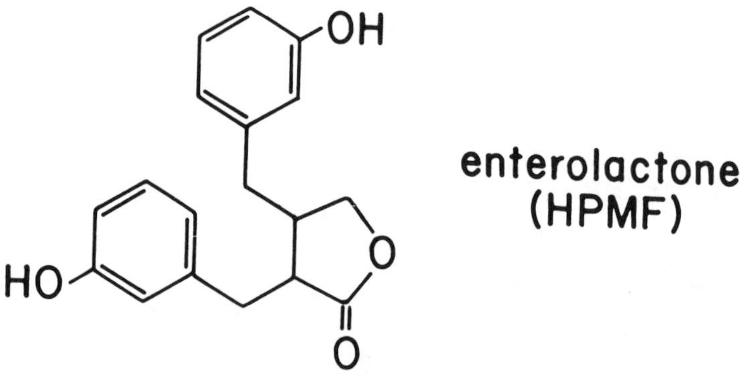

enterolactone (HPMF)

Fig. 11. The structure of the compound enterolactone.

microbial metabolic transformation in the intestine [36,39]. In testing
this compound we detected no estrogenic properties in a 3-day Rubin test
using immature female rats and no ability to inhibit [^{3}H]estradiol
binding to uterine estrogen receptors. However, we made two interesting
observations that might have clinical implications. The non-steroidal
antiestrogen, tamoxifen, inhibits estradiol-stimulated prolactin
synthesis by immature rat pituitary cells _in vitro_ [16]. Enterolactone
does not affect estradiol-stimulated prolactin synthesis, but is significantly estrogenic at 10 μM [40]. In another test that uses growth of
MCF7 breast cancer cells as an endpoint, tamoxifen alone inhibits the
growth of the cells, but this can readily be reversed with estradiol
[41]. Enterolactone (10 μM) can also reverse the inhibitory effect of
tamoxifen on the growth of MCF7 cells [40]. Clearly, high circulating
levels of enterolactone might be detrimental to patients undergoing
antiestrogen therapy for breast cancer.

ACKNOWLEDGEMENTS

These studies were supported by grants RO1-CA-32713, PO1-CA-20432
and P30-CA-14520 awarded by the National Institutes of Health. We would
like to thank Professor Herman Adlercreutz, University of Helsinki, for
providing the sample of equol, Dr. E.R. Clark, University of Leeds for
providing the tamoxifen derivatives and Dr. G.W. Woods, Organon, for
providing the sample of enterolactone.

REFERENCES

1. J.M. Fromson, S. Pearson, and S. Bramah. Xenobiotica _3_, 693-709
    (1973).
2. J.M. Fromson, S. Pearson, and S. Bramah. Xenobiotica _3_, 711-713
    (1973).
3. H.K. Adam, E.J. Douglas, and J.V. Kemp. Biochem. Pharmacol. _27_,
    145-147 (1979).
4. V.C. Jordan. Breast Cancer Res. Treat. _2_, 123-138 (1982).
5. R.R. Brown, R. Bain, and V.C. Jordan. J. Chromatog. _272_, 351-358
    (1983).
6. M.J.K. Harper and A.L. Walpole. Nature (Lond) _212_, 87 (1966).
7. V.C. Jordan, L. Rowsby, C.J. Dix, and G. Prestwich. J. Endocrinol.
    _78_, 71-81 (1978).
8. V.C. Jordan, C.J. Dix, K.E. Naylor, G. Prestwich, and L. Rowsby. J.
    Toxicol. Environ. Health _4_, 364-390 (1978).
9. R.L. Sutherland, J. Mester, and E.E. Baulieu. Nature (Lond) _269_,
    434-435 (1977).
10. B.J.A. Furr and V.C. Jordan. Pharmacol Ther. _25_, 127-205 (1984).
11. S.D. Lyman and V.C. Jordan. Biochem. Pharmacol. (in press).

234

12. B.S. Katzenellenbogen, H.S. Bhakoo, E.R. Ferguson, N.C. Lan, T. Tatee, T.L.S. Tsai, and J.A. Katzenellenbogen. Recent Prog. Horm. Res. 35, 259-300 (1979).

13. V.C. Jordan, M.M. Collins, L. Rowsby, and G. Prestwich. J. Endocrinol. 75, 305-316 (1977).

14. K.E. Allen, E.R. Clark, and V.C. Jordan. Br. J. Pharmacol. 71, 83-91 (1980).

15. M.E. Lieberman, R.A. Maurer, and J. Gorski. Proc. Natl. Acad. Sci. 75, 5946-5949 (1978).

16. M.E. Lieberman, V.C. Jordan, M. Fritsch, M.A. Santos, and J. Gorski. J. Biol. Chem. 258, 4734-4740 (1983).

17. M.E. Lieberman, J. Gorski, and V.C. Jordan. J. Biol. Chem. 258, 4741-4745 (1983).

18. V.C. Jordan, M.E. Lieberman, E. Cormier, R. Koch, J.R. Bagley, and P.C. Ruenitz. Mol. Pharmacol. 26, 272-278 (1984).

19. V.C. Jordan and M.E. Lieberman. Mol. Pharmacol. 26, 279-285 (1984).

20. B. Belleau. J. Med. Chem. 7, 776-784 (1964).

21. N.R. Farnsworth, A.S. Bingell, G.A. Cordell, F.A. Crane, and H.H.S. Fong. J. Pharm. Sci. 64, 717-754 (1975).

22. P.M. Martin, K.B. Horwitz, D.S. Ryan, and W.L. McGuire. Endocrinology 103, 1860-1867 (1978).

23. E.M. Bickoff, A.N. Booth, R.L. Lyman, A.L. Livingston, C.R. Thompson, and F. DeEds. Science 126, 969-970 (1957).

24. M. Shemesh, H.R. Lindner, and N. Ayalon. J. Reprod. Fert. 29, 1-9 (1972).

25. D.A. Shutt and R.I. Cox. J. Endocrinol. 52, 299-310 (1972).

26. E.M. Bickoff, A.L. Livingston, and A.N. Booth. J. Pharm. Sci. 53, 1411-1412 (1964).

27. R.B. Bradbury and D.E. White. Vit. & Horm. 12, 207-233 (1955).

28. E. Cheng, Y. Yoder, C.D. Storg, and W. Burrough. Science 120, 575-577 (1954).

29. D.A. Shutt. Endeavour 35, 110-113 (1976).

30. H. Adlercreutz, T. Fotsis, R. Heikkinen, J.T. Dwyer, M. Woods, B.R. Goldin, and S.L. Gorbach. Lancet 11, 1295-1299 (1980).

31. C. Bannwart, T. Fotsis, R. Heikkinen, and H. Adlercreutz. Clinica Chim. Acta. 136, 165-172 (1984).

32. K.D.R. Setchell, S.P. Borriello, P. Hulme, D.N. Kirk, and M. Axelson. Am. J. Clin. Nut. 40, 569-578 (1984).

33. M. Axelson, T. Sjövall, B.E. Gustafsson, and K.D.R. Setchell. J. Endocrinol. 102, 49-56 (1984).

34. D.W. Hahn, J.L. McGuire, F.C. Greenslade, and G.D. Turner. Proc. Soc. Exp. Biol. Med. 137, 1180-1185 (1971).

35. A. Eisenfeld. Endocrinology 94, 803-807 (1974).

36. S.R. Stich, J.K. Toumba, M.B. Groen, C.W. Funke, J. Loemhius, J. Vink, and G.F. Woods. Nature (Lond) 287, 738-740 (1980).

37. K.D.R. Setchell, A.M. Lawson, F.L. Mitchell, H. Adlercreutz, D.N. Kirk, and M. Axelson. Nature (Lond) 287, 740-742 (1980).

38. K.D.R. Setchell, S.P. Barriello, H. Gordon, A.M. Lawson, R. Harkness, D.M.L. Morgan, D.N. Kirk, H. Adlercreutz, L.C. Anderson, and M. Axelson. Lancet 11, 4-7 (1981).

39. M. Axelson, J. Sjovall, B.E. Gustafson, and K.D.R. Setchell. Nature (Lond) 298, 659-660 (1982).

40. V.C. Jordan, S. Mittal, B. Gosden, R. Koch, and M.E. Lieberman. Environ. Health Perspect. (in press).

41. M.E. Lippman and G. Bolan. Nature (Lond) 256, 592-595 (1975).

DISCUSSION

SETCHELL: Your data on enterolactane are intriguing but leave me very confused in light of our speculations for the role of these lignans in man. How accurately does your in vitro assay reflect the in vivo situation? Because if I heard you correctly, your in vivo testing of enterolactane showed no estrogenic effects. When we first described the structure of these lignans, we tested for in vivo estrogenic activity but could find no effect. At that time, because of an inefficient chemical synthesis we had insufficient sample to complete the testing at high levels. How do you explain the differences between your in vitro and in vivo systems?

JORDAN: I am sorry to confuse you and complicate your hypothesis by presenting experimental data. We developed the assay system in vitro to avoid complications of pharmacokinetics and metabolism. Our aim was to have a biological end-point (estrogen-stimulated prolactin synthesis) which could be regulated directly by potential binding ligands. I believe the studies in vivo were unsuccessful to induce estrogenic responses because we could not achieve high levels of enterolactone in the area of the target tissue for prolonged periods.

PASQUALINI: Do you have any idea of the plasma protein binding to tamoxifen or to N-demethyl tamoxifen in humans or other species?

JORDAN: We have no precise data except to say that tamoxifen is almost entirely protein bound.

SONNENSCHEIN: Using charcoal-dextran stripped human serum-supplemented media, we consistently see an increase in cellular proliferation yield when we add tamoxifen, 4'hydroxytamoxifen, N-demethyl tamoxifen, metabolite E and Y, and cis tamoxifen to the media. This effect is serum-concentration dependent. In the talk presented at this meeting by Dr. K. S. Korach and in previous reports from our labs and others, evidence is emerging suggesting a dichotomy of the effect of estradiol on specific protein synthesis on the one hand and cell proliferation on the other. Would you care to comment on the possibility that a similar phenomenon of dual mechanism of action of so called "antiestrogens?" Do you consider that the available data is fully compatible with the notion that the therapeutic effect of tamoxifen in breast cancer patients is mediated by an estrophilin-mediated mechanism?

JORDAN: Yes, I have found your studies with antiestrogens very interesting and, indeed, I think I am correct in saying that you can rank the compounds with cis tamoxifen being more of a proliferative agent than the trans isomer. Frankly, I am unclear about the precise mechanism of cell proliferation with steroids. However, the separation of proliferation and protein synthesis has been observed in many systems. Antiestrogens, for example, increase progesterone receptor induction in the rat uterus without drastically increasing mitotic activity in the luminal epithelial cells (Dix and Jordan, J. Endocrinol. 85, 393, 1980). Certainly, it is possible that estrogens cause growth by an autocrine mechanism and antiestrogens cause a reduced synthesis of growth factors. Rochefort has provided evidence to support a position that antiestrogens can regulate the synthesis of selected proteins. Thus, some are induced and others are not. Overall, I support a role for the estrogen receptor in the mechanism of action of antiestrogens in breast cancer. Whether the receptor mechanism is directly or indirectly involved in the events leading to proliferation remains to be resolved.

NAFTOLIN: What was tne content of your culture medium?

JORDAN: The media for pituitary cell cultures is 83% DMEM, 1% insulin penicillin/fungizone and 15% 3-times charcoal stripped horse:fetal calf serum (6:1). The methodology has been published (Liebeman et al., J. Biol. Chem. 258, 4734, 1983).

NAFTOLIN: What is the effect of tamoxifen on prolactin in humans?

JORDAN: Tamoxifen produces an interesting series of effects on the human pituitary. In premenopausal patients, tamoxifen reduces the mid-cycle estradiol-stimulated peak of prolactin. In post-menopausal patients, there are reports of reduced levels of prolactin and others that demonstrate no change. Our own studies indicate slight decreases but these are probably not significantly below no treatment. These results are markedly different from the effect of tamoxifen on LH and FSH levels in post-menopausal patients. There is a general decrease in circulating gonadotropin levels thus indicating an estrogen-like action. Therefore, different cells in the pituitary gland interpret the interaction of tamoxifen with the estrogen receptor differently.

NAFTOLIN: Please explain the apparent lack of enterolactone's interaction with estrogen receptor while there are induced "classical estrogen receptor" actions such as progesterone receptor--can this be blocked by antiestrogens such as tamoxifen or progesterone?

JORDAN: The fact that we do not observe an inhibition of $[^3H]$-estradiol binding to the estrogen receptor with enterolactone suggests to me that this assay method is inadequate to determine interaction of weak binding ligands to the receptor. In the assays in vitro, we are seeing a different sequence of events. The ligand, if it is in sufficient concentration, can impinge upon the receptor in the nuclear compartment and program the receptor to initiate a subsequent biochemical event. Very few of these imprintings may be required to cause the production of mRNAs and subsequent protein synthesis.

RAYNAUD: To further investigate which is the respective role of receptor binding and metabolism, have you tried to extend your pituitary cell culture model for prolactin output and uterus cell culture model for progesterone receptor into different species?

JORDAN: Yes. Carolyn Camper, a graduate student in Dr. Jack Gorski's laboratory has been working with us to develop a similar drug-receptor model for the induction of progesterone receptor in primary cultures of immature rat uterine cells. We have been surprised to find that, whereas estradiol can induce progesterone receptor, all antiestrogens are not active and only block estradiol stimulated progesterone receptor induction. Mouse uterine cells respond similarly. These data will be published in the June issue of Endocrinology, and we are currently developing new assay methods to extend these studies. These structure-activity relationship experiments will be conducted by Cathy Murphy in my laboratory.

TUCHMANN-DUPLESSIS: Tamoxifen is certainly a very complex and fascinating compound. How does it compare biologically to clomiphen, particularly in its action on the pituitary-hypothalamic axis?

JORDAN: Tamoxifen and clomiphene are both triphenylethylenes, but you should note that tamoxifen is the antiestrogenic trans isomer whereas the commercially available clomiphene is a 60:40 mixture of geometric isomers, one of which is fully estrogenic and the other is antiestrogenic. The effects of both compounds on the hypothalamopituitary axis are similar.

TUCHMANN-DUPLEISSIS: Does tamoxifen induce ovulation?

JORDAN: Tamoxifen is available in some countries for the induction of ovulation in subfertile women. I have recently reviewed the clinical pharmacology and endocrinology of the drug (Furr and Jordan, Pharmac. Ther. 25, 127, 1984).

CUNHA: Since tamoxifen or clomid stimulate proliferation of the human fetal vagina grown in athymic nude mice, are normal adult human estrogen target tissues stimulated or suppressed by tamoxifen when grown in athymic nude mice? Can you comment on the sensitivity of tumor versus normal human cells to tamoxifen?

JORDAN: I am unaware of any studies with normal target tissues grown in athymic mice to examine the effects of tamoxifen. I can say that tamoxifen does not support the growth of MCF-7 breast cancer cells growth in athymic mice. This has been demonstrated by Osborne, Lippman and recently by my laboratory. The result is interesting because the nude mouse host uterus is stimulated suggesting a target and species specificity for the drug. A recent study done using human endometrial carcinoma grown in athymic mice has demonstrated that tamoxifen produces a partial initiation of tumor growth. I believe that these results support the view that tamoxifen-receptor complexes are interpreted differently by different tissues.

MCLACHLAN: Does an additional para-hydroxyl on the bis-phenols (triphenol) enhance estrogenic activity?

JORDAN: No. We have tested a series of trihydroxy derivatives in the pituitary cell assay. There is not an increase in estrogenic activity and all of the compounds are partial agonists (Jordan and Lieberman, Mol. Pharmacol., 26, 279, 1984).

KOLB-MEYERS: To prove the existence of two-conformation models ("crocodile jaw model," "molecular perturbation model"), did you try to use SH cross-linking reagents of NEM? The latter reagents should affect the binding of estradiol and tamoxifen differently, or estradiol and tamoxifen should protect against these agents differently if the two-conformation models are operating.

JORDAN: That is a very good idea, but what we have been interested in describing is a model of hormone action based upon structure-activity relationships using a functional assay of estrogen action. What you suggest is a biochemical approach to determine the shape of the isolated receptor. This approach, however, may not resolve the issue of the actual shape of the ligand receptor complexes. I am concerned about a biochemical approach to drug action that is divorced from the functional role of the receptor. In the future, crystalization of the receptor with various ligands may resolve the hypothesis, but this is a long way off.

238

METABOLISM OF ZEARALENONE TO A MORE ESTROGENICALLY ACTIVE FORM

Mark E. Wilson* and Winston M. Hagler, Jr.*
*Mycotoxin Laboratory, Department of Poultry Science, N. C. State
University, Raleigh, NC 27695

ABSTRACT
    Zearalenone is a polyketide (resorcylic acid lactone) secondary
metabolite of several species of the fungal genus Fusarium. It exhibits
estrogenic and anabolic activities in animals. This compound has attracted
research attention as a contaminant of feedstuffs because it causes
hyperestrogenism in swine, apparently the most sensitive food animal
species. The relatively strong anabolic activity of zearalenone with its
relatively weak estrogenic activity led to commercial development of alpha-
zearalanol (zearanol or Ralgro) as a hormonally active anabolic agent in
cattle and sheep. There are several additional metabolites closely related
to zearalenone which have been found in cultures of Fusarium. Usually found
at much lower concentrations, some also have estrogenic and anabolic
properties; however, their importance as contaminants of feedstuffs is
unknown. The overall significance of zearalenone to agriculture and public
health is that: 1) zearalenone serves as the synthetic precursor to Ralgro,
and 2) zearalenone is often a naturally occurring contaminant of moldy feeds
and feed ingredients (primarily corn in the "corn belt" and grain sorghum in
the southeast). The metabolism and excretion of zearalenone and zearalanone
by animals is discussed comparatively with the metabolite by Fusarium,
Candida tropicalis, and rumen protozoans. In animals, zearalenone is
generally converted into a metabolite having greater estrogenic activity,
while zearalanol is metabolized to compounds having lower hormonal activity.

INTRODUCTION
    Zearalenone [2,4-dihydroxy-6-(10-hydroxy-6-oxo-trans-1-undecenyl)-beta-
resorcyclic acid-mu-lactone] is a secondary metabolism of several species of
the fungal genus Fusarium. Fusarium graminearum (perfect stage, Gibberella
zeae) is probably the best known of the zearalenone-producing Fusaria but
several other species such as F. moniliforme, F. equiseti, F.
sporotrichoides, and F. culmorum [1,2,3] have also been documented to
produce zearalenone. Figure 1 depicts the structures of zearalenone and
related compounds which have been reported, to date, in cultures of
zearalenone-producing isolates. Zearalenone and several other closely
related naturally produced metabolites have estrogenic and anabolic

activities in mammalian systems [4,5,6]. Urry et al. [7] accomplished the structural elucidation of zearalenone in 1966. Since then, the chemistry and biological activities of zearalenone and its derivatives have received considerable attention for two primary reasons. First, the occurrence of zearalenone in moldy feedstuffs has long been associated with various infertility and other health and production problems in agricultural animals. The most characteristic of these problems has been hyperestrogenism in swine. Other problems correlated with zearalenone contamination of feedstuffs may be due, at least in part, to the presence of other Fusarium metabolites such as some of the tricothecene mycotoxins. This reemphasizes the concept of "multiple causality" of mycotoxicoses [8]. Second, it was discovered that, in controlled doses, alpha-zearalanol, a synthetic derivative of zearalenone, exibited useful growth promoting anabolic activity in cattle and sheep [4]. Figure 2 illustrates the structural configuration of zearalanol and zearalanone.

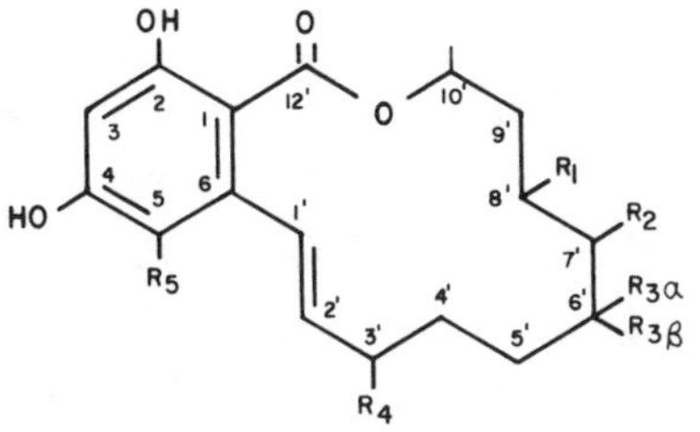

	R_1	R_2	R_3	R_4	R_5
α-Zearalenol	H_2	H_2	OH(α)	H_2	H
β-Zearalenol	H_2	H_2	OH(β)	H_2	H
Zearalenone	H_2	H_2	O	H_2	H
8'-hydroxyzearalenone	OH	H_2	O	H_2	H
6',8'-dihydroxyzearalene	OH	H_2	OH	H_2	H
3'-hydroxyzearalenone	H_2	H_2	O	OH	H
5-formylzearalenone	H_2	H_2	O	H_2	CHO
7'-dehydrozearalenone	H	H	O	H_2	H

Fig. 1. Trans configuration of zearalenone and its derivatives. (With permission)

The natural occurrence of zearalenone as a contaminant in moldy grain is very well documented by now. The list of commodities which have periodic contamination at harvest or after improper storage with zearalenone is rather extensive. Zearalenol has also been reported to occur naturally.

Hay, corn, wheat, barley, grain sorghum, and other substrates have been reported as contaminated with zearalenone [9,10,11,12]. Because grain is the major ingredient for most livestock and poultry feeds, research directed toward defining and alleviating the impact of moldy feedstuffs on agriculture has been growing steadily.

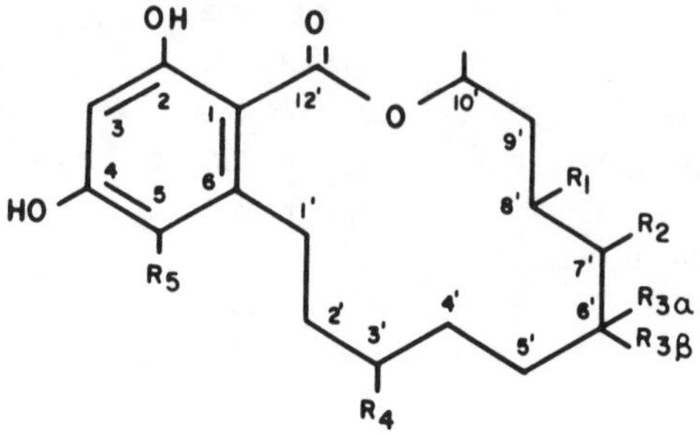

	R_1	R_2	R_3	R_4	R_5
α - Zearalanol	H_2	H_2	OH(α)	H_2	H
β - Zearalanol	H_2	H_2	OH(β)	H_2	H
Zearalanone	H_2	H_2	O	H_2	H

Fig. 2. Structure of zearalanol and zearalanone. (With permission)

The chronology of some discoveries related to zearalenone as a contaminant is interesting. Hyperestrogenism in swine had been reported earlier, but McNutt et al. (1928) [13] in the United States showed that sows fed moldy corn developed signs of hyperestrogenism. These signs included enlarged vulvas and mammary glands with a few individual animals having prolapses of the vagina and rectum. Then in 1952, McErlean in Ireland reported that swine fed barley infected with Fusarium showed similar signs [14]. In 1962, Stob et al. [6] first isolated a zearalenone-producing Fusarium from corn causing hyperestrogenism in swine. Cultures of this fungus on autoclaved corn were extracted with ethanol, and portions of the extracts were injected subcutaneously into mice; uterotropic activity was produced in the mice by this treatment, and the major active principle was partially purified and characterized. Christensen et al. (1965) [15] in Minnesota isolated and partially characterized the same active principle from cultures of an isolate of Fusarium and from samples of corn and feed associated with these outbreaks of hyperestrogenism. The Minnesota group also described a series of several similarly fluorescing compounds, with decreasing magnitudes of TLC retention factors, which were suspected of being derivatives of zearalenone because five of these exhibited estrogenic activity. Isolation and characterization of new zearalenone derivatives produced by Fusarium spp. has continued.

Von Bolliger and Tamm [16] isolated several other compounds related to zearalenone almost concurrently with the Minnesota group [17]. Some of these zearalenone derivatives were subsequently found to exhibit uterotropic activity while others seemed inactive. Relative biological activities and chemistry have been extensively reviewed [2,4,5,18]. 5-Formylzearalenone, 7'-dehydrozearalenone, 8'-hydroxyzearalenone, 6',8'-dihydroxyzearalene, 3'-hydroxyzearalenone, 6'-hydroxyzearalene (zearalenol), 4'5'-dihydroxyzearalene, cis-zearalenone, cis-zearalenol, trans-zearalanone, and zearalanol have now been reported in cultures of zearalenone-producing Fusaria [1,3,4,12,17,19,20]. The cis configuration of zearalenone and zearalenol is shown in Figure 3.

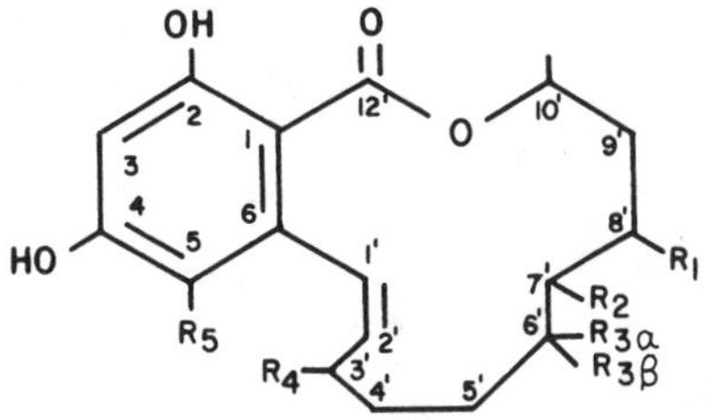

	R_1	R_2	R_3	R_4	R_5
α-Zearalenol	H_2	H_2	OH(α)	H_2	H
β-Zearalenol	H_2	H_2	OH(β)	H_2	H
Zearalenone	H_2	H_2	O	H_2	H

Fig. 3. Cis configuration of zearalenol and zearalenone. (With permission)

Steele et al. [21] showed that zearalenone arises biogenetically as an acetogenin through the acetate-malonate pathway. Later, by chemical degradation of biosynthetically labeled C-14-zearalenone, the alternate labeling pattern expected of the polyketide was confirmed [22]. Steele et al. [21] also 'trained' a zearalenone-producing strain to grow in the presence of high concentrations of zearalenone so that the metabolism of zearalenone by the producing fungus could be more easily investigated. By multivariate statistical analysis of gas chromatographic data obtained from this fungus when grown under different cultural conditions, they identified an array of prospective metabolites. The primary products of zearalenone metabolism were identified as 8'-hydroxyzearalenone and 6',8'-dihydroxyzearalene [21]. Identification of other products showed that opening and degradation of the macrocylic ring also occurred.

DISCUSSION

A discussion of the naturally produced metabolites of zearalenone-producing Fusaria is important to understanding the metabolism of zearalenone and zearalanone by animals. It is interesting that zearalenol was not detected earlier in cultures of Fusarium. Steele et al. [22] anticipated that zearalenol, because it is the reduction product of zearalenone, might be important in the biosynthesis or metabolism of zearalenone; they did not find zearalenol in this work. Richardson et al. [23] showed that C-14-alpha- and beta-zearalenol were oxidized to C-14-zearalenone by F. equiseti (F. roseum 'Gibbosum'). These two studies seem to indicate that alpha- and beta-zearalenol are precursors in the biosynthesis of zearalenone by Fusarium.

The first report of naturally produced zearalenol in Fusarium cultures was apparently that of Stipanovic and Schroeder [12]. Later, Hagler et al. [19] reported alpha-zearalenol in rice cultures of F. equiseti (F. roseum 'Gibbosum'. This isolate of F. equiseti has since been shown to produce both alpha- and beta-zearalenol under somewhat different culture conditions [1,31]. This is consistent with other reports of the natural occurrence of zearalenone and both alpha- and beta-zearalenol as natural contaminants of feedstuffs and plant material [1,24]. Bottalico et al. [1] found zearalenone and both alpha- and beta-zearalenol associated with stalk rot in corn, and Richardson et al. [3,20] found zearalenone, cis-zearalenone, zearalanone, alpha- and beta-zearalanol, and both cis and trans alpha- and beta-zearalenols in several zearalenone-producing Fusaria. The implications of having multiple contamination of feedstuffs is clear.

Mirocha et al. [25] determined the uterotropic activity of cis and trans diastereomers of both zearalenone and zearalenol (diastereomeric mixtures) in white rats. The compounds were administered either orally or topically in acetone to the freshly shaved skin of rats. Uterotropic activity was expressed as an increase in the fresh weight of rat uteri compared to the weight of controls. They found that cis-zearalenone was significantly more active than trans-zearalenone. There was no statistical difference in the activities of cis and trans-zearalenol. Also, trans-zearalenol (diastereomeric mixture) had more uterotropic activity than trans-zearalenone.

Zearalanone, (chemically produced from zearalenone) and the diastereomers of zearalanol were important compounds in the development of a commercial growth promoter for cattle and sheep. Alpha-zearalanol (zeranol) is marketed as Ralgro and is used as a subcutaneous implant in cattle and sheep. Beta-zearalanol, apparently a component of the original product, is also called taleranol. The anabolic and estrogenic activities of alpha-zearalanol are greater than that of either taleranol or zearalenone [4]. Experiments comparing alpha-zearalanol to diethylstilbestrol (DES) in cattle indicated equal anabolic activity of the two compounds; however, alpha-zearalanol had only about one three-thousandths (0.003) of the oral uterotropic activity of DES [5]. Also, there has been no tissue residue problem with Ralgro after administration in the approved fashion.

The differences in metabolism of zearalenone and by various biological systems is striking. While certain aspects of metabolism are common to several systems, some of the details are different. The metabolism of zearalenone by: 1) Fusarium graminearum [22], 2) the yeast Candida tropicalis [26], 3) rumen microorganisms [27], 4) laying hens [28], 5) Fisher rats [4,29], 6) dairy cattle, 7) swine, 8) rabbits, 9) non-human primates, 10) Guinea pigs, and 11) man [30] has been investigated. Oversimplified, with the exception of Fusarium, the metabolism of zearalenone in these biological systems entails reduction of the 6' keto functionality to the corresponding hydroxyl. In animals, zearalenone and zearalenol are rapidly conjugated with glucuronic acid and to a lesser extent with sulfate. Excretion is via urine and feces. Bilary conjugates in the gut probably result in enterohepatic circulation of the compounds [31].

In mammalian systems, zearalenol is the primary metabolite of zearalenone with proportions of alpha - to beta - varying among species. The 1'-2' double bond of zearalenone seems to be biologically stable to the metabolic apparatus of animal systems. No reductions of this bond or double bond introductions at this position have been reported from animal metabolism studies. In urinary excretion by most animals, zearalenone and zearalenol are conjugates giving more solubility in water. Hidy et al. [4] orally dosed rats with carbon-14 labelled zearalenone and found 70-80% excreted in the feces and 20-30% in the urine. Zearalenol was found in this and other studies to be the major metabolite. They also found the ratio of zearalenol:zearalenone in sheep feces to be 2:1. The in vivo metabolism of zearalenone in the urine of the cow, the pig, the rabbit, the rat, and man was studied by Mirocha et al. [30]. In general, the major products were free and glucuronide conjugates of zearalenone, alpha-zearalenol, and beta-zearalenol. In most species, the amount of zearalenone and alpha-zearalenol in the urine was much greater than the amount of beta-zearalenol. The cow showed the highest proportion of beta-zearalenol in urine, 51%, and small amounts of sulfate conjugates of zearalenone and beta-zearalenol were found in the milk. Of particular interest is man, where most of the zearalenone was excreted in 24 hr in the urine as the glucuronide conjugate of alpha-zearalenol. Dailey et al. [28] examined distribution of C-14 zearalenone in laying hens and found that ca. 94% of the radioactivity administered orally was excreted within 72 hr. About 33% of the dose was eliminated as zearalenone and another third as a more polar metabolite, possibly zearalenol. Egg yolks contained radioactivity accounting for the equivalent of 2 µg/g of zearalenone, while edible muscle did not contain major amounts of radioactivity.

Data obtained in an in vitro rat liver assay [32] using liver homogenates, microsomes, and isolated hepatocytes indicates two pathways for the metabolism of zearalenone. One pathway was the conjugation of zearalenone with glucuronic acid (added as uridine diphosphate glucuronic acid). The second reaction was thought to be catalyzed by a NADH-dependent hydroxysteroid dehydrogenase that later proved to be 3-alpha-hydroxysteroid dehydrogenase [33,34] and involved the reduction of zearalenone to alpha-zearalenol. Tashiro et al. [29] purified an enzyme responsible for the reduction of zearalenone to alpha-zearalenol which they called zearalenone dehydrogenase. The molecular weight of the enzyme was greater than 200,000 and the activity was dependent on the prescence of the reduced cofactors NADPH or NADH. Tashiro et al. [35] obtained data indicating probable conversion of alpha-zearalenone to zearalenone and beta-zearalenol; however, the enzymatic activity responsible was not described.

In an in vitro assay involving bovine, swine, and goats, Kiessing et al. [36] found that bovine liver homogenates had the least ability to form conjugated forms of zearalenone, while swine and goats had the greatest ability to do so. When Olsen and Kiessling [37] investigated the relative abilities of fractionated liver homogenates from female pigs, goats, sheep, hens, and cows to convert zearalenone to zearalenol, they found rather striking differences. Microsomes of the female pig and the goat converted zearalenone into both alpha-and beta-zearalenol while those of the cow and hen produced alpha-zearalenol. These species produced alpha- and beta-zearalenol in the cytosols when NADPH was the added cofactor. Moreover, the incubation of zearalenone with added NADPH resulted in the greatest conversion to alpha-zearalenol.

The metabolism of zearalenone by Candida tropicalis was studied because the yeast had been shown to cause disappearance of zearalenone from liquid culture media. Palyusik et al. [26] then found that Candida tropicalis was able to reduce about 80% of the added zearalenone to zearalenol yielding about 70% beta-zearalenol and about 10% alpha-zearalenol. 20% of the zearalenone remained unchanged.

The metabolism of zearalenone by rumen fluid, rumen protozoa, and rumen bacteria of bovine and sheep was studied by Kiessling, et al. [27]. They found that the protoza in intact rumen fluid quickly converted zearalenone to alpha-zearalenol and beta-zearalenol, however, only small amounts of beta-zearalenol were detected. Rumen bacteria had almost no zearalenone-reducing activity. There were only slight differences in the reducing activity of rumen fluid of sheep as compared to cows. These data and the results of Mirocha et al. [30] imply extensive conversion of alpha-zearalenol to zearalenone, with subsequent reduction to alpha- and beta-zearalenol, may occur.

The metabolism and excretion of zearalanone and zearalanol was reviewed by Migdalof et al. [31]. This metabolism of in animal systems follows essentially the same pattern as the metabolism of zearalenone and zearalenol. The keto function of zearalanone is partially reduced to the diastereomeric alcohols and these, along with the intact original compound, are conjugated to glucuronic acid or, to a lesser extent, converted to sulfates for excretion. Animal systems were apparently able to oxidize alpha-zearalenol to zearalanone, as beta-zearalanol was also detected as a metabolite of alpha-zearalanol. The details of this metabolism are presently unknown, but it was postulated that the beta-zearalanol arose through oxidation of alpha-zearalanol followed by reduction to alpha- and beta-zearalanol [31].

Olsen and Kiessling [37] concluded that there were two likely explanations for the estrogenic activity of zearalenone. First is the ability of zearalenone to bind with estrogen receptors [38,39]. Kaing et al. [38] demonstrated that zearalenone and some of its derivatives have a high affinity for and compete with estradiol-17-beta for estrogen binding sites. Secondly, available data as yet do not eliminate the possibility of disruption of hormone metabolism [34,40]. Relative estrogenicity of estradiol and zearalenone however, places zearalenone at approximately 400-fold less estrogenic than estradiol. Within the zearalenone series, there is a wide range of relative activities. Alpha-zearalenol is 3 to 4 times more estrogenic than zearalenone [19]. However, beta-zearalenol is less estrogenic than zearalenone [4].

The estrogenic activity of this series of compounds apparently is dependent on possession of three dimensional configuration which mimics endogenous estrogens such as estradiol-17-beta to the extent that they will have a reasonable affinity for the receptors. Variation in magnitude of estrogenic activities among derivatives implies configurations resulting in greater or lesser affinities for these binding sites and comparative experiments have supported this hypothesis.

SUMMARY

The metabolism of zearalenone has been extensively investigated in several animal systems both in vivo and in vitro. The magnitude of affinity of zearalenone and its derivatives for binding sites, overall, has given an excellent correlation with relative estrogenicity. The ranking of the compounds by increasing strenytn of binding affinities for estrogen receptor proteins in vitro coincides reasonably with ranking the compounds by uterotropic response in vivo.

Much of a dose of zearalenone is modified by the animal. In vivo and in vitro experiments again have been mutually supportive. Zearalenol is the major metabolite of zearalenone produced in the species tested to date. There are interesting and probably important differences in the details of this modification of zearalenone to zearalenol. All species tested seem to produce alpha-zearalenol as the major zearalenone metabolite. This could be considered a metabolic activation because alpha-zearalenol is nearly four-fold more estrogenic than zearalenone. There are considerable species differences in the details of conjugation of zearalenone and zearalenol to glucuronic acid and in patterns of excretion. Most of zearalenone and zearalenol are excreted in the urine and feces of animals. Many of the details of the metabolism of these compounds await further research. The ratios of metabolites as they relate to estrogenic activity may be important. Differences in species sensitivity and modes of action may, in the future, be rationalized on this basis.

REFERENCES

1. Bottalico, A., A. Visconti, A. Logrieco, M. Solfrizzo, and C. J. Mirocha, Appl. Environ. Microbiol. 49, 547-551 (1985).
2. Mirocha, C. J. and C. M. Christensen, in: Mycotoxins, I.F.H. Purchase, ed. (Elsevier, Amsterdam 1974) pp. 129-148.
3. Richardson, K. E., W. M. Hagler, Jr., and C. J. Mirocha, J. Ag. Food Chem., (In press).
4. Hidy, P. H., R. S. Baldwin, R. L. Greasham, C. L. Keith, and J. R. McMullen, Adv. Appl. Microbiol. 22, 59-82 (1977).
5. Hurd, R. N. in: Mycotoxins In Human and Animal Health, C. M. Hesseltine, J. V. Rodricks, and M. A. Mehlman, eds. (Pathotox, Park Forest South, IL. 1977) pp. 379-391.
6. Stob, M., R. S. Baldwin, J. Tuite, F. N. Andrews, and K. G. Gillette, Nature 196, 1318 (1962).
7. Urry, W. H., H. L. Wehrmeister, E. B. Hodge, and P. H. Hidy, Tetrahedron Letters 27, 3100-3114 (1966).
8. Mirocha, C. J., personal communication.

9. McMillian, W. W., D. M. Wilson, C. J. Mirocha, and N. W. Widstrom, Cereal Chem. 60, 226-227 (1983).
10. Mirocha, C. J., J. Harrison, A. A. Nichols, and M. McClintock, Appl. Microbiol. 16, 797-798 (1968).
11. Pathre, S. V., and C. J. Mirocha in: Estrogens in the Environment, J. A. McLachlan, ed. (Elsevier, North Holland 1979) pp. 265-278.
12. Stipanovic, R. D., and H. W. Schroeder, Mycopathologia 57, 77-78 (1975).
13. McNutt, S. H., P. Purwin, and C. Murray, J. Am. Vet. Med. Assoc. 73, 484 (1928).
14. McErlean, B. A., Vet. Record 64, 539 (1952).
15. Christenson, C. M., G. H. Nelson, and C. J. Mirocha, Appl. Microb. 13, 653-659 (1965).
16. von Bolliger, G., and Ch. Tamm, Helv. Chim. Acta 55, 3030-3048 (1972).
17. Jackson, R. A., S. W. Fenton, C. J. Mirocha, and G. Davis, J. Agric. Food Chem. 22, 1015-1019 (1974).
18. Shipchandler, M. T., Heterocycles 3, 471-520 (1975).
19. Hagler, W. M., C. J. Mirocha, S. V. Pathre and J. C. Behrens, Appl. Environ. Microbiol. 37, 849-853 (1979).
20. Richardson, K. E., W. M. Hagler, Jr., and C. J. Mirocha, Assoc. Offic. Anal. Chem. Abstr. 135, 14 (1984).
21. Steele, J. A., J. R. Lieberman, and C. J. Mirocha, Can. J. Microbiol. 20 531-534 (1974).
22. Steele, J. A., C. J. Mirocha, and S. V. Pathre, J. Agric. Food Chem. 24, 89-97 (1976).
23. Richardson, K. E., W. M. Hagler, Jr., and P. B. Hamilton, Appl. Environ. Microbiol. 47, 1206-1209 (1984).
24. Mirocha, C. J., B. Schauerhamer, C. M. Christensen, and T. Kommedahl, Appl. Environ. Microbiol 38, 3, 557-558 (1979).
25. Mirocha, C. J., S. V. Pathre, J. Behrens, and B. Schauerhamer, Appl. Environ. Microbiol. 35 986-987 (1978).
26. Palyusik, M., W. M. Hagler, Jr., L. Horvath, and C. J. Mirocha, Acta Vet. Acad. Sci. Hung. 28, 2, 159-166 (1980).
27. Kiessling, K. H., H. Pettersson, K. Sandholm, and M. Olsen, Appl. Environ. Microbiol. 37, 849-853 (1984).
28. Dailey, R. E., R. E. Reese, and E. A. Brouwer, J. Ag. Food Chem. 28, 286-291 (1980).
29. Tashiro, F., N. Nishimura, and Y. Ueno, Maikotokishin (Proc. Jap. Assoc. Mycotoxicol., Tokoyo) 11, 37-40 (1980).
30. Mirocha, C. J., S. V. Pathre and T. S. Robison, Food Cosmet. Toxicol. 19, 25-30 (1981).
31. Migdalof, B. H., H. A. Dugger, J. G. Heider, R. A. Coombs, and M. K. Terry, Xenobiotica 13, 209-221 (1984).
32. Kiessling, K. H. and H. Pettersson, Acta Pharmacol. et Toxicol. 43, 285-290 (1978).
33. Olsen, M., H. Pettersson, K. H. Kiessling, Toxicon 17, 134 (1979).
34. Olsen, M., H. Pettersson, and K. H. Kiessling, Acta Pharmacol. et Toxicol. 48, 157-161 (1981).
35. Tashiro, F., A. Shibata, N. Nishimura, and Y. Ueno, J. Biochem. 93, 1557-1566 (1983).
36. Kiessling, K. H., H. Pettersson, K. Tideman, and I. L. Andersson, Proceedings of the IV International IUPAC Symposium on Mycotoxins and Phycotoxins (In press).
37. Olsen, M. and K. H. Kiessling, Acta Pharmacol. et Toxicol. 52, 287-291 (1983).
38. Kiang, D. T., B. J. Kennedy, S. V. Pathre, and C. J. Mirocha, Cancer Res. 38, 3611-3615 (1978).
39. Tashiro, F., Y. Kawabata, M. Naoi, and Y. Ueno in: Medical Mycology, Zbl. Bakt. Suppl. 8, Preusser, ed. (Gustav Fiscker Verlag 1980) pp. 311-320.
40. James, L. J. and T. K. Smith, J. Anim. Sci. 55, 110-118 (1982).

248

DISCUSSION

NAFTOLIN: What is the function of fungal estrogens?

HAGLER: The usefulness of these compounds to the fungus is, as is the case with most fungal secondary metabolites, unknown. However, there are some data which suggest that zearalenone may play a role in the sexual reproduction of the fungus.

NAFTOLIN: Is the localization reported for zearalenone in the "early pregnant rat placenta" in the trophoblast or yolk sac?

HAGLER: I'm sorry, I don't remember.

MEYERS: The stereochemistry of α- versus β-zearalenols is similar enough that I believe differentiation between them by spectrometric means would be very difficult, let alone determining the absolute characterization of their α- versus β-stereochemistry by spectrometric means. How did you differentiate between these two isomers?

HAGLER: The absolute configurations for these diastereomers were established by X-ray crystallography. Fortunately, separation of α- and β-zearalenols is easy and convenient by TLC, GLC, and HPLC. Therefore, each can be quantitatively determined in the presence of the other at the nanogram level. Absorbance and fluorescence are very useful for these compounds, and confirmation typically employs capillary GC/MS.

MEYERS: How certain are you of the precision of your determinations and, therefore, of the comparison of their estrogenic activity?

HAGLER: Purification is achieved by these chromatographic means or by fractional crystallization. Because very pure preparations of each of these compounds are easy to handle, comparison of activities with precision and accuracy is routine.

Developmental Biology of Estrogens

Published 1985 by Elsevier Science Publishing Co., Inc.
Estrogens in the Environment, John A. McLachlan, Editor

DEVELOPMENTAL BIOLOGY OF ESTROGENS: INTRODUCTORY COMMENTS

JOHN A. MCLACHLAN
Laboratory of Reproductive and Developmental Toxicology, National
Institute of Environmental Health Sciences, National Institutes of
Health, Research Triangle Park, North Carolina 27709

Estrogens are associated with the differentiation and proliferation
of their target tissues. These processes are usually reversible in the
tissues of mature individuals. In younger animals, changes associated
with estrogens may persist and, in some cases, appear to be irreversible.
Thus, aspects of sex differentiation and genital tract or mammary gland
development may be influenced by estrogens early in life.

These considerations raise several questions to be answered. For
example:

Are the estrogen-response mechanisms the same in fetal or immature
tissues as they are in differentiated tissues? Are there estrogen receptors and are they physically the same? Do developing tissues respond to
estrogens like adult tissues or are there unique sets of differentiation-
specific responses? Can mature genes be stimulated in immature cells?

Are the metabolic patterns for estrogens (both endogenous and exogenous) the same in young and old individuals? Are prohormones activated
in immature tissues?

Does the relative distribution of environmental estrogens within the
body or organ change over time? Are exogenous estrogenic compounds
excreted more slowly early in life?

What are the threshold levels of hormone required for estrogenic stimulation of developing target tissues?

Certainly the answers to this small subset of research questions
should start to provide the information necessary for understanding the
role, both normal and abnormal, for estrogens in developing systems.

252

BIOLOGICAL EFFECTS OF ESTROGENS AND ANTIESTROGENS IN THE FETUS
AND NEWBORNS

Jorge R. PASQUALINI, Charlotte SUMIDA and Nora GIAMBIAGI
C.N.R.S. Steroid Hormone Research Unit,
Foundation for Hormone Research, 26 Boulevard Brune,
75014 Paris, France

I. INTRODUCTION

It is generally accepted that the biological effects of
steroid hormones are mediated by specific, high affinity receptor proteins. In different model systems of various animal species a correlation has been observed between an increase and
long-term retention in the specific nuclear binding of the hormone and the biological response(s). The presence of estrogen
receptors in the reproductive organs has been widely established
but these receptors are also found in non-classical target
tissues such as : kidney, lung, liver, spleen and thymus. Most
of the studies on receptors and the mechanism of action of
steroid hormones were carried out in immature or adult animals.
In 1971, in this laboratory, the presence of specific binding
for steroid hormones in the fetal compartment of guinea pigs
was observed for estradiol in the fetal brain [1] and for aldo-
sterone in the fetal kidney [2]. At present, much information
has been accumulated in different animal species on the existence of steroid hormone receptors in the fetal and placental
compartments, as well as the correlation of these receptors
with the biological effects.

Triphenylethylene derived substances (e.g. : MER 25, clomiphene, CI 628, Nafoxidine, Tamoxifen) are extensively used as
antiestrogens. In the last few years, Tamoxifen, due to its
very limited side effects, has been widely used in the treatment of breast cancer, particularly during the post-menopausal
period [3,4]. However, it has been observed that these triphenylethylene derivatives can act as agonists or partial agonists during the perinatal periods [5-8].

We summarize here different aspects of the action of
estrogens and antiestrogens during the fetal and neonatal
periods.

II. ESTROGEN AND PROGESTERONE RECEPTORS IN THE FETAL COMPARTMENT

A) Physico-chemical Characteristics of Estrogen (ER) and
Progesterone (PR) Receptors

For many years the guinea pig fetus has been used as a
model system for the study of receptors, the mechanism of
action and the biological responses of steroid hormones during
fetal life. After the first demonstration that receptors of
estrogens were present in the whole fetal brain of this species,
these receptors were also found in other fetal tissues which include : uterus, lung, kidney, testis, thymus, hypothalamus, hypophysis [9-13] and recently in the fetal vagina [14]. The
physico-chemical properties of ER are similar in the various
fetal tissues but since in the fetal uterus the number of specific binding sites is 10-300 times higher than in the other
fetal tissues (see Section II, B) this tissue was particularly
used for the studies of the different properties of the interaction of the hormone with the receptor protein. Table I summarizes the physico-chemical characteristics of the estrogen receptor in the fetal and neonatal uterus of the guinea pig.

Most of the estrogen receptor (90-95%) in the fetal
uterus of guinea pig is present in the cytosol and about 80% is
not occupied by endogenous estrogens [15]. The quantitative
evaluation of the concentration of endogenous estrogens in the
fetal uterine tissue showed values which correspond to the
levels of the receptor sites occupied by the hormone [22].

Specific binding sites for progesterone have been detected in the fetal uterus and ovary of this animal species [23,
24]. At the end of gestation, the number of specific binding
sites for progesterone in the fetal uterus is 136 ± 35 (SD)
fmoles/mg protein and in the fetal ovary 72 ± 12 fmoles/mg protein.

During gestation in the guinea pig, progesterone binds
with high affinity to a specific plasma protein (Progesterone
Binding Globulin : PBG) which was discovered by Diamond et al.
in 1969 [25] ; this protein was also detected in fetal plasma
[26]. Since the concentration of PBG is very high : 1-1.5 g/liter
in maternal plasma and 1-3 mg/liter in fetal plasma, it is important to differentiate between the physico-chemical characteristics of the PBG-progesterone complex and the progesterone-

TABLE I. Physico-chemical properties of the estrogen receptor in the fetal and newborn uteri of the guinea pig.

		Fetus (55-65 days)	Newborn (6 days)
Number of sites (Total : occupied + non-occupied)	pmoles/mg protein	1-2	0.4-0.9
	pmoles/mg DNA	12-19	5-6
	pmoles/g tissue	60-100	29-39
	pmoles/uterus	4-7	4-7
	sites/cell	43,000-67,000	18,000-22,000
Dissociation constant (K_d : x 10^{-9}M, 4°C)		0.13-0.4	0.3
Association rate constant k_{+1} (x 10^5 $M^{-1}sec^{-1}$) 4°C		0-6	-
Dissociation rate constant k_{-1} (x 10^{-4} sec^{-1}) 4°C		1-9	2-6
Sedimentation coefficient	low salt :	8S	8S
	high salt :	4S	4S
Isoelectric point		6.1-6.2	-
Ammonium sulfate precipitation		36%	-
Temperature effect		Thermolabile	Thermolabile
Immunorecognition		Binds specifically to monoclonal antibody against human ER	

Data from references : 11, 13, 15-21.

TABLE II. Comparative physico-chemical properties of the specific binding of ^{3}H-progesterone (^{3}H-P) and ^{3}H-R5020 in fetal uterine cytosol and in the fetal plasma of guinea pig.

	Fetal uterus		Fetal plasma	
	^{3}H-P	^{3}H-R5020	^{3}H-P	^{3}H-R5020
Dissociation constant K_d (x 10^{-9}) 4°C	3.3 ± 1.7	0.7 ± 0.3	0.88 ± 0.35	No specific binding
Sedimentation coefficient	6-7 ; 4	6-7 ; 4	4.6	-
Isoelectric point	5-5.5	-	<3	-
Thermal stability[a]	Thermolabile	Thermolabile	Thermolabile	No specific binding

[a]Aliquots of fetal uterine cytosol fraction or diluted fetal plasma (1/10-1/50 v/v) were preheated for 1h at 37°C in the absence of the hormone and then reincubated with ^{3}H-progesterone or ^{3}H-R5020 (4 x 10^{-9}M) with or without a 100-fold excess of the unlabeled steroids to measure the number of specific binding sites after adsorbing the unbound radioactive steroids with dextran charcoal.
From references 24 and 27.

receptor complex. Table II summarizes these data. It is to be remarked that in the cytosol or nuclear fraction of the fetal uterus only binding with the characteristics of the progesterone receptor is present and PBG is not detectable in the tissue.

B) The Ontogeny of Estrogen and Progesterone Receptors in the Uterus and Other Tissues of the Guinea pig

     In the fetal guinea pig, estrogen receptors can be detected relatively early in development. As seen in Figure 1, the fetal uterus, testis and thymus already contain significant amounts of receptors at least by 34 to 35 days of gestation (mid-gestation in this animal species). In the uterus, lung, kidney and thymus, receptor concentrations tend to increase during fetal development and decline after birth in the uterus, kidney and thymus [9-11].

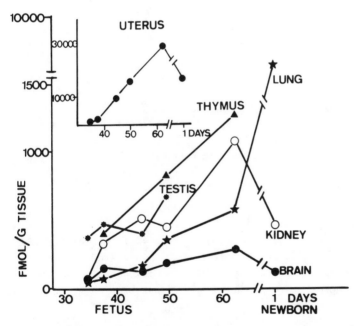

FIG. 1. Ontogeny of estrogen receptors in the uterus and other organs of the guinea pig fetus and newborn.
Cell suspensions of 1 g of tissue were incubated with 5×10^{-8}M ^{3}H-estradiol (± a 300-fold excess of unlabeled estradiol) at 37°C for 15 min. The values represent the sum of cytosol and nuclear binding. The uterus is indicated in the inset.

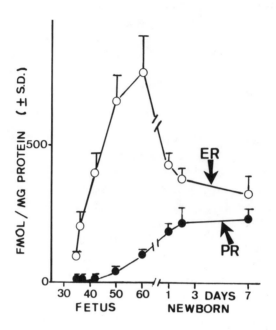

FIG. 2. Ontogeny of estrogen and progesterone receptors in
fetal and neonatal guinea pig uterus.
Receptor binding was measured by incubating uterine cytosol
with 4×10^{-9}M ^{3}H-estradiol or ^{3}H-progesterone ($\pm$ a 100-fold
molar excess of unlabeled steroid) at 4°C for 4h. Bound and unbound radioactivity was separated with dextran-coated charcoal.

  In the fetal uterus progesterone receptors only appear
10-15 days after the estrogen receptor and they rise until after
birth, parallel with the decline in estrogen receptor (Fig. 2).
  The delay in the appearance of the PR suggests that in
the fetus its control depends on the action of estrogens (and/
or ER), as established in immature or adult animals [28,29].
Experiments in which estradiol was administered to pregnant
guinea pigs confirmed that this control mechanism of progesterone receptor synthesis also operates in the fetal compartment
(see Section III, A).

C) Immunorecognition of the Fetal Estrogen Receptor by a Monoclonal Antibody

  Using a monoclonal antibody (D547Spγ) developed against

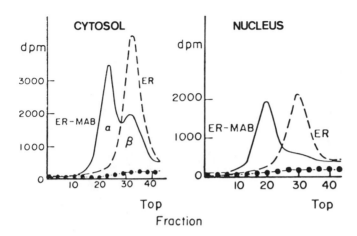

FIG. 3. Sucrose density gradients of the cytosol and nuclear estrogen receptor of fetal guinea pig uterus.
Aliquots of cytosol were incubated with 10^{-8}M [^{3}H]-E$_2$ and with (——) or without (- -) the monoclonal antibody D547Spγ for 18h at 4°C. Minced uteri were incubated with 5×10^{-8}M [^{3}H]-E$_2$ for 1h at 30°C and then, after homogenization and subcellular fractionation, the 0.6 M KCl nuclear extract was incubated with (——) or without (- -) the antibody for 18h at 4°C. Samples were centrifuged through 10-30% w/v sucrose - 0.4 M KCl gradients for 105 min at 400,000 g using a vertical rotor VTi 65. Nonspecific binding ($\cdot$ $\cdot$) was determined by adding a 100-fold excess of unlabeled estradiol.

the estrogen receptor from the MCF-7 human breast cancer line [30], two forms of the estrogen-receptor complex, with different immunological characteristics, were observed in the cytosol fraction of fetal guinea pig uterus. One of them (α Form) was recognized by the antibody, increasing its sedimentation coefficient in high-salt sucrose gradient (10-30% w/v sucrose, 0.4 M KCl) from 4.5S to 7.4S ; the other (β Form), not recognized by the antibody, sedimented at 4.5S. In contrast, only one form, which could be totally bound to the antibody, was found in the nucleus (Fig. 3) [20].

These two forms of the estrogen receptor were also found in uterine cytosol from newborn and immature animals, even if the receptor concentration was sharply decreased after birth [21].

Dynamic studies of the "in vitro" translocation of the estradiol receptor complex to the nucleus have shown that the α Form disappeared rapidly from the cytosol fraction while the

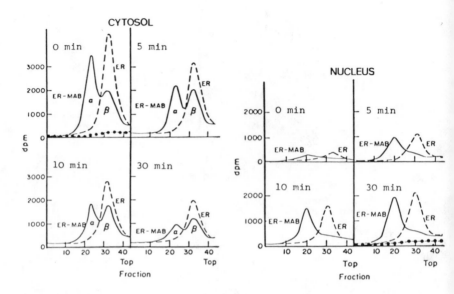

FIG. 4. Sucrose density gradients of the cytosol and nuclear fractions of fetal guinea pig uterus during the "in vitro" translocation of the cytosol estrogen receptor to the nucleus. Aliquots of cytosol were incubated with $10^{-8}M$ [^3H]-E_2 for 2h at 4°C then added to the nuclear suspension and reincubated for different times at 25°C. Tubes were centrifuged and aliquots of cytosol and of the 0.6 M KCl nuclear extract were incubated with (——) or without (--) the monoclonal antibody D547Spγ for 18h at 4°C. Samples were centrifuged through 10-30% w/v sucrose - 0.4 M KCl gradients for 105 min at 400,000 g using a vertical rotor VTi 65. Non-specific binding (· ·) was determined by adding a 100-fold excess of unlabeled estradiol.

β Form was only slightly affected when cytosol was incubated with nuclei at 25°C. The estrogen receptor found in the nuclear extract was always recognized by the antibody (Fig. 4) [21].

Further studies of the cytosol estrogen receptor showed that the α Form was not detectable in short (2-3h) preparations of the estradiol-receptor complex ; all the receptor was initially found as the β Form. A transformation of the β Form to the α Form was induced by different factors such as time (20h, 4°C), temperature (15 min, 25°C) and high ionic strength (0.4 M KCl), which also induced estrogen receptor activation, determined by an increase in its binding to nuclei and DNA cellulose.

On the other hand, sodium molybdate inhibited both the receptor activation and the transformation to the α Form induced by time and temperature [31].

The correlation observed between the appearance of the α Form and the activation of the receptor together with the different behavior of the α and β Forms in the translocation process suggest that the α Form, which is recognized by the monoclonal antibody, is the activated form of the estrogen receptor of fetal uterus of guinea pig.

III. BIOLOGICAL RESPONSES TO DIFFERENT ESTROGENS AND PROGESTE-
RONE IN THE UTERUS OF THE FETUS AND NEWBORN

A) Estrogens

In the fetal guinea pig uterus, progesterone receptors are detectable only 10 to 15 days after the appearance of estrogen receptors, suggesting responsiveness to endogenous estrogens by this fetal organ since the progesterone receptor is known to be an estrogen-inducible protein. Two parameters of estrogen action were studied more particularly in response to the exogenous administration of estrogen. As shown in Figure 5A, fetal uterine wet weight increases by 70% after 3 daily injections of 1 mg estradiol/kg body weight to the mother and 6 daily injections lead to a 3-fold increase in weight [19]. The uterotrophic effect does not depend on fetal age [32] but it develops further after birth. By 6 days after birth, the uterus responds with a 2.75-fold increase in weight to 3 daily injections of estradiol [33].

Figure 5B shows that progesterone receptor concentrations can be increased by as much as 10 times by estradiol treatment. Progesterone receptor can even be induced by estradiol at ∿40 days of gestation when its concentration is otherwise negligible. Unlike the uterotrophic response, the degree of sensitivity of this parameter to estradiol is much higher in the fetus than in the newborn [34,35].

Progesterone receptor can also be induced in organ culture of explants of fetal uterus but its concentration rises spontaneously in the absence of any added estrogen or other steroid [36].

260

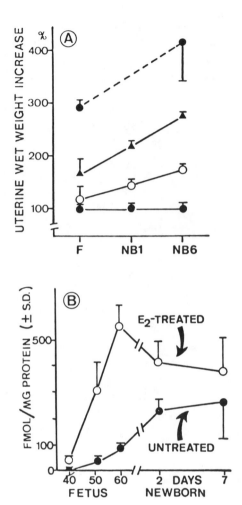

FIG. 5. Uterotrophic and progesterone receptor responses to
estradiol in fetal and neonatal guinea pig uterus.
Pregnant guinea pigs were injected with 1 mg estradiol/kg body
weight. After birth animals received 1-100 μg estradiol.
A. Uterine weight gain is expressed as a percent of weights of
untreated animals assigned the value of 100%.
F : fetuses ; NB1 : one-day-old newborns ; NB6 : 6-day-old newborns ; ●-● : untreated animals ; O-O : single injection ;
▲-▲ : 3 daily injections ; ●---●: 6 daily injections.
B. Progesterone receptor binding was measured in the cytosol
fraction by incubation with 4 nM ³H-progesterone (± a 100-fold
molar excess of unlabeled progesterone) at 4°C for 18h. Fetuses
received 3 daily injections. Newborns received a single injection.

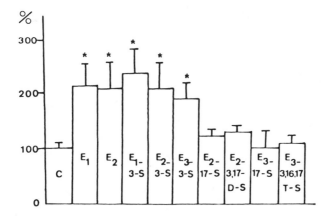

FIG. 6. Effect of seven different estrogen sulfates, as well
as unconjugated estrone and estradiol on the weight of the fetal
uterus of guinea pig.
Pregnant guinea pigs (55-65 days of gestation) were injected
subcutaneously with 1 mg/kg/day of estrone (E_1), estradiol (E_2)
or with 1.4-2.1 mg/kg/day of the following sulfates : estrone-
3-sulfate (E_1-3-S), estradiol-3-sulfate (E_2-3-S), estriol-3-
sulfate (E_3-3-S), estradiol-17-sulfate (E_2-17-S), estriol-17-
sulfate (E_3-17-S), estradiol-3,17-disulfate (E_2-3,17-DS),
estriol-3,16,17-trisulfate (E_3-3,16,17-TS) (dissolved in 20%
v/v ethanol-saline solution) for 3 days and sacrificed on day 4.
Uteri were excised, stripped of adhering fat and weighed.
Control (C) animals received the vehicle alone. Values represent the mean ± S.D. of 5-21 determinations.
*$p < 0.001$ (p calculated versus non-treated animals).

The uterotrophic response has been shown to be correlated with long-term retention of significant quantities of estrogen receptor in the nucleus in the fetal guinea pig uterus
but progesterone receptor stimulation could not be clearly related to the subcellular distribution of the estrogen receptor
[19]. From these observations and the ontogenetic studies of
these two responses, we have concluded that these parameters
are dissociated from one another and that the increase in progesterone receptor in the fetal uterus is controlled by other
multiform factors, some of which may be peculiar to the fetus.

B) Effects of Different Estrogen Sulfates in the Fetal and Newborn Uteri

Estrogen sulfates represent quantitatively one of the

most important forms of estrogens circulating in the fetal compartment of humans and in other mammalian species such as the cow, sheep, guinea pig and Rhesus monkey. In the fetal compartment of the guinea pig, sulfokinase activity is very intense. It was demonstrated that 30 min after s.c. injection of radioactive estradiol "in vivo" and "in situ" to the fetus, most of the radioactivity (50-70%) circulating in the fetal plasma was found to be estrone and estradiol sulfates [37]. An attractive hypothesis has been put forward whereby these sulfates serve to protect the fetus from the biological action of the hormone or that they can act as a pre-hormone which becomes active after hydrolysis.

Figure 6 shows the effect on fetal uterine weight of the administration of three estrogen sulfates in C_3 (estrone-3-sulfate, estradiol-3-sulfate and estriol-3-sulfate) and of four estrogen sulfates in C_{17} (estradiol-17-sulfate, estradiol-3,17-disulfate, estriol-17-sulfate and estriol-3,16,17-trisulfate) after 3 consecutive days of treatment to the pregnant guinea pig (55-65 days of gestation). Only the C_3 sulfates provoked a significant uterotrophic effect in the fetal uterus. Similarly, this type of sulfate stimulated (7-10 times) the number of specific progesterone binding sites (Table III) [38].

The radioimmunoassay of the unconjugated and conjugated estrogens in the fetal plasma after the different treatments [38] indicated that : 1) there was a transplacental transfer of both C_3 and C_{17} estrogen sulfates from the mother to the fetus ; 2) the estrogens with the sulfate in the C_3 position were partially hydrolysed ; 3) very little or no hydrolysis was found in the treatment with the estrogen-17-sulfates. In conclusion, estrogen-3-sulfates can be used as pre-hormones which become active after hydrolysis or they can serve as protective or reserve material of the active hormone.

C) Progesterone as an Antiestrogen in the Fetus and Newborn

In the fetal guinea pig uterus, progesterone inhibits the estrogen-induced increase in wet weight (Fig. 7A) and diminishes the concentration of its own receptor (Fig. 7B). Progesterone appears to act in the fetus by rapidly clearing the estrogen receptor from the nucleus [39] and has no effect on

TABLE III. Effect of seven different sulfates, as well as of
unconjugated estradiol and estrone on the concentration of the
specific binding sites of progesterone in the fetal uterus of
guinea pig.

| | pmoles/mg DNA | |
	Cytosol	Nucleus
Control (non-treated)	1.97 ± 0.67	0.10 ± 0.07
Estrone-3-sulfate	15.20 ± 2.90^{a}	0.71 ± 0.25^{a}
Estradiol-3-sulfate	16.50 ± 7.00^{a}	1.39 ± 0.60^{a}
Estriol-3-sulfate	18.40 ± 3.34^{a}	1.64 ± 0.56^{a}
Estradiol-17-sulfate	1.45 ± 0.60	0.09 ± 0.05
Estriol-17-sulfate	2.27 ± 0.18	0.19 ± 0.08
Estradiol-3,17-disulfate	1.96 ± 0.91	0.03 ± 0.01
Estradiol-3,16,17-trisulfate	1.85 ± 0.60	ND
Estrone	18.10 ± 3.50^{a}	0.75 ± 0.22^{a}
Estradiol	18.90 ± 2.50^{a}	1.00 ± 0.14^{a}

$^{a}P < 0.001$ (P calculated vs non-treated animals).
Pregnant guinea pigs (55-65 days of gestation) were injected
with 1.4-2.1 mg/kg/day of the different estrogen sulfates or
with 1 mg/kg/day of unconjugated estrone or estradiol for 3
consecutive days and sacrificed on day 4. Fetal uteri were
separated and progesterone receptors were measured in cytosol
and nuclear fraction (0.6 M KCl). Aliquots of these fractions
were incubated with [³H]-R5020 (5 x 10⁻⁹M) with or without a
100-fold molar excess of non-labeled R5020 for 14h at 4°C.
Bound and unbound steroids were separated with dextran-coated
charcoal mixture and specific [³H]-R5020 binding was calculated
by the difference between the total and non-saturable binding.
The values represent the mean ±SD of 5-11 determinations.
Data from ref. 38.

the replenishment of cytosol estrogen receptor [40]. Progesterone also antagonizes both of these estrogen responses in the
newborn uterus but, unlike the fetal uterus, cytosol estrogen
receptor replenishment is impaired [41].

Progesterone decreases the concentration of its own
receptor even under organ culture conditions. As long as progesterone is present in the culture medium, the spontaneous rise
in progesterone receptor does not occur. When progesterone is
removed, the fetal uterine explants are again capable of synthesizing progesterone receptor in high amounts [42].

IV. SPECIFIC BINDING AND BIOLOGICAL RESPONSES OF ANTIESTROGEN
    IN THE FETAL AND NEWBORN UTERI OF THE GUINEA PIG

The interaction of [³H]-tamoxifen with specific macro-

264

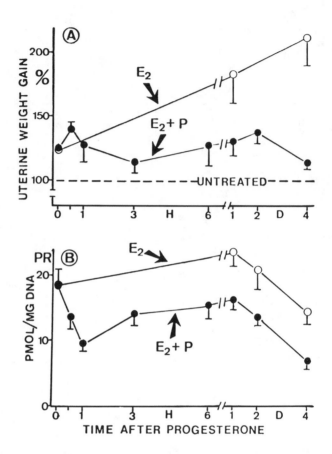

FIG. 7. Antagonistic effects of progesterone in the uterus of
the estradiol-primed fetal guinea pig.
Pregnant guinea pigs were injected subcutaneously with 1 mg of
estradiol (E_2) and one day later half of the group received 5 mg
of progesterone ($E_2 + P$).
A. Uterine weight is expressed as a percent of weights of untreated animals assigned the value of 100%.
B. Progesterone receptors (PR) were measured in the cytosol and
nuclear fractions by incubation with 5 nM [^{3}H]-R5020 ($\pm$ a 100-
fold molar excess of unlabeled R5020) at 4°C for 18h.
Means $\pm$ S.E.

molecules was explored in the fetal uterus of the guinea pig
where two specific binding sites were found : Site A which corresponds to the estrogen receptor and Site B which binds to
antiestrogens with the triphenylethylene structure (nafoxidine,
tamoxifen) [43,44]. The physico-chemical characteristics of

TABLE IV. Physico-chemical characteristics of [^{3}H]-tamoxifen
binding in the cytosol of the fetal guinea pig uterus.

	Estrogen Receptor Site A	Site B
K_d at 4°C (x 10^{-9})	1.8 ± 0.4	0.39 ± 0.04
Number of sites (pmol/mg DNA)	12 ± 1.8	5.5 ± 0.1
k_{-1} at 4°C (x $10^{-4}sec^{-1}$)	8.3 ± 2	0.81 ± 0.14
Binding specificity	Natural and synthetic estrogens	Triphenylethylene derivatives
Temperature effect	Thermolabile	Thermoresistant
Precipitation by ammonium sulfate (%)	36	36
Effect of proteolytic treatment	Destroyed	Destroyed
Nuclear transfer	Yes	No

Data from ref. 43.

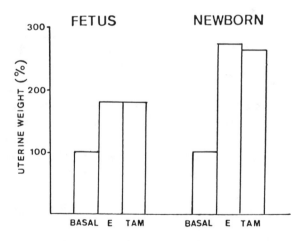

FIG. 8. Uterotrophic effect of estradiol (E) and tamoxifen
(TAM) administration in fetal and newborn guinea pig.
Tamoxifen and estradiol (1 mg/kg body weight) were injected for
3 consecutive days to pregnant animals (55-65 days of gestation)
and the uterotrophic response in fetuses was evaluated on the
fourth day. Estradiol (30 ng/g body weight) and tamoxifen
(0.6 µg/g body weight) were injected daily for 3 days to 6-day-
old newborn guinea pigs, and the uterotrophic effect was determined 24h after the last administration. The results are expressed as a percentage of basal values (assigned the value of
100%).

these two binding sites of tamoxifen are summarized in Table IV.
It is to be remarked that this multiple interaction of antiestrogens was also observed in other animal species : chick
oviduct [45], rat uterus [46], as well as in the human myometrium [47].

The biological responses to tamoxifen and nafoxidine
were studied in the fetal uterus after administration of these
triphenylethylene derivatives to the pregnant guinea pig. As
indicated in Figure 8, the uterotrophic response is similar for
antiestrogens and for estrogens in both the fetal and neonatal
periods [7,43,44]. Concerning the effect on progesterone receptors, the stimulatory action provoked by nafoxidine or tamoxifen in the fetal uterus is limited, representing only 1/4-1/2
of the effect induced by the estrogens, but in newborns the
effect is similar [7,48].

Recent studies in newborn guinea pigs subjected to a
long treatment (12 days) with tamoxifen, estradiol or with the
mixture of these compounds have shown that : 1) the effect on
uterine weight is similar for both estradiol and tamoxifen,
2) the effect is much more intense when the two compounds are
administered together, 3) tamoxifen stimulates the specific
progesterone binding sites and does not block the effect of
estradiol when administered together [49].

Figure 9 gives an example of the histological modifications provoked after these treatments. The effect is particularly intense on the height of the epithelium of the endometrium, as well as on the epithelium of the uterine glands
[50]. In conclusion, tamoxifen acts in both the fetal and newborn uteri of the guinea pig as a real agonist.

IV. COMMENTS AND CONCLUSIONS

The experimental information accumulated during the
last decade indicates the presence of steroid hormone receptors
in various organs of the fetus and also shows the evolution in
the concentration of the receptor during fetal and postnatal
development. Further evidence also shows that a good correlation exists between receptor binding, nuclear translocation and
biological responses elicited by the hormone during fetal de-

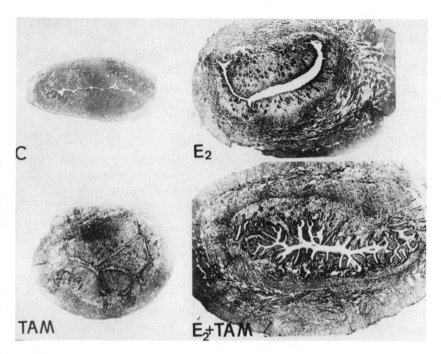

FIG. 9. Histological general view of transversal section of
the uterine horns of newborn guinea pig treated during 12 days
with estradiol, tamoxifen or with a mixture of tamoxifen +
estradiol.
Newborn (2 days old) guinea pigs received s.c. injection of
estradiol (E_2) (20 µg/animal/day) ; tamoxifen (TAM) (100 µg/
animal/day) or a combination of [E_2 + TAM] in the amounts given
above, for 12 days. C : control (non-treated animals).
Data from ref. 50.

velopment and in the newborn. The biological responses themselves are sometimes much more intense during fetal life than
after birth (e.g. : stimulation of progesterone receptor by
estrogens).

The fact that gonadal hormone receptors and biological
responses are present during fetal life suggests that many of
the processes of the programming of maturation of the reproductive organs are initiated during fetal life. However, the
full understanding of the physiological impact of these biological responses present in fetal life on puberty or on the
reproductive period remains to be acquired. In addition, the
presence of estrogen receptors in the fetal hypothalamus and
hypophysis also suggests that many of the interactive functions

of the hypothalamo-hypophyseal-gonadal axis are already operational during fetal life.

It can also be remarked that estrogens provoke in the fetal uterus other biological responses such as the very rapid (10-20 min) acetylation of nuclear histones [51], an increase in RNA polymerase I and II activities [52] and protein synthesis [53].

Interesting data have also been obtained showing that estradiol receptor is present in organs which are not classical target organs (e.g. : lung, kidney, thymus) indicating that hormones can have polyvalent actions in the fetus which may even be different from those in extra-uterine life.

Besides the fetal guinea pig, estrogen receptors have also been found in the Müllerian ducts and in the uterus of rat fetuses [54,55] and, using autoradiographic techniques, in the mesenchyme surrounding the Müllerian and Wolffian ducts and the urogenital sinuses of fetal mice [56]. Progesterone receptors have been found in the fetal uterus of rat [55] and progesterone-binding proteins with characteristics similar to those of progesterone receptor were localized in the placenta of rats [57], rabbits [58] as well as in the human [59,60].

Another attractive aspect during fetal life is the biological action of the estrogen-3-sulfates, which can have two main functions : 1) as a pre-hormone, which becomes active after hydrolysis ; 2) as a protective mechanism controlling the excess of the active hormone. This can be of broad interest because estrogen sulfates are present in different mammalian species.

Finally, another important conclusion is that substances which are considered as antiestrogens (e.g. : tamoxifen, nafoxidine) can be real agonists during fetal life and in newborns. Not only do these "antiestrogens" act as estrogens but they also enhance the effect of estradiol when administered together with the hormone. This poses the question of the use of these drugs during the reproductively active period of life and particularly in the treatment of breast cancer during pregnancy.

ACKNOWLEDGEMENTS

Part of the expenses of this work was defrayed by the

'Centre National de la Recherche Scientifique', France (Unité
Associée C.N.R.S. N° 548) and by the 'Fondation pour la Recherche Médicale Française'.

REFERENCES

1. J.R. Pasqualini,and M. Palmada, Endocrinology, Supp. Vol.
   88, A242 (1971).
2. J.R. Pasqualini,and C. Sumida, C.R. Acad. Sci. (Paris) 273,
   1061-1063 (1971).
3. H.W.C. Ward, Brit. Med. 1, 13-14 (1973.
4. H. Mouridsen, T. Palshof, J. Patterson,and L. Battersby,
   Cancer Treat. Rev. 5, 131-141 (1978).
5. L. Terrenius, Acta Endocr. (Copenh.) 66, 431-447 (1971).
6. J.H. Clark,and E.J. Peck Jr. in: Monographs on Endocrinology, Vol. 14 F. Gross, M.M. Grumbach, A. Labhart, M.B.
   Lipsett, T. Mann, L.T. Samuels and J. Zander, eds.
   (Springer-Verlag, Berlin 1979) pp. 99-134.
7. J.R. Pasqualini, C. Sumida, A. Gulino, B.-L. Nguyen, J.
   Tardy,and C. Gelly in: Hormones and Cancer S. Iacobelli,
   R.J.B. King, H.R. Lindner and M.E. Lippman, eds. (Raven
   Press, New York 1980) pp. 53-64.
8. J.R. Pasqualini, A. Gulino, C. Sumida,and I. Screpanti,
   J. Steroid Biochem. 20, 121-128 (1984).
9. J.R. Pasqualini, C. Sumida, C. Gelly,and B.-L. Nguyen, J.
   Steroid Biochem. 7, 1031-1038 (1976).
10. J.R. Pasqualini, C. Sumida, B.-L. Nguyen,and C. Gelly, J.
    Steroid Biochem. 9, 443-447 (1978).
11. I. Screpanti, A. Gulino,and J.R. Pasqualini, Endocrinology
    111, 1552-1561 (1982).
12. J. Tardy, and J.R. Pasqualini, Clin. Neuropharmacol. 7,
    312-319 (1984).
13. J.R. Pasqualini, and B.-L. Nguyen, C.R. Acad. Sci. (Paris)
    283, 413-416 (1976).
14. B.-L. Nguyen, and J.R. Pasqualini, unpublished data (1985).
15. C. Sumida, and J.R. Pasqualini, Endocrinology 105, 406-413
    (1979).
16. C. Sumida, and J.R. Pasqualini, J. Steroid Biochem. 11,
    267-272 (1979).
17. J.R. Pasqualini, and C. Cosquer-Clavreul, Experientia 34,
    268-269 (1978).
18. A. Gulino, and J.R. Pasqualini, Cancer Res. 42, 1913-1921
    (1982).
19. A. Gulino, C. Sumida, C. Gelly, N. Giambiagi, and J.R.
    Pasqualini, Endocrinology 109, 748-756 (1981).
20. N. Giambiagi, and J.R. Pasqualini, Endocrinology, 110,
    1067-1069 (1982).
21. N. Giambiagi, J.R. Pasqualini, G. Greene, and E.V. Jensen,
    J. Steroid Biochem 20, 397-400 (1984).
22. C. Gelly, C. Sumida, A. Gulino, and J.R. Pasqualini, J.
    Endocr. 89, 71-77 (1981).
23. J.R. Pasqualini, and B.-L. Nguyen, J. Endocr. 81, 144P-
    145P (1979).
24. J.R. Pasqualini, and B.-L. Nguyen, Endocrinology, 106,
    1160-1165 (1980).
25. M. Diamond, N. Rust, and U. Westphal, Endocrinology, 84,
    1143-1151 (1969).

270

26. R. Castellet, and J.R. Pasqualini, C.R. Acad. Sci. (Paris) 276, 1205-1208 (1973).

27. A. Millet, and J.R. Pasqualini, C.R. Acad. Sci. (Paris) 287, 1429-1432 (1978).

28. P. Corvol, R. Falk, M. Freifeld, and C.W. Bardin, Endocrinology 90, 1464-1469 (1972).

29. P.D. Feil, S.R. Glasser, D.O. Toft, and B.W. O'Malley, Endocrinology, 91, 738-746 (1972).

30. G.L. Greene, C. Nolan, J.R. Engler, and E.V. Jensen, Proc. Nat. Acad. Sci. 77, 5115-5119 (1980).

31. N. Giambiagi, and J.R. Pasqualini, Biochem. J., in press (1985).

32. C. Sumida, and J.R. Pasqualini, J. Receptor Res. 1, 439-457 (1980).

33. A. Gulino, I. Screpanti, and J.R. Pasqualini, Biol. Reprod. 31, 371-381 (1984).

34. J.R. Pasqualini, and B.-L. Nguyen, Experientia 35, 1116-1117 (1979).

35. C. Sumida, C. Gelly, and J.R. Pasqualini, J. Endocr. 85, 429-434 (1980).

36. C. Sumida, C. Gelly, and J.R. Pasqualini, Biochim. Biophys. Acta 755, 488-496 (1983).

37. J.R. Pasqualini, C. Sumida, and C. Gelly, Acta Endocr. (Copenh.) 83, 811-828 (1976).

38. J.R. Pasqualini, A. Lanzone, A. Tahri-Joutei, and B.-L. Nguyen, Acta Endocr. (Copenh.) 101, 630-635 (1982).

39. C. Sumida, C. Gelly, and J.R. Pasqualini, J. Receptor Res. 2, 221-232 (1981).

40. C. Sumida, C. Gelly, and J.R. Pasqualini, Steroids 39, 431-444 (1982).

41. A. Gulino, and J.R. Pasqualini, Endocrinology 112, 1871-1873 (1983).

42. C. Sumida, C. Gelly, and J.R. Pasqualini, J. Endocr. 105, in press (1985).

43. A. Gulino, and J.R. Pasqualini, J. Steroid Biochem. 15, 361-367 (1981).

44. A. Gulino, and J.R. Pasqualini, Cancer Res. 40, 3821-3826, (1980).

45. R.L. Sutherland, and M.S. Foo, Biochem. Biophys. Res. Commun. 91, 183-191 (1979).

46. J.C. Faye, B. Lasserre, and F. Bayard, Biochem. Biophys. Res. Commun. 93, 1225-1231 (1980).

47. O.L. Kon, J. Biol. Chem. 258, 3173-3177 (1983).

48. J.R. Pasqualini, C. Sumida, A. Gulino, J. Tardy, B.-L. Nguyen, C. Gelly, and C. Cosquer-Clavreul in: Progesterone and Progestins C.W. Bardin, E. Milgrom and P. Mauvais, Jarvis, eds. (Raven Press, New York 1983) pp. 77-90.

49. J.R. Pasqualini, B.-L. Nguyen, and F. Lecerf, Proc. 67th Meeting Amer. Endocr. Soc. (1985).

50. J.R. Pasqualini, B.-L. Nguyen, C. Mayrand, and F. Lecerf, unpublished data (1985).

51. J.R. Pasqualini, C. Cosquer-Clavreul, G. Vidali, and V.G. Allfrey, Biol. Reprod. 25, 1035-1039 (1981).

52. F. Lauré, and J.R. Pasqualini, Experientia 39, 209-210 (1981).

53. C. Sumida, and J.R. Pasqualini, Experientia 37, 782-783 (1981).

54. G.J. Sömjen, A.M. Kaye, and H.R. Lindner, Biochim. Biophys. Acta 428, 787-791 (1976).

55. B.-L. Nguyen, J.R. Pasqualini, R. Hatier, and G. Grignon, unpublished data (1985).

271

56. W.E. Stumpf, R. Narbaitz, and M. Sar, J. Steroid Biochem. 12, 55-64 (1980).
57. T.S. Ogle, Endocrinology 106, 1861-1868 (1980).
58. J. Guerne, and F. Stutinsky, Hormone Metab. Res. 10, 548-553 (1978).
59. E.S. Kneusll, I.G. Ances, and E.D. Albrecht, Proc. 63rd Meeting Amer. Endocr. Soc., Abs. 854 (1981).
60. M.A. Younes, N.F. Besch, and P.K. Besch, Am. J. Obstet. Gynec. 141, 170-174 (1981).

DISCUSSION

DEGEN: You showed that the estrogen-receptor (ER) goes up at birth in the lung. What is the "estrogenic response" of this tissue, or simpler: what is the ER doing there?

PASQUALINI: The number of specific binding sites for estrogen in the fetal lung of the guinea pig is relatively high and this increases after birth. In other animal species, ER are also found in lung tissues. The presence of these receptors during fetal life in this organ could be related to the fetal lung maturation, but this possibility is to be explored.

RAYNAUD: When you manipulate the concentration of steroid in pregnant guinea pigs by injection of exogenous hormone, have you verified what role progesterone binding globulin can play?

PASQUALINI: Progesterone binding globulin (PBG) concentration levels in the maternal serum is around 1 g/liter and in the fetal plasma is 2-4 mg/liter. In different studies, we demonstrated that no PBG is present inside of uterine cells because, generally, it does not interfere with the progesterone receptor present in this tissue. However, we agree that the high concentration of this protein controls the plasma progesterone concentration and probably the fraction of the hormone necessary to elicit the biological response.

BIGSBY: We find that uteri taken from neonatal mice continue their rapid rate of cell proliferation when transplanted under the kidney capsule of ovariectomized adult animals. These grafted uteri also develop glands. This suggests that there is, indeed, an intrinsic fetal factor carried over with the tissue which is responsible for continuation of its maturation. Also, concerning the effects of progesterone which you showed us, when we inject progesterone into these hosts, the grafted epithelial cell DNA synthesis is specifically blocked. This, we suggest, indicates that the antiuterotrophic action of progesterone does not involve the estrogen receptor mechanism, as you and many others have suggested. What the progesterone mechanism is remains to be defined.

PASQUALINI: I agree with your findings. We think that during fetal life progesterone receptor (PR) can be controlled by other factors independent of estrogen action; in this situation estrogens could be necessary but not sufficient. On the other hand, progesterone can be the main parameter which controls it own receptor.

NAFTOLIN: Were there mitosis or simply very long columnar cells in your estradiol and tamoxifen treated fetuses?

PASQUALINI: We think that both effects are present after estradiol and tamoxifen treatment.

NAFTOLIN: Did the tamoxifen induce desmosomes/gap junctions or nucleolar channels as appeared the case from the few EM's you showed?

PASQUALINI: This is an interesting suggestion to explore.

NAFTOLIN: Is the lung binder a receptor, i.e., could it be an enzyme or other binder? Is it translocated?

PASQUALINI: In the lung, estradiol binds to macromolecule with the typical characteristic of the receptor as we prove by K_d, Scatchard, and ultracentrifugation analysis.

MCLACHLAN: Is there a time during development of the guinea pig uterus in which there is no ER and yet an estrogen response?

PASQUALINI: ER appears in the fetal uterus at least by 30 days of gestation and PR 10-13 days later, suggesting the PR could be controlled by estradiol and/or ER, which we demonstrate after s.c. administration to the pregnant guinea pig. At the present, we do not have information if all the different biological responses of estrogen in the fetal tissues are mediated by the intermediate action of ER. We have one example in the fetal uterus in which the estrogen effect could be independent of ER, that is nuclear histone acetylation; this effect occurs very quickly (10 min after hormone injection). Probably this action could be a direct effect of estradiol and independent of ER.

FORSBERG: We have just published a paper where we have compared the effects of tamoxifen, clomiphene, naphoxidine hydrochloride, and MER-25 with those of DES and estradiol-benzoate in the neonatal period of mouse life. Except MER-25, the antiestrogens are very potent inducers of abnormal epithelia in the genital tract; in fact, more active than DES and estradiol-benzoate. In contrast to this, the clomiphene-treated females have normal ovaries and are fertile. Thus, we conclude that the antiestrogens could be very potent estrogens in peripheral target organs but less so than DES and estradiol in the hypothalamic-pituitary region. Except MER-25, the antiestrogens also have a pronounced effect on uterine wet weight.

PASQUALINI: This is an interesting comment.

STANCEL: In the experiments when PR increases 3x in vitro, what happens to the cell numbers of the cultured tissue?

PASQUALINI: In this tissue culture, PR increases 10-20 times in 16-24 hrs, ER decreases very significantly, and there is no increase in DNA content.

STROMAL-EPITHELIAL INTERACTIONS IN THE DETERMINATION OF HORMONAL
RESPONSIVENESS

GERALD R. CUNHA, ROBERT M. BIGSBY, PAUL S. COOKE, AND YOSHIKI SUGIMURA
Department of Anatomy,
University of California, San Francisco
San Francisco, CA 94143

INTRODUCTION

The importance of mesenchymal-epithelial interactions in
development of the genital tract and mammary gland is now well
established [1,2]. The developmental processes required to attain full
epithelial maturation and functional activity include morphogenesis,
growth, expression of specific hormone receptors, and specific patterns
of epithelial cytodifferentiation. Mesenchyme plays a central role in
all of these processes. Although evidence is more extensive and
compelling for this conclusion in the male genital tract, close
parallels between developmental events in male and female genital tracts
suggest that the basic regulatory processes are similar if not identical
for both androgen- and estrogen-target organs.

THE DEVELOPING PROSTATE AS A MODEL FOR ANDROGEN-INDUCED MORPHOGENESIS

The prostate is a compound tubular gland whose development, growth,
and functional activity is androgen dependent. Its development is
initiated when solid epithelial cords grow from the hollow, tubular
urogenital sinus into the surrounding mesenchyme. In the mouse this
occurs on the 17th day of gestation, which is about 4 days after the
initiation of testosterone synthesis by the fetal testes [3,4,5]. The
solid prostate buds elongate and branch within the mesenchyme
surrounding the urogenital sinus. Ductal morphogenesis occurs over an
extended period, mostly during the first month postnatally [6,7]. As in
all other exocrine glands, this morphogenetic process is specifically
dependent upon association of the epithelium with its mesenchyme;
however, ductal morphogenesis will also occur if urogenital sinus
epithelium is associated with the mesenchyme of a closely related gland,
the seminal vesicle [8,9]. Glandular morphogenesis fails to occur in
the absence of mesenchyme or when mesenchyme from a non-urogenital organ
is utilized [9-11]. Prostatic ductal morphogenesis can be induced by
urogenital sinus mesenchyme (UGM) in epithelium of the urogenital sinus
(UGE), fetal or adult urinary bladder (BLE), postnatal vagina (VE) or
prostate [1,8,12-15]. All of these epithelia share a common
developmental history, being derived in total or part from the primitive
urogenital sinus, the ventral division of the cloaca [16-18]. Tissue
recombinants prepared with UGM plus any of the above epithelia show vast
increases in wet weight, DNA content, and amount of epithelial tissue
during 1 month of in vivo growth (renal subcapsular grafts) in response
to endogenous levels of androgens in the male hosts [1,19,20]. Thus,
ductal morphogenesis and the associated epithelial growth are only
observed when two conditions are met: 1) when intact male hosts are
employed and 2) when urogenital mesenchyme is utilized.

As branching morphogenesis proceeds within the developing prostate,
the solid epithelial cords canalize, and the epithelial cells
differentiate into a tall simple columnar epithelium. Secretory
cytodifferentiation only occurs if the UGE is associated with urogenital
mesenchyme [9]. Moreover, UGM elicits prostatic secretory

cytodifferentiation in epithelium of the urinary bladder or vagina [4,12,13]. Although this remarkable induction of secretory cytodifferentiation in vaginal or bladder epithelium implies a major change in epithelial functional activity, it does not prove that the induced epithelial cells are actually prostatic. This question has been specifically addressed in tissue recombinants composed of urogenital sinus mesenchyme and adult bladder epithelium (UGM + BLE). These recombinants produce fully differentiated prostate-like glands when grown for 1 month in intact male hosts [14]. The resultant glands resemble prostate by a variety of criteria (Table I).

TABLE I

EPITHELIAL CHARACTERISTICS IN PROSTATE, URINARY BLADDER AND HETEROTYPIC TISSUE RECOMBINANTS*

Type of Analysis or Feature	Specimen		
	Bladder	Prostate	UGM + BLE
Histology	Transitional	Glandular	Glandular
Electron Microscopy	Non-Secretory Asymmetric Membrane	Secretory Symmetric Membrane	Secretory Symmetric Membrane
Histochemistry			
Alkaline Phosphatase	+	-	-
Alcian Blue	-	+	+
Nonspecific Esterase	±	+	+
Prostate Antigens	-	+	+
Androgen Receptors	-	+	+
Androgen-dependent DNA Synthesis	-	+	+
Protein Synthesis (2-D gels)	bladder	prostate	prostate-like

*From Cunha et al, [21]; Neubauer et al, [22]

Most significantly the epithelial cells express androgen receptors, prostate-specific antigens, and androgen-dependency for DNA synthesis. Also, mapping of gene products of the UGM + BLE recombinants by two-dimensional gel electrophoresis demonstrates a distinctly prostatic pattern. From this body of evidence we have concluded that urogenital sinus mesenchyme induces and specifies prostatic epithelial morphogenesis, growth, cytodifferentiation, and gene expression.

Analysis of tissue recombinants composed of epithelium and mesenchyme from urogenital sinuses of wild-type and Tfm (Testicular feminization) mice has indicated that androgens act indirectly through the mesenchyme to promote epithelial growth [4,27,28]. Androgens are absolutely essential for eliciting prostatic development and also for regulating prostatic growth and secretion in adulthood [23-26]. For this reason Tfm males which are genetically insensitive to androgens due to a defect in the androgen receptor, never develop a prostate [29-31] As indicated by tissue recombination studies (Figure 1), the expression of androgenic effects (prostatic development) is dependent upon the presence of wild-type mesenchyme. The androgenic sensitivity of the epithelium is irrelevant. Thus, an androgen-insensitive Tfm epithelium can be induced by wild-type UGM to form prostatic glands. In the course of this process the following occur: prostatic ductal morphogenesis, epithelial growth, and secretory cytodifferentiation. All of these processes are induced by androgens, but are expressed in androgen-insensitive Tfm epithelium lacking androgen receptors [20]. This suggests that mesenchyme is the target and mediator of androgenic effects upon the epithelium, an interpretation corroborated by Tfm/wild-type recombination studies in the mammary system [32,33], and by autoradiographic studies of androgen binding in the developing prostate and mammary gland in which specific nuclear binding is confined to the mesenchyme [34,35].

The concept of mesenchymal mediation of androgenic effects, derived from analysis of developing systems, also appears to be applicable to the adult prostate. The adult prostate has androgen receptors in both epithelial and stromal cells [36], whereas nuclear androgen binding sites are present only in the mesenchyme of the urogenital sinus [34]. The presence of intra-epithelial androgen receptors in the adult prostate suggests that proliferation of prostatic epithelial cells could be regulated by direct androgenic action. However, evidence to date indicates that the presence of intra-epithelial androgen receptors is

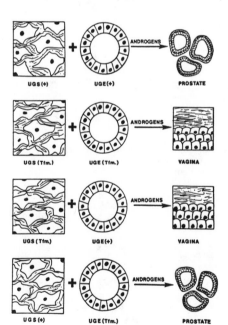

Fig. 1. Recombination experiments between epithelia and mesenchyme of urogenital sinuses from Tfm and wild-type mouse embryos. Wild-type mesenchyme (UGS +) induces prostatic morphogenesis in the epithelium (UGE), irrespective of the source (Tfm or +, wild-type). Conversely, wild-type epithelium does not develop prostate-like structures when associated with Tfm mesenchyme (UGS Tfm), but rather exhibits a vaginal-type morphology.

neither necessary nor sufficient for regulation of prostatic epithelial growth by androgens. This conclusion is based upon three lines of evidence. First, primary cultures of normal prostatic epithelial cells (free of stroma) proliferate at similar rates in the presence or absence of androgens [37-39]. Second, when tissue recombinants composed of wild-type UGM plus a single adult wild-type prostatic duct (UGM + PR) are grown for 1 month in an intact male host, prostatic ductal mass increases several hundred fold. By contrast, if a wild-type prostatic duct is grown under identical conditions but in association with Tfm UGM (Tfm UGM + PR), the duct is maintained but does not grow [5]. Third DNA synthesis in recombinants composed of UGM + Tfm BLE is stimulated by androgens administered to castrated hosts. The kinetics of this induction are similar to that reported for wild-type prostate [40]. More recently, these findings have been extended and refined through parallel autoradiographic analysis utilizing labelling index as the measure of epithelial cell growth (Table II).

TABLE II
TRITIATED-THYMIDINE LABELLING INDEX OF PROSTATIC EPITHELIAL
CELLS IN HETEROTYPIC TISSUE RECOMBINANTS*

RECOMBINANTS	TREATMENT	EPITHELIAL LABELLING INDEX*
UGM + BLE	TP	19.6 ± 1.78
	OIL	1.0 ± 0.57
	TP + CA	0.8 ± 0.50
UGM + TFM-BLE	TP	17.7 ± 1.41
	OIL	0.4 ± 0.23
	TP + CA	1.2 ± 0.63

TP = testosterone propionate; CA = cyproterone acetate
*Data (mean ± SEM) based upon analysis of 1000-2000 cells/group. From Sugimura and Cunha [41].

Epithelial proliferation (labelling index) is androgen-dependent and virtually identical in mature prostate-like ducts in both UGM + wild-type BLE and UGM + Tfm BLE recombinants [41]. Since Tfm epithelial cells of UGM + Tfm BLE recombinants lack androgen receptors [20], prostatic epithelial proliferation cannot be regulated directly via intra-epithelial androgen-receptors. Instead, these data favor an indirect mechanism involving trophic factors or regulators produced by androgen-receptor-positive stromal cells.

THE DEVELOPING FEMALE GENITAL TRACT AS A MODEL FOR ESTROGEN-INDUCED MORPHOGENESIS

Many lines of evidence suggest that the basic regulatory mechanisms are the same for both androgen- and estrogen-target organs. As in the male genital tract, epithelial morphogenesis, cytodifferentiation, and functional activity are induced and specified by the stroma [9,42]. For example, uterine stroma (UtS) induces neonatal vaginal epithelium (VE) to undergo uterine differentiation, while vaginal stroma (VS) induces neonatal uterine epithelium (UtE) to undergo vaginal differentiation

[42]. Grafts that express vaginal differentiation (VS + UtE) synthesize proteins that give a profile on two-dimensional gel electrophoresis very similar to that of the vagina. By contrast, UtS + VE recombinants (which express uterine differentiation) produce a uterine profile of proteins [43]. Moreover, in VS + UtE recombinants grown in intact cycling female hosts, the epithelium alternates from a cornified to a mucified state through the estrous cycle in concert with the host's vaginal epithelium [42,44]. This cyclical change in epithelial phenotype is one of the unique functional characteristics of vaginal epithelium. Thus, in developing estrogen-target organs, the mesenchyme induces specific patterns of epithelial morphogenesis, cytodifferentiation, and functional activity.

Although estrogens do not appear to be required for early morphogenesis, the fetal and neonatal female genital tract of many species is sensitive to exogenous estrogens. In the mouse, perinatal administration of large doses of estrogen leads to ovary-independent hyperplasia of the vaginal epithelium during adulthood [45]. When epithelium from a normal adult vagina is recombined with vaginal stroma from an adult that was neonatally estrogenized, the epithelium exhibits ovary-independent hyperplasia; the reciprocal recombination (normal vaginal stroma + neonatally estrogenized vaginal epithelium) also yields an ovary-independent hyperplastic epithelium [46]. Such results indicate that not only are vaginal tissues of the neonatal mouse sensitive to estrogenic stimulation but that growth regulation of vaginal epithelium involves the stromal component of the organ. In mature animals estrogen also stimulates growth and regulates differentiation of both uterine and vaginal epithelia [47]. The role of stroma in regulating these responses is unclear.

Vaginal and uterine epithelia of neonatal mice appear to be devoid of estrogen receptors, yet they respond to estrogenic stimulation. Autoradiographic analysis of estrogen uptake after exposure to ^{3}H-estradiol (^{3}H-E$_2$) or ^{3}H-moxestrol in vitro or in vivo indicates that vaginal and uterine epithelia of newborn animals do not have nuclear binding sites (estrogen receptors) [48]. In contrast, uterine and vaginal stromal cells possess nuclear estrogen receptors throughout fetal, neonatal, and adult periods (Figure 2) [36,48,49]. These autoradiographic findings have been recently confirmed by biochemical uptake studies. When epithelial cells of 4- and 5-day-old mice are incubated with ^{125}I-E$_2$ over a concentration range of 0.15-10 nM, binding is neither saturable nor specific. However, parallel analysis of epithelial cells derived from 20-day-old animals demonstrates saturable, specific uptake of the radiolabelled steroid (Figure 3). In agreement with the autoradiography, uterine stromal cells of both age groups exhibit estrogen receptor activity [50].

Even though the uterine epithelium of the 4-day-old mouse is devoid of estrogen receptor, these cells respond to exogenous estrogen in vivo by increasing their rate of proliferation (Figure 4). The lag between estrogen administration and increased DNA synthesis is identical to that in the ovariectomized adult mouse [51]. In addition, neonatal vaginal and uterine epithelial cells that have expressed an estrogenic response continue to lack estrogen receptors [35,50]. These results suggest that estrogen-induced proliferation of uterine epithelium is mediated by mesenchymal estrogen receptors in the neonatal mouse. Since the time course of estrogen response is similar in the adult, it is possible that the proliferative response of adult epithelium is also mediated by the same mechanism.

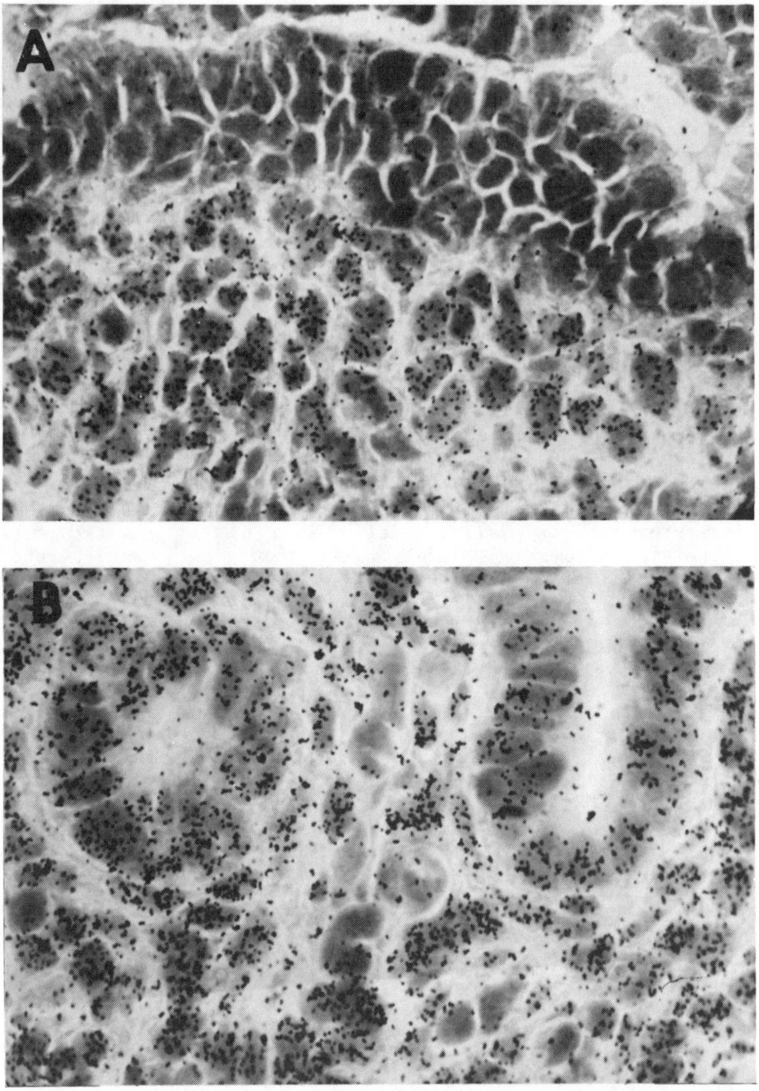

Fig. 2. Autoradiographic demonstration of uterine ^{3}H-estradiol uptake. Note the lack of any concentration of silver grains over the nuclei of the epithelial cells of the 4-day-old uterus compared to the intense labelling of the stromal component (A). Also, note the nuclear localization of labelling for both epithelial and stromal cells in the 20-day old uterus (B).

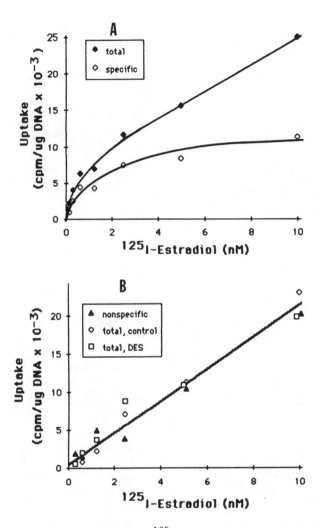

Fig. 3. Whole cell uptake of ^{125}I-estradiol by uterine epithelial cells. A. Depicted are the "total" and "specific" uptake by uterine epihtelium isolated from 20-day-old mice. Scatchard analysis of the specific uptake yields a K_D of 1.2 nM and a cellular binding capacity of 9.3 fmol/ug DNA. B. "Total" and "nonspecific" uptake by epithelial cells isolated from uteri of 5-day-old mice are depicted. The mice had been treated with diethylstilbestrol (DES) or oil vehicle (control) 12 h before the epithelium was harvested. Note that there is no difference between nonspecific or total uptake of either group of animals (a single straight line was drawn through the data points for simplicity).

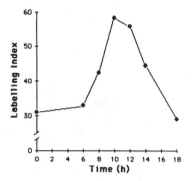

Fig. 4. Estrogen induction of DNA synthesis in uterine epithelium of neonatal mice. At various times after 5 ug/g DES was administered, 1.5 uCi/g ³H-thymidine was injected ip into each animal. The percent labelled epithelial cells (labelling index) at each time is depicted; at least 1000 cells were counted for each time point.

USE OF CULTURED CELLS TO STUDY CELL-CELL INTERACTIONS

Epithelial cells in culture exhibit marked changes in shape, protein synthetic patterns, hormone responsiveness, etc. compared to intact epithelia in vivo [52-54]. One of the most puzzling aspects of cell growth in culture is that hormones which are potent mitogens in vivo frequently have no proliferative effect on their target cells in vitro. Estradiol (E_2) is the primary mitogen for the epithelium of the female reproductive tract in vivo [47,55]. However, previous work has shown that E_2 is not mitogenic for isolated mammary, uterine, or vaginal epithelial cells grown in culture [56-58]. Several explanations for the paradoxical dichotomy between E_2 effects in vivo and in vitro have been suggested. Among these are that E_2 acts indirectly on target epithelia through the stroma; thus, isolated epithelia are incapable of a direct mitogenic response to E_2. Conversely, epithelial cells could become transformed in culture so that they no longer are dependent on E_2 for growth, or culture conditions could result in the selective growth of a subpopulation(s) of epithelial cells which are able to grow without E_2. To test these possibilities, we examined the ability of cultured uterine and vaginal epithelium (UtE and VE, respectively) to re-express their normal morphology and hormone responsiveness when recombined with homologous stroma and transplanted in vivo.

VE and UtE from ovariectomized (OVX) 40-day-old mice were grown in collagen gels for 6 to 10 days using serum-free medium [56]. Total DNA content of the VE and UtE cultures increased 4- and 4-to 8- fold, respectively, in the absence of E_2 and was not stimulated by E_2 [57,58]. Following exposure to E_2 in vitro, these cultured epithelia show decreased cytosolic estrogen receptor (ER), increased nuclear ER, and increased cytosolic progesterone receptors, indicating that the lack of proliferation in response to E_2 is not due to a non-functional ER system [58,59]. Both epithelia form stellate colonies in the collagen gel, but VE does not stratify or keratinize in vitro.

Cultured VE and UtE were recombined with homologous vaginal or uterine stroma (VS and UtS, respectively) and grown under the renal capsule of intact female hosts for 4 weeks. Upon recovery, the epithelium of the VS + cultured VE recombinants showed a normal

stratified morphology and alternating keratinized and mucified layers
characteristic of the normal histological changes that occur through the
estrous cycle (Fig. 5). The epithelium in the UtS + cultured UtE
recombinants was also morphologically normal.

Proliferation of both UtE and VE in the recombinants was E_2-dependent. VS + cultured VE and UtS + cultured UtE recombinants were
grown in intact female hosts for three weeks. The hosts were then OVX
and one week later were injected with either E_2 or oil. Cell
proliferation was examined 24 hours later by 3H-thymidine
autoradiography. The epithelium of the VS + cultured VE recombinants in
E_2-injected hosts was stratified, and showed very intense labelling in
the basal cells indicative of rapid cell proliferation. Conversely, the
VE of recombinants in oil-injected hosts was atrophic, consisting of 1-2
cell layers which were very sparsely labelled (Fig. 6). The epithelium
in UtS + cultured UtE recombinants in E_2-injected hosts was also highly
labelled, while that in oil-injected controls showed very little
labelling.

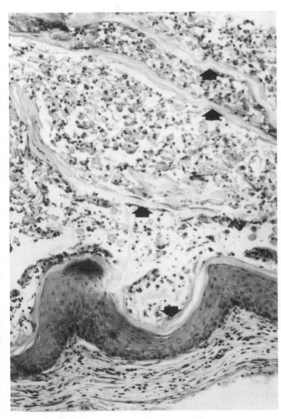

Fig. 5. A recombinant
of VS + cultured VE
grown for 4 weeks in an
intact female host.
Note that the epithelium
has a normal stratified
morhpology. In addi-
tion, the alternating
keratinized and mucified
layers in the lumen
indicate that the
epithelium (arrows) has
undergone the normal
changes typically seen
in vaginal epithelium
during the estrous
cycle.

282

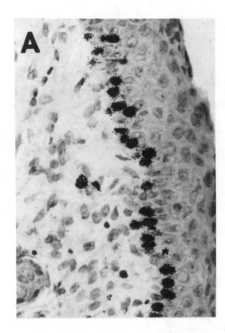
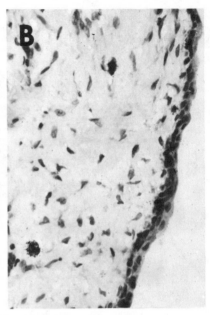

Fig. 6. Thymidine labelling of VS + cultured VE recombinants in OVX
hosts. The hosts had been injected with either 100 ng of E_2 in oil (A)
or oil above (B) 24 hours perviously. Recombinants in E_2-injected hosts
had a stratified epithelium with very heavy labelling of the basal cells
indicative of a high rate of proliferation. Conversely, the epithelium
of recombinants in oil-injected controls was atrophic and showed very
sparse labelling.

These results indicate that cultured VE and UtE can re-express
their normal phenotype when grown with homologous stroma <u>in vivo</u>. In
addition, the epithelia of the recombinants again become dependent on E_2
for proliferation, a characteristic which was not expressed <u>in vitro</u>.
Thus, the lack of E_2 responsiveness <u>in vitro</u> is not due to a
transformation of the cells, and likewise is not due to the selection of
a non-dependent subpopulation(s) by the culture regimen. These data
emphasize the importance of stroma for normal epithelial growth and
function, and suggest that the lack of E_2 responsiveness of isolated
epithelia <u>in vitro</u> may be due to separation from their stroma.

CONCLUSION

A basic concept that has influenced thinking on the mechanism of
sex hormone action is that a cell must have a specific receptor in order
to respond to its trophic hormone. This idea has emerged from numerous
investigations of the mammary gland, and the male and female genital
tracts.   For estrogen-target organs the following example can be
given.   The chronic administration of E_2 to ovariectomized females
elicits generalized uterine growth, while a single dose specifically
stimulates uterine epithelial proliferation. Myometrium, endometrial
stroma, and epithelium of the mature uterus all have high affinity
estrogen receptors. It is tempting to conclude from these facts that

estrogen receptors within a given cell mediate the proliferative response of that cell to estrogen. However, it is of paramount importance to realize that the data obtained are merely correlative and that no causal relationship has ever been proved between epithelial estrogen receptors and estrogen-induced epithelial proliferation. The same can be also stated for epithelial androgen receptors and androgen-induced epithelial proliferation in the male genital tract.

Until recently the role of stromal cells relative to regulation of epithelial proliferation had been ignored. In the prostate it is now clear that the stroma is the mediator of many androgenic effects upon the epithelium in both the developing and mature prostate. Evidence is now sufficiently strong to postulate the existence of growth-regulatory substances of stromal origin in the prostate. Evidence of this nature is still somewhat inconclusive for estrogen target organs, but clear parallels between the male and female genital tracts do exist as described above. Clearly, stromal cells are of fundamental importance in the development and differentiation of epithelia of both the male and female genital tracts. A fuller understanding of the true functional role of prostatic, uterine, and vaginal stromal cells is likely to resolve many of the long-standing paradoxes that have confounded investigators for years.

ACKNOWLEDGMENTS

The authors wish to thank Gary L. Myers and Ed Cleary for typing the manuscript and Simona Ikeda for preparation of the figure. This study was supported in part by the following grants: March of Dimes, 1-837; NIH, HD 17491, 1F32 HD06520, 5 F32 HD06580.

1. G.R. Cunha, L.W.K. Chung, J.M. Shannon, O. Taguchi, H. Fujii, Rec. Prog. Horm. Res. 39, 559 (1983).
2. K. Kratochwil, Mod. Probl. Pediat. 15, 1 (1975).
3. G.R. Cunha, Anat. Rec. 175, 87 (1973).
4. G.R. Cunha, B. Lung in: Accessory Glands of the Male Reproductive Tract. E. Spring-Mills and E.S.E Hafez, eds. (Ann Arbor Science Publishers, Ann Arbor 1979). pp. 1-28.
5. J-P. Weniger, A. Zeis. C.R. Acad. Sci. Paris 275, 1431 (1972).
6. B. Lung, G.R. Cunha, Anat. Rec. 199, 73 (1981).
7. Y. Sugimura, G.R. Cunha, A.A. Donjacour, Biol. Reprod. (Submitted).
8. G.R. Cunha, Anat. Rec. 172, 179 (1972).
9. G.R. Cunha, Int. Rev. Cytol. 47, 137 (1976).
10. G.R. Cunha, Anat. Rec. 172, 529 (1972).
11. G.R. Cunha, Anat. Rec. 173, 205 (1972).
12. G.R. Cunha, B. Lung, J. Exp. Zool. 205, 181 (1978).
13. G.R. Cunha, Endocrinology 95, (1975).
14. G.R. Cunha, B. Lung, B. Reese, Invest. Urol. 17, 202 (1980).
15. J.T. Norman, G.R. Cunha, Y. Sugimura, Prostate (Submitted).
16. W. Felix in: Manual of Human Embryology, R. Keibel and F.P. Mall, eds. (Lippincott Co., Philadelphia 1912) pp. 869-972.
17. J.G. Forsberg, Am. J. Obstet. Gynecol. 115, 1025 (1973).
18. G.R. Cunha in: Urologic Endocrinology, J. Rajfer, ed. (W.B. Saunders, Philadelphia 1985) (In Press).
19. L.W.K. Chung, G.R. Cunha, Prostate 4, 1983).
20. J.M. Shannon, G.R. Cunha, Biol. Reprod. 31, 175 (1984).
21. G.R. Cunha, H. Fujii, B.L. Neubauer, J.M. Shannon, L. Sawyer, and B.A. Reese, J. Cell Biol. 96, 1662 (1983).
22. B.L. Neubauer, L.W.K. Chung, K. McCormick, O. Taguchi, T.C. Thompson, G.R. Cunha, J. Cell Biol. 96, 1671 (1983).
23. A. Jost in: Organogenesis, R.L. DeHaan and H. Ursprung, eds. (Holt, Rinehart, and Winston, New York 1965) pp. 611-628.
24. D.S. Coffey in: Male Accessory Sex Organs: Structure and Function in Mammals. D. Brandes, ed (Academic Press, New York 1974) pp. 307-328.
25. N. Bruchovsky, B. Lesser, E. Van Doorn, S. Craven, Vitamins and Hormones 33, 1 1975).
26. W.I.P. Mainwaring, (Springer-Verlag, New York 1977).
27. G.R. Cunha, L.W.K. Chung, J.M. Shannon, B.A. Reese, Biol. Reprod. 22, 19 (1980).
28. I. Lasnitzki, T. Mizuno, J. Endocrinol. 85, 423 (1980).
29. B. Attardi, S. Ohno, Cell 2, 205 (1974).
30. S. Ohno, (Springer-Verlag, New York 1979).
31. J.D. Wilson, J.E. Griffin, M. Leshin, F.W. George, Human Genetics 58, 78 (1981).
32. K. Kratochwil, P. Schwartz, Proc. Natl. Acad. Sci. 73, 4041 (1976).
33. U. Drews, U. Drews, Cell 10, 401 (1977).
34. J.M. Shannon, G.R. Cunha, Prostate 4, 367 (1983).
35. G.R. Cunha, J.M. Shannon, O. Taguchi, H. Fujii, L.W.K. Chung, J. Animal Sci. 55 (Suppl): 14 (1982).
36. W.E. Stumpf, M. Sar in: Receptors and Mechanism of Action of Steroid Hormones, J.R. Pasqualini ed. (Marcel Dekker, New York 1976) pp. 41-84.
37. S. Chevalier, G. Bleau, K.D. Roberts, A. Chapdelaine, Mol. Cell. Endocrinol. 24, 1 (1981).
38. W.L. McKeehan, P.S. Adams, M.P. Rosser, Cancer Res. 44, 1998 (1984).
39. W.L. McKeehan, H.A. Glass, M.P. Rosser, P.S. Adams, Prostate 3, 231 (1984).
40. G.R. Cunha, L.W.K. Chung, J. Steroid Biochem. 14, 317 (1981).
41. Y. Sugimura, G.R. Cunha, Endocrinology (Submitted)

285

42. G.R. Cunha, J. Exp. Zool. 196, 361 (1976).
43. G.R. Cunha, J.M. Shannon, O. Taguchi, H. Fujii, B.A. Meloy in: Epithelial-Mesenchymal Interactions in Development, R.H. Sawyer and J.F. Fallon, eds (Praeger Scientific Press, New York 1983) pp. 51-74.
44. G.R. Cunha, B. Lung, In Vitro 15, 50 (1979).
45. N. Takasugi, Int. Rev. Cytol. 44, 193 (1976).
46. G.R. Cunha, B. Lung, K. Kato, Dev. Biol. 56, 52 (1977).
47. L. Martin, In: Estrogens in the Environment, J.A. McLachlan, ed. (Elsevier/No. Holland, New York 1980) pp. 103-170.
48. G.R. Cunha, J.M. Shannon, K.D. Vanderslice, M. Sekkingstad, S.J. Robboy, J. Steroid Biochem. 17, 281 (1982).
49. W.E. Stumpf, R. Narbaitz, M. Sar, J. Steroid Biochem. 12, 55 (1980).
50. R.M. Bigsby, G.R. Cunha, Endocrinology (Submitted).
51. L. Martin, C.A. Finn, G. Trinder, J. Endocrinol. 56, 133 1973).
52. V.D. Sobel, R. Tchao, J. Bozzola, M.E. Levison, D. Kaye, In Vitro 15, 993 (1979).
53. E.Y-H Lee, G. Parry, M.J. Bissell, J. Cell Biol. 98, 146 (1984).
54. D. Gospodarowicz, V.P. Tauber, Endo. Rev. 1, 201 (1980).
55. P. Galand, F. Leroy, J. Chretien J. Endocrinol. 49, 243 (1971).
56. S. Nandi, W. Imagawa, Y. Tomooka, M.F. McGrath, M. Edery, Arch Toxicol 55, 91 (1984).
57. T. Iguchi, F-D.A. Uchima, P.C. Ostrander, H.A. Bern, Proc. Natl. Acad. Sci., USA 80, 3743 (1983).
58. F-D.A. Uchima, M. Edery, L.I. Sewell, H.A. Bern, Program of the 67th Annual Meeting of the Endocrine Society, Baltimore, MD 1985).
59. F-D.A. Uchima, M. Edery, L.I. Sewell, H.A. Bern, Proc. Am. Assoc. Cancer Res. 25, 206 (1984).

DISCUSSION

STUMPF: You probably misspoke yourself when you said "autoradiography is not a quantitative technique." Not only can we count silver grains and determine labeling indices, but also silver grains can be converted into number of molecules, provided several requirements are met and the specific silver grain yield has been determined (Stumpf et al., J. Histochem. Cytochem. Suppl., Jan. 1981). Since in your recombination studies with Tfm derived epithelium, the wild-type connective (androgen target) tissue is capable of inducing "androgen-specific" cell proliferation and differentiation in the Tfm derived epithelium, why should it not be possible to induce receptors! Apparently you controlled for negative chemography, which is sometimes present in epithelium, especially uterine luminal epithelium. Also, ligand-receptor binding could be diminished or inconspicuous during certain functional states and hormonal conditions, while it may be conspicuous under conditions different from those studied.

CUNHA: Yes, I agree autoradiography can be quantified although that is quite tedious. It is possible to induce androgen receptors in urogenital sinus mesenchyme and bladder epithelium (UGM+BLE) recombinants provided the bladder epithelium is derived from wild-type embryos (Neubauer et al., J. Cell Biol. 96, 1671, 1983). Under identical conditions, when UGM + Tfm BLE recombinants are analyzed, specific nuclear androgen binding is not observed in the Tfm epithelium even when exposures are utilized which are 120 weeks (30 times that required to detect nuclear binding in wild-type cells). These data are consistent with Ohno's idea that the Tfm mutation may be the gene for the androgen receptor. We conclude that Tfm cells are incapable of expressing androgen receptors. I might add that in a variety of tissues taken directly from Tfm mice, androgen receptors are not exposed (Cunha, unpublished).

FORSBERG: How long a time is it necessary to have epithelial-stroma contact in a heterocombinant to change the development of the epithelium?

CUNHA: We see evidence of an inductive response in UGM + BLE recombinants in 3 to 4 days.

FORSBERG: Is the stromal-induced epithelial differentiation reversible or irreversible? Is it possible to make secondary heterocombinants? Could you, for instance, after a primary vaginal stroma-uterine epithelium interaction make a new combinant with this epithelium and some other type of stroma and again change epithelial development?

CUNHA: We have not determined whether the stromal-induced epithelial differentiation is reversible. It is technically possible to construct "secondary recombinants" as you suggest, but this has not been done.

FORSBERG: How do you explain that neonatal genital epithelial cells, in spite of lacking estrogen receptors, demonstrate an estrogen response as evidenced by proliferation increase and specific protein synthesis?

CUNHA: I do not believe that uterine epithelial proliferation is regulated by intra-epithelial estrogen receptors (ER). Instead, I believe that epithelial proliferation is regulated indirectly via growth regulatory substances from stroma. In support of this idea are the following observations: (a) Estrogen- (or androgen) receptor-positive epithelial cells do not exhibit a proliferative response to estrogen (or androgen as for prostate epithelium) in vitro; (b) Neonatal uterine epithelium in situ, which appear to lack ER, proliferate in response to estrogen; (c) Tfm prostatic epithelial cells in prostates constructed from wild-type mesenchyme and Tfm epithelium proliferate in response to injected androgen despite the fact that they lack androgen receptors.

TOMOOKA: Is influence from stroma on epithelial cell growth due to cell-cell contact or a diffusible factor?

CUNHA: We don't know as yet, but transfilter experiments to answer this question are now in progress.

STANCEL: Have you been able to grow recombinants in vitro or simply culture pieces of tissue (i.e., organ culture) and get epithelial cell division in response to estrogen?

CUNHA: These experiments which you suggest have not been done as yet.

EROSCHENKO: All that I have heard during this meeting is receptor mediation. Is it possible that during the first few days of life estrogen may enter these cells either without combining with a specific estrogen-receptor or combining with a different, non-specific receptor?

CUNHA: Certainly this is a possibility. We need to know more about non-receptor mediated effects of steroids and more about indirect effects.

NAFTOLIN: If proliferation was built into the differentiation of, e.g., vaginal stem cells, you would now require receptors in the induced epithelial cells at the outset. Is this not true?

CUNHA: This is possible.

NAFTOLIN: Do you find this mesenchymal-epithelial interaction in apparently steroid insensitive tissues?

CUNHA: Non-urogenital organs whose development is not influenced by sex hormones, e.g., the integumental, gastrointestinal, respiratory, and urinary systems, develop via epithelial-mesenchymal interactions. For the most part, these organs lack hormone receptors.

SONNENSCHEIN: I am personally rewarded to hear that you are now entertaining the possibility that the regulatory effect of mesenchyme on epithelial cells may be mediated by inhibitory factors.

CUNHA: Yes, you have opened our minds to this possibility.

Published 1985 by Elsevier Science Publishing Co., Inc.
Estrogens in the Environment, John A. McLachlan, Editor

DIETHYLSTILBESTROL ASSOCIATED DEFECTS IN MURINE GENITAL TRACT DEVELOPMENT

RETHA R. NEWBOLD AND JOHN A. McLACHLAN
Developmental Endocrinology and Pharmacology Section, Laboratory of
Reproductive and Developmental Toxicology, National Institute of
Environmental Health Sciences, National Institutes of Health, Research
Triangle Park, NC 27709

INTRODUCTION

For decades, estrogens have been reported to elicit teratogenic and

carcinogenic changes in the reproductive tracts of experimental animals

following exposure during critical periods of development [1-3]. Since

many chemicals, such as insecticides, drugs, and natural compounds in

our environment have estrogenic activity [4], concern has developed

regarding the biological effects of these estrogenic compounds on the

developing fetus. The dramatic and well-known effects of in utero expo-

sure to the potent synthetic estrogen, diethylstilbestrol (DES),

illustrates this problem.

For almost thirty years, DES was used as a therapeutic agent for

threatened abortion. In 1971, an association between the use of DES

during pregnancy and an increased incidence of vaginal and cervical adeno-

carcinoma in female offspring was reported [5]. While the full extent of

DES use is unknown, it is estimated that at least 2 million pregnant

women may have been treated with the drug [6]. Although DES is no longer

used clinically to prevent threatened abortion, the number of progeny at

risk will peak in this decade. Hormonal teratogenesis and carcinogenesis

on the scale of the DES episode constitutes a potentially serious health

problem which may persist even after the passing of the original

DES-exposed population.

The DES episode has focused attention on the role of estrogens in

genital tract development. Future assessment of the defects resulting

from prenatal exposure to estrogenic substances, such as DES, will

require knowledge of the mechanisms of development of the genital tract.

To this end, we have developed an animal model to study the long-term effects of developmental exposure to DES. Although our published studies have primarily focused on prenatal exposure to DES [7-11], many of the principles and ideas established with the prenatal mouse model were pioneered using the estrogen-exposed neonatal mouse [12,13]. Close comparison of abnormalities induced by neonatal DES exposure may give a better understanding of the developmental events that are disturbed by exposure to potent estrogenic compounds during critical stages of sex differentiation. This chapter will review female and male genital tract abnormalities found in mice prenatally exposed to DES.

PRENATAL DES EXPOSURE

To study the effects of prenatal exposure to DES, outbred CD-1 mice were treated subcutaneously with DES on days 9 through 16 of gestation. The doses of DES ranged from 0.01 to 100 µg/kg during pregnancy. These doses of DES are less than that given therapeutically to pregnant women. Mice were born on day 19 of gestation, and both male and female offspring were studied. The time of DES exposure encompasses the major events of organogenesis of the genital tract in the mouse. The developmental events in the genital tract that occur prenatally and neonatally in the mouse occur prenatally in humans. Mice exposed to DES in utero during the time that reproductive organs are forming have different abnormalities than those described in mice exposed to DES during neonatal life when the structures have formed.

Early in the normal development of the reproductive tract of an embryo, there is an undifferentiated stage in which the sex of the embryo cannot be determined. At this stage, the gonads have not developed into either testis or ovary, and all embryos have a double set of genital ducts, Müllerian ducts (paramesonephric) and the mesonephric (Wolffian) ducts. In the female, as sex differentiation occurs, the Müllerian ducts

develop into the oviduct, uterus, cervix, and upper vagina, while the
mesonephric duct regresses. In the male, under the influence of testicular secretions, the mesonephric ducts form the epididymis, vas deferens
and other tissues such as the seminal vesicles, while the Müllerian ducts
regress. Exposure to DES during this critical period of sex differentiation results in alterations in both female and male reproductive tract,
including the retention of the opposite duct system in both sexes.

FEMALE GENITAL TRACT ABNORMALITIES

Ovary

In a group of animals 4 weeks to 10 months of age that were exposed
prenatally to 100 µg/kg of DES, prevalence of inflammation in the ovary
of DES-treated females varied from 17 to 46%. Oophoritis was not observed
among control animals in the same study [11].

In addition to the high incidence of inflammation, at 6 months of age
the cross-sectional areas of various ovarian components differed between
control and animals exposed prenatally to 100 µg/kg DES; more interstitial
tissue relative to other ovarian components was seen in ovaries from
DES-treated animals. Whether there was quantitatively more interstitial
tissue (ovarian rete) in the DES-exposed animals as compared to controls
was difficult to determine, since decreases in the other ovarian components may have simply made the ovarian rete appear more prominent. For
example, the DES-treated and control animals appeared to have comparable
numbers of follicles at 2 months of age; however, from 2 to 4 months of
age, there was an increase in the number of large follicles in the
DES-treated animals as compared to controls. By 6 months of age, the
ovaries of all the DES-treated animals were largely composed of interstitial tissue with only a few well-defined corpora lutea in some animals
and few remaining follicles in all DES-treated animals. This reduction
in other ovarian components (i.e., oocytes, follicles, and corpora lutea)

resulted in a prominent ovarian rete. This abnormality could not be described in DES-treated animals older than 6 months because large ovarian cysts left little tissue to evaluate.

Ovarian cysts were observed in control and DES-treated animals at 2 months of age. The ovarian bursa was the site of cyst formation in control animals. However, cysts in the DES-treated animals appeared to be from prominent mesonephric remnants since the irregular lining epithelium of the cysts resembled cells of mesonephric origin rather than ovarian surface epithelium. In fact, dilated mesonephric remnants (intra- and connecting ovarian rete) were common in the young DES-treated animals and enlarged in the older animals, forming such large cysts that there was little remaining ovarian tissue to evaluate. Strands of ovarian tissue were frequently found in the walls of the larger cysts. Often the cysts were large, multilocular, and lined by cuboidal or flattened epithelium. The prevalence of ovarian cysts, from mesonephric origin, in the animals exposed to DES in utero was 60% at 8 months and 50% at 10 months. The control animals had ovarian cysts but the location of the cysts was different, the prevalence of cysts was much lower (10% to 20%), and the cysts were smaller in the control animals as compared to the DES-exposed animals.

Oviduct

The association of prenatal exposure to DES and the subsequent development of abnormalities in the oviduct was not surprising since other structures arising from the Müllerian ducts had been reported to be affected in both humans and experimental animals. One example of a teratogenic defect in the oviduct, noticeable at birth in the female DES-exposed offspring, was a malformation.

Marked differences were observed when oviductal development in DES-exposed animals was compared to untreated animals (Fig. 1).

292

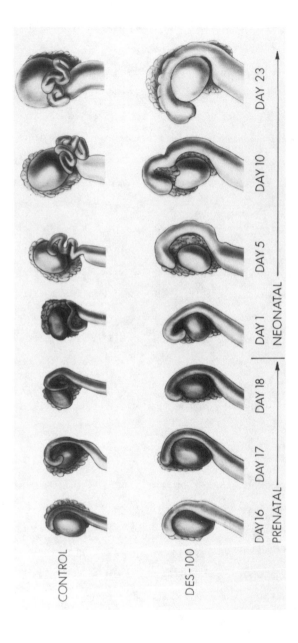

FIG.1. Schematic drawing of oviductal development. Composite drawing from control females and females exposed to DES (100 ug/kg) on days 9-16 of gestation demonstrate oviductal morphogenesis. Each drawing represents three to five females from different litters examined at each age [15].

The oviductal segment normally differentiated late on gestational day 16 with a narrowing of the cranial portion of the Müllerian duct (Fig. 1, upper panel). On day 17, the Müllerian duct developed slight undulations in the oviductal region and then a series of loose, wavy folds were formed, followed by deep coils. By day 1 of neonatal life, the oviduct was identifiable as a discrete region of the Müllerian duct, and its caudal limits were demarcated by an enlargement of the uterine segment. By postnatal day 10, the ovary rotated into the position it had in adult life, and the oviduct increased in length and diameter resulting in tightly packed coils which partially covered the ovary.

In contrast, DES treatment retarded oviductal morphogenesis in mice exposed in utero (Fig. 1, lower panel). Differences were readily apparent by neonatal day 1 when normal Müllerian duct coiling was absent in DES-treated female offspring. Differences became more obvious during postnatal development of the reproductive tract because the oviduct in DES-treated mice failed to lengthen or coil and retained a fetal-like appearance. In those animals exposed to DES in utero the ovary did not rotate, and there was little or no demarcation between the oviduct and the uterus. Also, the angle of entry of the oviduct into the uterus was altered; the oviduct appeared to join the uterus at its apex and formed a straight tube. This malformation of the oviduct was observed in 100% of the females treated prenatally with 100 µg/kg of DES but was not observed in any control animals.

This oviductal malformation persisted throughout the animal's life (Fig. 2) and distorted the anatomical relationships with the uterus, oviduct, and ovary. The retention of this fetal anatomical relationship suggested the term "developmentally arrested oviduct", which we have used to describe this phenomenon [15]. The use of this term was supported by the relative lack of growth of the oviductal segment. Although the body weights of mature (11 to 12 week old) DES-treated and control offspring

were similar (38 grams vs. 36 grams respectively), the average length of
the oviducts of the DES-treated females was only about half that of
control females (8 mm vs. 16 mm).

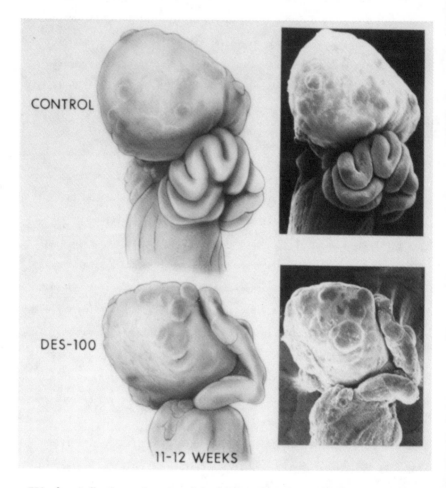

FIG. 2. A drawing and a scanning electron micrograph (SEM) from a 11 to
12 week-old control offspring and an offspring exposed to 100 μg/kg/day
of DES on days 9-16 of gestation. Note the relationship of the ovary,
oviduct, and uterus in the control as compared to the DES-exposed structures. The oviductal coils in the control form regular loops which are
uniform in diameter whereas the DES-exposed oviduct is closely adherent
and wrapped around the ovary [15].

The experimental animal model clearly establishes the oviduct as a target for a teratogenic effect of DES. Moreover, the arrest in development resulting from prenatal exposure to DES suggests a role for estrogens in the normal morphogenesis of the mouse oviduct. It is possible that an increase in estrogen levels during oviductal development may play a role in the ultimate structural or functional integrity of this organ in humans as well as mice. In fact, some of the salient features of the "developmentally-arrested oviduct" in mice exposed prenatally to DES, such as decreased oviductal length, relative lack of fimbriae, and abnormal anatomical location are described in 16 women exposed to DES during gestation [16]. Thus, altered or arrested development of the mammalian oviduct may be a general biological consequence of prenatal exposure to DES.

Prenatal exposure to DES was also associated with functional alterations of the oviduct [15]. Dye injected into the uterine lumen of DES-treated females passed readily into the oviduct and ovarian bursa. However, when the dye was injected into the uterus of control animals, only one out of 17 demonstrated penetration of the dye into the lumen of the oviduct. The dye experiment indicated that the uterotubal junction did not function in the DES-exposed animals to retain the dye in the uterus. Considering the extensive malformation of the oviduct and uterus in the mice exposed prenatally to DES, the passage of dye from the lumen of the uterus to the oviduct was not surprising. Scanning electron microscopy (SEM) of the area of the uterotubal junction of control mice demonstrated a papillary projection where the oviduct entered the uterus. This papillary structure was absent in more than half of the DES-treated animals; and when it was present, it did not function to prevent retrograde flow of uterine fluids.

Defects, on the cellular level, in the oviduct of DES-exposed mice contributed to functional abnormalities. Microscopic alterations of the oviductal epithelium accompanied the teratogenicity associated with prenatal DES treatment [11]. In the control animals, the histologic differentiation coincided with the morphogenetic development. The epithelium showed an increase in cell height, pseudostratification, and evidence of secretory activity. In contrast, the histological differentiation was halted in DES-treated mice. One example was the fimbriae which only minimally developed. Also, in the ampulla of both control and treated animals, there were ciliated and secretory cells. However, in DES-treated animals, the arrangement of the columnar cells lining the lumen and the mucosal folds was irregular. In addition, gland formation was observed in the DES animals which extended through the muscularis, a feature never observed in control mice. Epithelial hyperplasia was also noted, and inflammatory changes were more prevalent in all segments of the oviduct of DES-treated animals.

In the course of our developmental studies, it was determined that epithelial hyperplasia was also seen in mice treated with DES during the first five days of neonatal life, a time when cellular morphogenesis continued in the mouse genital tract. Neonatal female mice were each treated by subcutaneous injection of DES in corn oil on day 1-5 of age. Animals were sacrificed at various times following treatment and their oviducts examined. The induction of epithelial hyperplasia in the oviduct after neonatal treatment occurred in the absence of gross structural malformations induced by prenatal exposure to DES. The time dependent incidence of these staged oviductal alterations is seen in Table 1. The oviducts of control mice never developed epithelial hyperplasia or gland formation (Fig. 3a). However, females exposed neonatally to DES progressively developed proliferative changes in their oviducts which could be grouped into four categories related to the extent of growth disturbances (Table 1).

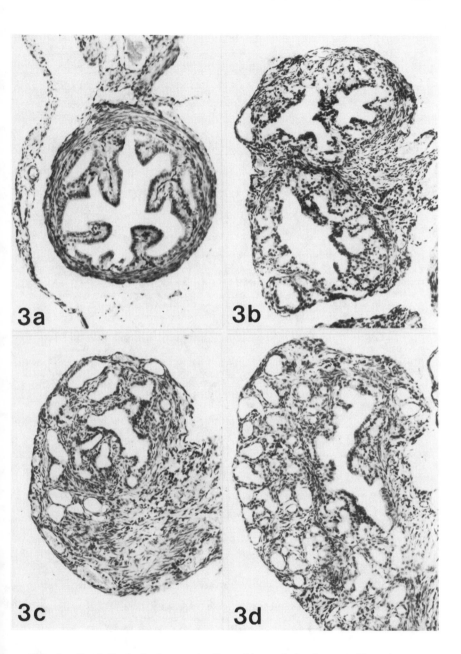

FIG. 3. Morphological changes in the oviduct of developmentally estrogenized mice. Experimental details and description of staging are given in
Table 1. a, Represents the histological appearance of a control oviduct;
b, stage 1; c, stage 3; d, stage 4 of oviductal progressive proliferative
lesion.

Table 1. Epithelial hyperplasia and gland proliferation in the oviduct.

Age after Treatment (months)	Number of Animals	Mice with Oviductal Lesions				
		No Lesion	Stage 1	Stage 2	Stage 3	Stage 4
1	18	2 (11)	16 (89)	0	0	0
4	10	1 (10)	0	9 (90)	0	0
6	12	0	0	0	12 (100)	0
12	30	0	0	0	10 (34)	20 (66)

Outbred CD-1 female mice were subcutaneously injected with DES (Sigma Chemical Co., St. Louis, MO) dissolved in corn oil on days 1-5 of neonatal life (2 μg/day). At 1 to 12 mo. of age, mice were sacrificed and examined for oviductal alterations. The results were summarized into four increasingly severe categories. Stage 1: focal epithelial hyperplasia with a single epithelial fold extended into the muscle wall. Stage 2: general epithelial hyperplasia with several mucosal folds extended through the muscularis; some folds split the muscle wall and sent another layer of connective tissue around the epithelial elements; "gland-like structures" connected with lumen. Stage 3: irregular oviductal serosal surface with marked adenomatous proliferation through the muscularis; no apparent connection of some glandular structures with lumen. Stage 4: cellular changes and degree of severity of folds increased to resemble adenocarcinoma. Glands were never seen in groups of 10 to 15 untreated mice evaluated at corresponding ages at various stages of the estrous cycle. Numbers in parentheses are percentages [17].

Within one month after treatment, changes were noticeable in 16 of 18 (89%) of the mice exposed prenatally to DES (Fig. 3b) and by six months, changes (Stage 3, Fig. 3c) were noted in all of the treated animals. One year after treatment, approximately one-third of the mice had Stage 3 and two-thirds had severe Stage 4 growth disturbances in terms of proliferation and altered differentiation. In DES-exposed mice at 1 month of age, focal epithelial folds extended into the muscle wall. These mucosal folds had an adenomatous (gland-like) appearance but maintained connection with the oviductal lumen. By 4 months, the entire epithelium was hyperplastic, while the muscle layer and stroma were thinner than that of corresponding controls. The number of adenomatous mucosal folds and the degree of extension through the muscle wall increased with age. When treated animals were one year-old, (Table 1: Stage 4), this prolifera- tive lesion, which was first observed in only the ampullary region of the oviduct, had progressed to include the entire length of the tube. The epithelium was markedly hyperplastic and the cells were irregular in size and shape (Fig. 3d). Epithelial proliferation in the wall of the oviduc- tal muscularis resembled adenocarcinoma although this lesion did not spread along the serosal surface and no metastases were observed. Figure 4 schematically represents the progressive proliferation of this oviductal lesion.

It is interesting to note that the histologic changes in mice treated developmentally with DES, i.e., epithelial hyperplasia and gland formation (diverticuli) of the oviductal mucosa which extend into the muscle wall, resembled the clinically described lesions, salpingitis isthmica nodosa (SIN). Since its description by Chiari in 1887, the etiology and patho- genesis of salpingitis isthmica nodosa had been the subject of much debate. Clinically, this lesion had been related to ectopic tubal pregnancy and infertility. The data obtained from our experimental ani- mal model raised the possibility that these clinically noted cases of salpingitis isthmica nodosa have resulted from an altered hormonal environment during early development. Moreover, it is interesting to note that a recent study described salpingitis isthmica nodosa in the oviducts of women exposed prenatally to DES [18].

The mechanisms for regulating epithelial cell proliferation of the reproductive tract are unknown; however, the alterations in the oviduct following neonatal exposure to DES provided a unique model to study epithelial hyperplasia. In addition, the oviduct demonstrated the ability to differentiate into gland-like structures. Thus, this experimental

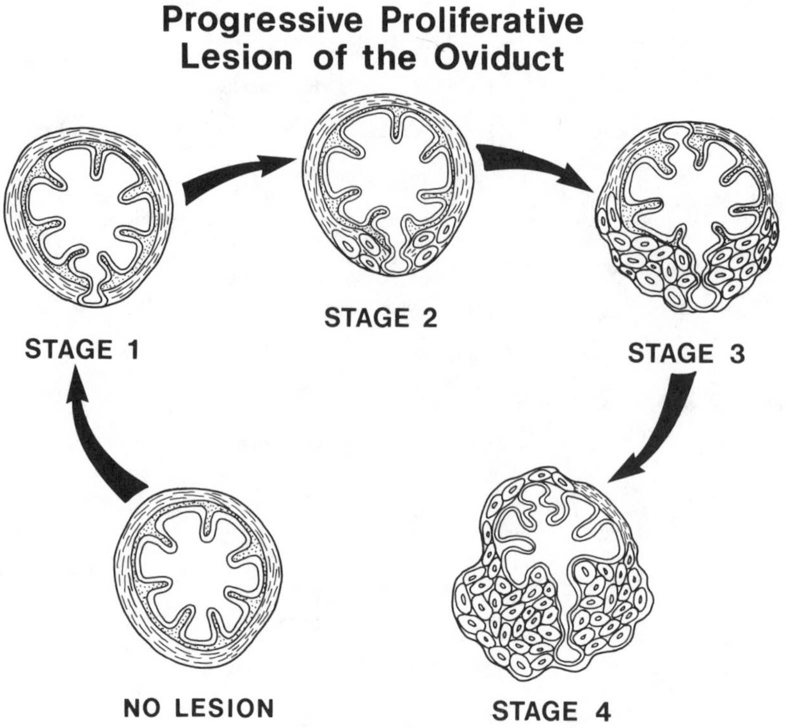

Progressive Proliferative
Lesion of the Oviduct

STAGE 1

STAGE 2

STAGE 3

NO LESION

STAGE 4

FIG. 4. Schematic representation of the progressive proliferative lesion of the oviductal epithelium following developmental exposure to DES. Description of staging is given in Table 1 legend.

model provides an opportunity to study the regulation and differentiation of Müllerian duct epithelium. While the observed changes resided in the epithelium, it is not clear whether the epithelium was responding independently or in combination with factors from the underlying stroma. Since the connective tissue in these DES-treated mice was relatively thin and hypoplastic, it might have been a defect in the stromal compartment that modified the epithelial response. Considering these observations in mice, it was apparent that the proliferative capacity of the epithelium in the Müllerian duct in different regions (uterus, oviduct) may be determined by hormonal exposure during development. If estrogen levels

301

were significantly elevated, as with prenatal DES treatment of animals and humans, the proliferative capacity may be altered. A similar situation may occur with the clinical lesion of salpingitis isthmica nodosa where the oviductal epithelium possesses an increased capacity for proliferation and forms gland-like structures that penetrate the muscle layer.

Mesonephric Duct Remnants

The mesonephric system, which normally regresses in the female, was also affected by prenatal DES exposure [8,11,19]. Figure 5 is a photomicrograph of cystic paraovarian structures between the ovary and oviduct; the cysts were predominantly localized in the region of the ovarian hilus which was consistent with the location of mesonephric remnants.

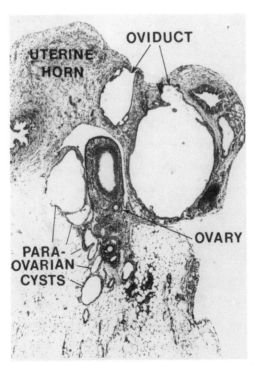

FIG. 5. Cystic paraovarian structures between the ovary and oviduct of a DES-exposed female (100 µg/kg) [19].

Histological variation was apparent in the cysts. The cyst in the upper portion of the photograph, surrounded by a muscle wall, was of meso-nephric duct origin; whereas, the thin-walled cysts located in the lower portion of the figure was of mesonephric tubule origin. Ciliated epithe-lial cells were seen in the upper cyst which is consistent with similarly derived structures in the male. Mesonephric cysts of this magnitude were never observed in our control series of animals. The arrangement of multiple cysts in this animal was similar to the multiple cysts described in a woman who was prenatally exposed to DES [19].

Uterus, Cervix, and Vagina

In addition to the oviduct, structural changes were observed in other regions of the reproductive tract. Following prenatal exposure to DES (100 µg/kg), the uterus was smaller in diameter and length as compared to control females. The muscle compartment of the DES animal was not well organized. At 21 days of age in response to estrogen stimulation, the prenatal DES-exposed mice had decreased uterine growth response, decreased uterine luminal fluid quantity and protein concentration, alterations in specific uterine luminal proteins, and altered cellular differentiation (squamous metaplasia) [20]. Table 2 summarizes the response of the uteri of prepubertal mice exposed prenatally to DES. In aged prenatal DES-exposed females, cystic endometrial hyperplasia was common. A low incidence of benign (leiomyomas) and malignant (adenocar-cinoma, stromal cell sarcoma) tumors was observed [8].

In the cervico-vaginal region of the DES-exposed animals, striking structural abnormalities were also observed. All of the DES animals (100 µg/kg) had hypertrophy of the cervical region. In the most severely affected cases, the Müllerian ducts did not fuse to form a common cer-vical canal. In other less severe cases, the cervix was short cranio-caudally but still had a relatively large diameter, both internal and external with increased stromal elements. The epithelial mucosa of the

cervix also had fewer folds and those that were present were less convoluted and shallower than were observed in control tissue. Also, the
vaginal fornix was always shallower as compared to controls; and, in a
low percentage of DES animals, the fornix was not present (Fig. 6).
Prominent mesonephric remnants were also observed in serial cross-sections
of the cervico-vaginal region [9].

Table 2. Estrogen response of the uteri of prepubertal mice exposed
prenatally to DES.

Prenatal Treatment	Estrogen-stimulated				
	BW (gm)	Ut. wt. (mg)	Apparent uterine luminal surface area (mm^2)	ULF vol (μl)	ULF protein (μg/ml)
Control	17.9 ± 1.0	89 ± 16	90 ± 9	106 ± 37	7559
DES	15.3 ± 2.2	46 ± 13	36 ± 3	29 ± 13	3285

Mice were the female offspring of CD-1 mice treated with either DES (100
μg/kg maternal BW day) or vehicle on days 9-16 of gestation. All mice were
stimulated with DES (100 μg/kg) on days 21-23 of life and killed on day 24.
Control = 21 animals and DES = 45 animals [20].

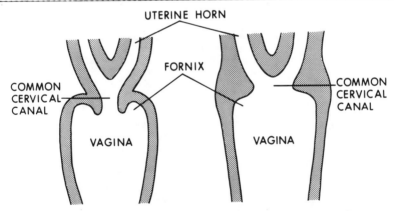

FIG. 6. Schematic drawing of female reproductive tracts. Control,
untreated females (left). Prenatal DES, females treated with DES 100
μg/kg day (right). Note shallow vaginal fornix and a short (craniocaudal)
cervical region. In some cases, there was lack of fusion of the Müllerian
duct to form the common cervical canal.

Aged DES-treated animals (100 μg/kg) had excessive vaginal keratinization which extended into the cervix. The vaginal epithelium of these
DES animals was composed of many layers of immature and mature cells
covered by sheets of keratin. Leukocytes were often seen in the superficial layers. In some animals, increased keratinization combined with
basal cell hyperplasia resulted in irregular pegs of epithelium which
extended into the subadjacent stroma. In 5 of 20 mice, aged 12 to 18
months, there were epidermoid tumors of the vagina [8]. Excessive keratinization, epithelial pegs, and vaginal epidermoid tumors were not seen
in animals exposed to doses of DES less than 100 μg/kg.

Urethral openings, abnormally located anterior to the vulva (persistent
urogenital sinus) were seen in the animals exposed to 100 μg/kg of DES
(female hypospadias). "Gland-like structures" were associated with this
abnormality and were assumed to be of urothelial origin.

Vaginal adenosis was seen in 75% of the mice exposed to DES during
neonatal life, but it was not a common finding in mice following treatment
with DES in utero. However, vaginal adenocarcinoma was observed in low
incidence after prenatal DES exposure; currently, there are 3 cases of
vaginal adenocarcinoma in 230 prenatal DES-exposed animals observed (Fig.
7). The development of vaginal adenocarcinoma was reported to originate
from an alteration in the differentiation of the Müllerian duct epithelium.
Since perinatal mouse studies described a high incidence of vaginal adenosis [21] but, to our knowledge, no cases of vaginal adenocarcinoma, the
demonstration of vaginal adenocarcinoma in the prenatal DES-exposed animal
suggested that the stage of cellular differentiation at the time of DES
exposure may be critical in the final expression of these abnormalities.
The stages of reproductive tract differentiation in mice that encompass
both prenatal and neonatal development occur entirely prenatally in the
human.

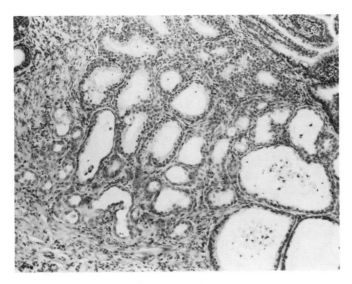

FIG. 7. Vaginal adenocarcinoma in a mouse treated prenatally with DES on days 9-16 of gestation. This lesion is characterized by glands in the vaginal fornix, nuclear pleomorphism, and invasion into the underlying tissue. These findings are consistent with well-differentiated adenocarcinoma.

Reproductive Tract Dysfunction

Studies from our laboratory showed that prenatal exposure to varying doses of DES (0.1 to 100 μg) resulted in a striking dose-related decrease in the fertility of the offspring (Table 3). Over the 32 week period that the animals were observed, the effects ranged from minimal subfertility (90% of control at the lowest dose) to essential sterility at the two highest doses. It should be pointed out that the highest daily dose used in that study (100 μg/kg) was roughly 1/20 the average daily dose based on body weight given therapeutically to pregnant women (100 mg/woman).

The mechanisms responsible for the subfertility in the female mice exposed to DES in utero were products of many problems: oviductal malformation; ovarian dysfunction; improper uterine environment and uterine secretions; uterine, cervical, and vaginal structural alterations. All of these parameters established the fact that exposure to DES, even at relatively low doses, impaired reproductive capacity throughout the animal's lifetime. In humans, infertility [22-24] and unfavorable pregnancy outcome [25-27] have also been reported in women prenatally exposed to DES.

Table 3. Fertility of female mice exposed to DES prenatally[a].

Maternal DES dose (μg/kg)	No. of Females	Total No. of live offspring per mouse	Total reproductive capacity of female offspring[b] (% control)
0	83	74	100
0.01	64	67	91
1	61	55	74
2.5	21	40	54
5	20	18	24
10	67	3	4
100	40	2	3

[a]Timed pregnant CD-1 mice (at least 20 animals per group) were treated subcutaneously with diethylstilbestrol from days 9 to 16 of gestation.

[b]Determined by repetitive force-breeding techniques and expressed as the total number of live young born per mouse over a 32-wk interval [10].

MALE GENITAL TRACT ABNORMALITIES

Arrests in genital tract differentiation and development in males exposed prenatally to DES are demonstrated in Fig. 8. In this schematic representation, the control male is in the left panel. By day 16 of fetal life, the testes of the CD-1 mouse were descending, and the development of the seminal vesicle and other accessory sex organs were seen. In the prenatal DES-exposed animal (right panel), however, the testes were retained. The testes remained in the position occupied during fetal development. In addition, the seminal vesicle did not grow and differentiate after prenatal exposure to DES. These abnormalities represented structural defects that can be seen early in the life of the male animal.

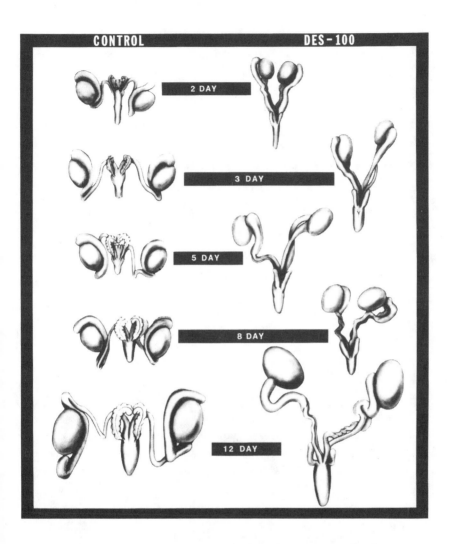

FIG. 8. Schematic representation of male reproductive tract development. Left panel – Control, untreated; note descended testes and development of seminal vesicles and other accessory sex organs. Right panel – Male treated prenatally with DES (100 µg/kg) on days 9–16 of gestation. Testes are retained and seminal vesicles do not grow and differentiate.

This particular structural defect was observed throughout the life of

the animal. Figure 9 is a photograph of an adult male mouse that was

given DES in utero. This animal had retained testes located high in the

308

abdominal cavity and nodular enlargement in the area of the prostatic

utricle. In addition, this animal had large epididymal cysts. As in the

female, the male also had retained the opposite duct system. Müllerian

duct remnants, which normally regressed in the male, contributed to the

formation of epididymal cysts. The regulation of the morphological

events involved in these defects in differentiation was unclear but the

lack of testicular descent and oviductal malformation could be compared

in males and females since it was probably a common phenomenon respon-

sible for the teratogenic effects in both. These were just two examples

of teratogenic changes in male and female mice following prenatal expo-

sure to DES. In addition to these gross structural defects, there were

examples of other abnormalities of the reproductive tract of mice exposed

prenatally to DES. The DES-exposed males experienced similar functional

problems as the females. The fertility of the males following prenatal

DES exposure was also reduced (Table 4).

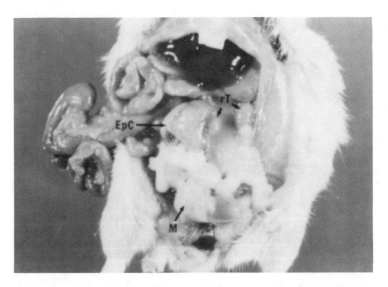

FIG. 9. Reproductive tract abnormalities in a 9 month-old male mouse
exposed prenatally to DES include retained testes (rT), an epididymal cyst
(EpC), and a mass (M) in the region of the seminal colliculus [7].

Table 4. Effect of prenatal exposure to DES on fertility of male offspring*.

Treatment (µg/kg/day)	Number of sterile males
Corn oil (Control)	0/10
DES	
0.01	0/10
1	0/10
10	1/10
100	6/10

*Males were the 20- to 25-week-old offspring of pregnant CD-1 mice treated with diethylstilbestrol (DES) on days 9 through 16 of gestation. Nonsterile males had the same breeding performance as controls [28].

In the prenatal DES-exposed mouse only the highest dose was associated with noticeable changes in the reproductive tract so far; 6 out of 10 of the male offspring treated with 100 µg/kg were sterile. The nonsterile males had the same breeding performance as controls. Several factors appeared to be related to this decreased fertility in the males. These included: (1) abnormal sperm morphology and motility, (2) lesions in the reproductive tract, (3) abnormal secretions and (4) inflammation [27]. Thus, there were many examples of abnormalities in both the male and female offspring which contributed to functional defects in the genital tract.

In the male, we also found a long-term, rare alteration that was apparently derived from a change in the mesonephric epithelium. During embryonic development the mesonephric duct system gives rise to the rete testis and other male structures.

Carcinoma of the rete testis is an exceptionally rare lesion. It has only been reported infrequently in the clinical literature [29] and three times in experimental animals [30-32]. But treatment of pregnant

CD-1 mice with DES (100 μg/kg) resulted in rete lesions resembling adenocarcinoma in 5% of their male offspring (Fig. 10) [33].

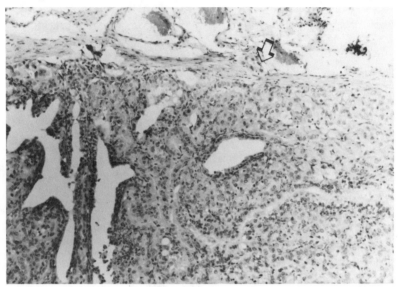

FIG. 10. Adenocarcinoma of the rete testis from a 16 month-old prenatally DES-treated mouse. While the papillary pattern is focally apparent,
the majority of the tumor has a tubular arrangement of pleomorphic
epithelial cells. Arrow shows an area of invasion.

Cryptorchidism has been implicated as a predisposing factor for
testicular neoplasms. The high incidence of retained testes in mice
(92%) following prenatal DES exposure and the occurrence of this specific
rare form of testicular cancer, rete adenocarcinoma, raised the possibility of an association between cryptorchidism, prenatal DES exposure and
rete testis cancer. Although cryptorchidism resulted in decreased or
lack of spermatogenesis in male mice, inactivity could not solely account
for higher prevalence of rete adenocarcinoma since several of the mice
with the lesion had spermatogenesis occurring in the same testis. Table
5 demonstrates the occurrence of rete hyperplasia and adenocarcinoma.
These results suggested an association between prenatal DES exposure and
the subsequent development of testicular lesions including neoplasia of
the rete testis in mice.

Table 5. Testicular lesions in male mice exposed prenatally to
diethylstilbestrol[a].

Lesion	Control	DES-100
Rete Testis Hyperplasia	$\frac{23}{96}$ (24)[b]	$\frac{130}{233}$ (56)[c]
Rete Testis Adenocarcinoma	$\frac{0}{96}$ (0)	$\frac{11}{233}$ (5)[d]

[a]Lesions in the testes of male mice exposed prenatally to DES. Males were
10 to 18 months old offspring of CD-1 mice treated with DES (100 μg/kg subcutaneously) on days 9-16 of gestation. Since there was not a statistically significant difference in prevalence of lesions with age, rete testis
hyperplasia and adenocarcinoma in each age group have been combined.

[b]Numbers in parentheses are percentages.

Statistical significance of DES-exposed animals to corresponding age-
matched controls by Fisher exact test.

[c]$p < .0001$ [d]$p < .05$

USEFULNESS OF THE PRENATAL DES MODEL

Although animal studies must be considered thoughtfully if extrapola-
tion to humans is to follow, the prenatal mouse model has provided some
useful comparisons to similarly DES-exposed women. These are summarized
in Tables 6 and 7.

A schematic representation of the early changes in the reproductive
tract of males and females exposed to DES during the critical stage of
sex differentiation is shown in Fig. 11. This figure demonstrates the
arrest in development common to male and female mice which results in
structural malformations in the genital tracts of both sexes which persist into adult life.

Vaginal adenocarcinoma in the female and rete adenocarcinoma in the
male, both extremely rare findings in experimental animals and humans,
represent only two examples of growth control derangements seen as long-
term defects in mice following prenatal DES exposure. By studying

alterations in both sexes, it gives us a better understanding of the developmental events and the mechanisms involved in these observed defects.

Table 6. Comparative developmental effects of prenatal exposure to diethylstilbestrol in mice and humans: Female offspring.

Structural Malformation of Oviduct

    Mouse (McLachlan et al., 1980; Newbold et al., 1983)
    Human (DeCherney et al., 1981)

Paraovarian Cysts (Mesonephric Origin)

    Mouse (Newbold et al., 1983)
    Human (Haney et al., submitted)

Salpingitis Isthmica Nodosa (SIN) of the Oviduct

    Mouse (Newbold et al., 1983; Newbold et al., 1984)
    Human (Shen et al., 1983)

Vaginal Adenocarcinoma

    Mouse (McLachlan et al., 1980; Newbold et al., 1982)
    Human (Herbst et al., 1971)

Table 7. Comparative developmental effects of prenatal exposure to diethylstilbestrol in mice and humans: Male offspring.

Cryptorchid Testes

    Mouse (McLachlan et al., 1975; McLachlan, 1981)
    Human (Bibbo et al., 1975; Gill et al., 1981)

Epididymal Cysts

    Mouse (McLachlan et al., 1975; McLachlan, 1981)
    Human (Bibbo et al., 1975; Gill et al., 1981)

Testicular Lesions

    Mouse (Newbold et al., submitted)
    Human (Gill et al., 1979; Conley et al., 1983)

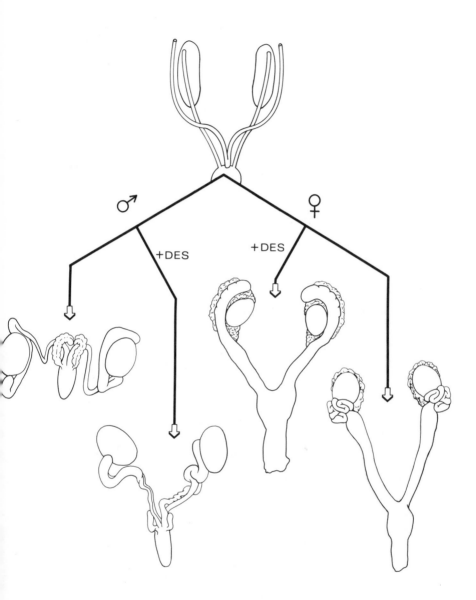

FIG. 11. Schematic representation of the early changes in the reproductive tract of males and females exposed to DES during the critical stage of sex differentiation.

SUMMARY

Prenatal exposure to the potent synthetic estrogen, DES, is associated with structural, functional, and long-term alterations in the male and female offspring. The changes that were seen have been associated with doses that are in the range of 1-100 micrograms per kilogram of maternal body weight. Whether these effects would be seen with other estrogenic compounds that may have different receptor or biological activity, or that remain in the fetus for a different length of time, or that are metabolized along reactive pathways is unknown, but it will provide many new subjects of investigation.

Finally, since some of these effects are apparently common to different species and experimental results can be both informative and predictive, continued close surveillance of the exposed human population seems warranted, especially in view of the young age of the patients.

REFERENCES

1. R.R. Greene, M.W. Burrill, and A.C. Ivy, Am. J. Anat. 67, 305 (1940).
2. T.B. Dunn and A.W. Green, J. Natl. Cancer Inst. 31, 425 (1963).
3. N. Takasugi, H.A. Bern, and K.B. De Ome, Science 138, 438 (1962).
4. J.A. McLachlan, Estrogens in the Environment (Elsevier/North Holland, New York 1980).
5. A.L. Herbst, H. Ulfelder, and D.C. Poskanser, N. Engl. J. Med. 284, 878 (1971).
6. DES Task Force Summary Report. Washington, D.C., United States Department of Health, Education and Welfare, U.S.1 Government Printing Office (1978).
7. J.A. McLachlan, R.R. Newbold, and B. Bullock, Science 190, 991 (1975).
8. J.A. McLachlan, R.R. Newbold, and B.C. Bullock, Cancer Res. 40, 3988 (1980).
9. R.R. Newbold and J.A. McLachlan, Cancer Res. 42, 2003 (1982).
10. J.A. McLachlan, R.R. Newbold, H.C. Shah, M.D. Hogan, and R.L. Dixon, Fert. Sterility 38, 364 (1982).
11. R.R. Newbold, B.C. Bullock, and J.A. McLachlan, Biol. Reprod. 28, 735 (1983).
12. H.A. Bern and F.J. Talamantes in: Developmental Effects of Diethylstilbestrol (DES) in Pregnancy, A.L. Herbst and H.A. Bern, eds. (Thieme-Stratton, New York 1981) pp. 129-147.
13. J.G. Forsberg, Natl. Cancer Inst. Mono. 51, 41 (1979).
14. H. Tuchmann-Duplessis, G. David, and P. Haegel, Illustrated Human Embryology, Vol. II (Springer Verlag, New York 1972).
15. R.R. Newbold, S. Tyrey, A.F. Haney, and J.A. McLachlan, Teratology 27, 417 (1983).
16. A.H. DeCherney, I. Cholst, and F. Naftolin, Fert. Steril. 36, 741 (1981).

17. R.R. Newbold, B.C. Bullock, and J.A. McLachlan, Terat. Carcino. Mut. (Submitted).
18. S.C. Shen, M. Bansal, R. Purrazzella, V. Malviya, and L. Strauss, Am. J. Surg. Path. 1, 293 (1983).
19. A.F. Haney, R.R. Newbold, B.F. Fetter, and J.A. McLachlan, Am. J. Path. (Submitted).
20. D.B. Maier, R.R. Newbold, and J.A. McLachlan, Endocrinology 116, 1878 (1985).
21. L. Plappinger and H.A. Berne, JNCI 63, 507 (1979).
22. A.L. Herbst, M.M. Hubby, R.R. Blough, and F. Azizi, J. Rep. Med. 24, 62 (1980).
23. M.J. Burger and D.P Goldstein, Ob-Gyn 55, 25 (1980).
24. G. Schmidt, W.C. Fowler, L.M. Talbert, and D.A. Edelman, Fertil. Steril. 32, 21 (1980).
25. L. Cousins, W. Karp, C. Lacey, and W.E. Lucas, Ob-Gyn 56, 70 (1980).
26. E.C. Sandberg, N.L. Riffle, J.V. Higdon, and C.E. Getman, Am. J. Obst. Gynecol. 14, 194 (1981).
27. A.B. Barnes, T. Colton, J. Gundersen, K.L. Noller, B.C. Tilley, T. Strama, D.E. Townsend, P. Hatab, and P.C. O'Brien, N. Engl. J. Med. 302, 609 (1980).
28. J.A. McLachlan, J. Toxicol. Env. Health 2, 527 (1977).
29. F.K. Mostofi and E.B. Price in: Atlas of Tumor Pathology, Second Series, Fascicle 8, Armed Forces Institute of Pathology, Washington, D.C. (1973).
30. J.E. Searson, Vet. Pathol. 17, 391 (1980).
31. K.C. Snell and C.F. Hollander, JNCI 49, 1381 (1972).
32. K. Yoshitomi and S. Morii, Vet. Pathol. 21, 300 (1984).
33. R.R. Newbold, B.C. Bullock, and J.A. McLachlan, Cancer Res. (Accepted).

DISCUSSION

NAFTOLIN: Tamoxifen (unpublished) and clomid (Moushita et al., 1975) induce a similar picture in the neonatally-treated rat, but the tubes are actually bloated by the accumulation of massive numbers of desquamated cells. Do your DES-treated mice have such a picture explaining their widely dilated tubes?

NEWBOLD: No.

NAFTOLIN: The treated mice undoubtedly had estrogen sterilization of the hypothalamus with constant high estrogen. Do you get such long-term adenomas of the tube in castrated or castrated/physiologic estradiol treated mice?

NEWBOLD: Proliferative lesions of the oviduct are not seen in mice which have been ovariectomized prepubertally. Estrogen treatment stimulates the expression of this lesion.

EROSCHENKO: As I understand it from current literature, prenatal DES
treatment induces a different type of cell surface in cornified vaginal
cells (lack of well-developed microridges). Have you seen any such
changes in your DES-treated animals? I have often compared the changes
in cornified vaginal cells in Kepone-treated females (also a lack of
well-developed microridges) to those reported in DES-treated females. I
wonder if such changes are still recorded in your work?

NEWBOLD: Such changes in the surface architecture have been seen in prenatally DES-treated mice (Lamb et al., Cancer Res., 41, 4057, 1981).

JONES: Have you transplanted these DES-exposed oviducts into nude mice?

NEWBOLD: Yes, and no tumors have been observed.

JONES: What effects have you seen in progesterone-treated animals?

NEWBOLD: Progesterone does not stimulate expression of these epithelial
proliferative lesions in the oviducts of DES-treated mice.

TUCHMANN-DUPLESSIS: First of all, I want to express to you my compli-
ments for your clear and elegant presentation. The experiments presented
raise many basic problems. I will however limit my questions to two:
(1) Is the cryptorchidism shown in your slide related to an action on the
pituitary hypothalamic axis? (2) How do you explain that even very small
doses of DES are capable to determine structural and functional lesions?

NEWBOLD: In answer to your first question, exposure to DES or other
estrogens early in development certainly has an effect on the establish-
ment of normal neural function. However, the maldescent of the testes is
recognized as early as day 16 of gestation in the mouse. Furthermore,
there are microscopically detectable defects in the fetal/neonatal guber-
naculum. With regard to the second question, it seems that DES overrides
the physiological mechanisms which protect the fetus from estrogenization
during normal pregnancies.

CUNHA: We have found that in human fetal reproductive tracts grown in
vivo in athymic mice DES stimulated the mesonephric duct in agreement
with your findings. Since mesenchyme in the developing genital tract is
definitely an estrogen target tissue, it may be that estrogen (DES)
impairs the normal differentiation of the mesenchyme in the uterus, or
oviduct into its two cell lineages, stroma versus smooth muscle. This
could account for many of the lesions that you and others have reported.

NEWBOLD: I agree. In fact, the uterus and oviduct of these animals
clearly display disorganization of the muscle layer as we have previously
reported (Newbold et al., Biol Reprod., 28, 735, 1983).

STUMPF: It would be of interest to know whether or not there is a relationship between the occurrence of lesion and local nuclear binding of
DES at the time of induction of the lesion. Have such kinds of studies
been done in conjunction with your morphological experiments?

NEWBOLD: As you know, your work (Stumpf et al., J. Steroid Biochem. 12,
55, 1980) in our mice have shown that DES is apparently localized in the
nuclei of mesenchymal cells in the genital tracts of 16 day fetal mice
treated in utero with ^{3}H-DES. We had earlier shown in a pharmacokinetic
study that the fetal genital tract accumulated DES associated radioactivity some 3-4 fold when compared to fetal plasma (Shah and McLachlan,

JPET, 197, 687, 1976). Of possibly greater importance than localization, we have recently demonstrated that the fetal mouse genital tract in organ culture is capable of oxidatively metabolizing DES (Maydl et al., Endocrinol, 113, 146, 1983.

BOYLAN: Regarding uniformity versus variability of response within or between litters, which parameters studied display the most uniformity/most variability of response? Are siblings more or less variable in response than pups within the treatment group? How do you treat siblings statistically?

NEWBOLD: With our current experimental design, this information is not available. Treated pups are Caesarian derived on day 19 of gestation, randomized between litters and foster mothered. In previous studies in which litter effects were rigorously studied (McLachlan et al., Fertil. Steril. 38, 364, 1982), their influence on reproductive performance was minimal.

NAFTOLIN: The DES effect on the human oviduct is the opposite of the mouse result. The tubes are long and thin "withered tubes" (DeCherney et al., Fertil. Steril. 36, 741, 1981). Please discuss the species differences. Furthermore, it is interesting that Turner Syndrome patients who have evidence of "minature" uteri can be made normal enough to carry IVF pregnancies to term and deliver normally. Therefore, there may be a broader spectrum of influences than previously known. The point made by Dr. Gerald Cunha concerning the lack of the muscle compartment on his DES-treated embryonic tracts is perhaps mirrored in the DES tube and uterus ("withered tube" and "T-shaped" uterus, respectively), which lack muscle but apparently not epithelium.

NEWBOLD: Developmental treatment with DES has a profound influence on muscle organization in the genital tract. The differences in the oviducts of mice or humans treated prenatally with DES may not be that great considering that one species (mouse) has an ovarian bursa to collect oocytes and the other (human) displays a well-developed fimbria. In the paper you mention, the "withered tube" is described as a foreshortened, sacculated, convoluted tube with a pinpoint os and constricted fimbria." The fimbria were described as withered. In both species, the tubes are apparently underdeveloped.

GOLDZIEHER: There are such differences in pharmacokinetics, pharmacodynamics and metabolism of estrogen in rodents versus man that comparisons on a mg/kg basis of administered dose are quite meaningless. In man, ability to conceive (as contrasted with ability to carry to term) is not impaired, contrary to your statement and contrary to events in the rodent, where the persistent estrus condition has no comparable phenomenon in women. Since ovarian function and, therefore, the endocrine environment in these mice is grossly altered, how have you taken this into consideration in the interpretation of your observations? Your table of similarities between mouse findings and similar clinical conditions is only half of the available data set. What about also tabulating the differences, e.g., the lack of effect on human cyclicity and ovulation versus the persistent estrus syndrome in rats, mice?

NEWBOLD: Obviously, there are differences in pharmacokinetics and metabolism between experimental animals and humans. That makes the species similarities in DES-associated defects all the more striking. It should further be pointed out that the major metabolite of DES, dienestrol, has been determined in many different species including mice and humans.

Although there seems to be general agreement among clinicians that, on average, prenatal exposure to DES has a somewhat adverse effect on pregnancy outcome, the influence of such treatment on human fertility is still controversial; however, at least three studies report increases in infertility in DES-exposed women (Herbst et al., J. Reprod. Med. 24, 62, 1980); Berger and Goldstein, OB-GYN, 55, 25, 1980; Schmidt et al., Fertil. Steril., 32, 21, 1980). With regard to altered cyclicity in humans and rodents, I don't think enough detailed studies have really been done on this subject in humans; although Bibbo and colleagues (OB-GYN, 49, 1, 1977) found a statistically significant increase in menstrual irregularities among 229 DES-exposed women, compared with 136 age-matched control patients, and Haney et al. (Fertil. Steril. 31, 142, 1979) also reported increased primary dysmenorrhea and menstrual irregularity in DES-exposed patients. Finally, it has recently been shown cytologically that women exposed to DES in utero have significantly higher frequencies of karatotic reaction as evidenced by vaginal smears than their corresponding controls (Woodhouse et al., Acta Cytologia, 28, 1984). These data taken together with those presented in the formal paper and described by others for neonatally treated mice speak more to species similarities than to dissimilarities.

SONNENSCHEIN: The incidence of lesions you described in these mice are comparable to those in humans. Are you aware of mice strains in which the incidence of these lesions is lower or absent? The implication of my question relates to the possibility that strains of mice in which the incidence of lesions is higher represent populations in which "inborn errors of control of cellular proliferation" are prominent.

NEWBOLD: Differences in sensitivity to tumor induction by estrogens is well known among mouse strains. The only studies dealing with strain differences in developmental induction of genital lesions by estrogens was that of Plapinger and Bern (JNCI, 63, 507, 1979) in which they, indeed, determined a more sensitive strain for induction of adenosis-like lesions.

ESTROGEN-ASSOCIATED DEFECTS IN RODENT MAMMARY GLAND
DEVELOPMENT

HOWARD A. BERN, KAREN T. MILLS AND MARC EDERY
Department of Zoology and Cancer Research Laboratory, University of California,
Berkeley, California 94720

INTRODUCTION

Prenatal and/or neonatal exposure of laboratory rodents to estrogens may lead to

alterations in mammary gland structure and function by two principal routes: (1)

changes resulting from the direct effect of early hormone exposure on the mammary

gland itself, and (2) changes resulting from an altered hormonal milieu and hence

indirect. In prior studies of cervicovaginal changes arising from exposure to steroids

during the early critical period [see 1], both ovary-independent (direct effects) and

ovary-dependent (indirect effects mediated by an altered hypothalamo-hypophysio-

ovarian axis) abnormalities are encountered. This paper will survey briefly the avail-

able experimental data on the mammary gland pointing to direct and indirect effects

of early hormone exposure. The literature in this field up to 1979 has been reviewed

in some detail [2; see also 1].

Table I summarizes briefly the nature of the effects that have been reported as

results of early exposure of rodents to estrogens including diethylstilbestrol (DES). It

is not always possible to state with certainty whether each of these effects is the

result of direct action of the initial hormonal treatment upon the epithelium and/or

stroma of the gland or whether the effect has been mediated by the altered endocrine

system which might involve continuous ovarian estrogen secretion and subsequent

continuous hypophysial prolactin secretion. However, the altered sensitivity to

carcinogen in the rat appears to be a direct effect [19].

The animal model systems used (Table 1) indicate that intrauterine exposure to

DES or other exogenous estrogens might be expected to have consequences on breast

tissue and/or on the endocrine axes involved in regulation of breast development and

function. All of the rodent data have indicated the likelihood of increased

hyperplasia, dysplasia and sensitivity to chemical or viral carcinogens and to hormones in the mammary tissue exposed to estrogens in early life, except for the neonatally exposed rat, where an inhibition in sensitivity to carcinogens has been reported [14-16]. However, Boylan and Calhoon [17-19] have now clearly shown that prenatal exposure of the developing rat to DES results in an increased carcinogenic response to later DMBA exposure. Possibly the critical period for the rat is earlier than for the mouse.

TABLE I. Mammary gland changes in rodents following prenatal or neonatal estrogen exposure

Mouse	Increased growth, secretory activity, dysplasia [3-6] Increased tumor incidence in presence of expressed mammary tumor virus [7-9] Increased sensitivity to carcinogen (dysplasias) [10] Increased sensitivity to hormones [11-13]
Rat	Decreased sensitivity to carcinogen (neonatal DES)[14-16] Increased sensitivity to carcinogen (prenatal DES) [17-19] Increased sensitivity to DES (prenatal DES) [20]
Hamster	Increased sensitivity to carcinogen [21]

EXPERIMENTAL STUDIES

Studies at Berkeley have delineated a number of effects on the mammary gland of exposure of mice to sex steroids. In our earlier studies using female BALB/c mice, we extended the pioneering observations of Mori by showing that neonatal exposure to estradiol (and to any other sex steroid) resulted in a significantly higher mammary tumor incidence in mammary tumor virus (MTV)-expressed (BALB/cfC3H) mice [7-8]. When MTV-unexpressed mice were used, tumors did not develop but hyperplasia and dysplasia were clearly evident [7,9]. Mammary tumorigenesis after neonatal sex hormone exposure requires the presence of both MTV and the ovary. Nodule-like structures were encountered in appreciable numbers in the neonatally exposed MTV-unexpressed mice, and similar structures have been seen after neonatal DES exposure (Bern, Mills, Kohrman and Mori, in preparation). However, when these "noduloids" were transplanted into the cleared mammary fat pads of syngeneic mice, only 3 out of 95 transplants produced appreciable hyperplastic lobuloalveolar outgrowth, arguing against their preneoplastic nature. Indeed, we presently interpret these structures as being residual lobules reflecting the excess stimulation of the mammary gland which occurs as a result of activation of the hypothalamo-hypophysial gonadotropin-ovarian estrogen-hypophysial prolactin axis.

There is some controversy as to whether neonatal treatment of mice with DES or other estrogens results in increased circulating prolactin (PRL) levels and in increased prolactin synthesis and/or release in adult life. The picture is confounded by the use of different mouse strains, the presence or absence of expressed MTV, and the neonatal dosage of hormone employed. Thus, the data of Nagasawa et al. [22] on BALB/c mice include some evidence of increased blood levels; pituitaries from estrogen-treated mice show a significantly greater number of prolactin cells [23]. Kalland et al. [24] found no increased levels in their mouse stock but an increased sensitivity of the pituitary prolactin cells to estrogen stimulation as a result of neonatal DES treatment. Huseby and Thurlow [25] found evidence for hyper-prolactinemia in C3HxBALB/c and BALB/c mice exposed prenatally to "low-dose" DES. Lopez et al. [26] found that high doses (2.5 μg daily) of DES given neonatally to C3H/MTV+ mice decreased circulatory levels of PRL and decreased PRL synthesis by the pituitary incubated in vitro (release was the same in the DES and control pituitaries). The decreased PRL levels at high DES dose levels are consistent with the minimal mammary development seen in BALB/c mice so exposed (Mills and Bern, unpublished).

When the 5-day neonatal estrogen treatment was begun after day 3, the mammary glands failed to show abnormalities [5]. There is thus a critical period for the later occurrence of mammary gland dysplasias, as there is for the occurrence of persistent vaginal cornification, in response to neonatal estrogen. Whether the critical period is at the hypothalamic level or at the mammary gland level, or both, is not known.

When quantification of immediate and postpubertal effects of early sex hormone exposure was attempted, following the technique of counting ductal branch-points used by Warner [3], we found that estradiol had an early inhibitory effect (at 6 days of age) and a later stimulatory effect (at about 5 weeks of age) on ductal development [4]. We interpret the former response as reflecting a direct action upon the mammary duct system and the latter as evidence of a precociously stimulated hypothalamo-hypophysio-ovarian complex.

We have recently examined the mammary glands from neonatally DES-exposed BALB/c males and found evidence for DES inhibition of the minimal ductal branching seen at 6 weeks and at 4 months of age (Table II). However, in the absence of the ovary and of estrogen, this experiment provided no real measure of altered responsiveness of the mammary gland.

TABLE II. Responses of mammary glands of intact BALB/c male mice exposed neonatally to DES.

Treatment	n	Glands absent	Binary branching or less	Tertiary branching
A. At 6 weeks				
Control	12	4	4	4
10^{-1} µg DES	12	8	4	0
1 µg DES	5	3	2	0
B. At 4 months				
Control	27	6	12	9
1 µg DES	22	11	10	1

The mammary glands of female mice exposed neonatally to DES show an increased sensitivity to later treatment with female sex hormones, as judged by increases in cystic alveolar adenosis, terminal duct hyperplasia and dilated ducts (Mills, Ostrander, Hatch and Bern, in preparation). Evidence for an increased sensitivity to hormones as is seen in the neonatally DES-exposed female mouse should also be sought in the neonatally DES-exposed male mouse; these data may have some relevance to the situation wherein young male humans may show breast hypertrophy after inadvertent exposure to estrogens both before and after puberty.

The receptor levels of breast tissue may be altered as a consequence of early exposure to hormones. When the mammary glands of BALB/c mice exposed to various neonatal doses of DES (from 10^{-5} µg to 1 µg daily for the first 5 days of life), a significant decrease (p < 0.01) in cytosolic estrogen receptor levels [see 27 for methods] was seen at the highest dose levels (10^{-1} and 1 µg) at 1, 2, 6 and 12 months of age (Table III). Inasmuch as a 2-µg dose of DES also results in inhibition of mammary growth by 5 weeks of age [4], and doses > 1 µg DES do the same when mice reach older ages (Mills and Bern, unpublished), the inhibition may be related to the decreased estrogen receptor level. Verhoeven et al. [28] found lower estrogen receptor levels in DMBA-induced mammary tumors in rats given estradiol antenatally compared with control rats. Antenatal DES exposure appeared to favor greater progestin binding by rat mammary tumors compared with tumors in control rats [29].

TABLE III. Effect of neonatal DES exposure on estrogen receptor level in mammary glands of female BALB/c mice.

DES dosage (µg)	Cytosolic Estrogen Receptor (fmol/mg protein)			
	1 month	2 months	6 months	12 months
1	25±4*	30±5*	22±6*	29±5*
10^{-1}	29+7*	31±4	24±5*	38±7
10^{-2}	39±8	35±9	39±5	44±3
10^{-3}	36±5	38±6	46±10	43±6
10^{-4}	42±10	39±3	42+7	40±7
10^{-5}	47±11	42±7	48±4	44±5
Control	52±7	43±5	45±8	41±6

*significantly different from control (p < 0.01); n = 4 experiments (4-6 mice per group)

The isolated mammary epithelial cells of female BALB/c mice treated neonatally with sex steroids show altered responses, when cultured in collagen gels in a defined serum-free medium, to growth factors such as Li^+ and epidermal growth factor [30]. There appears to be a lowered response to growth factors generally after early estrogen exposure.

PERSPECTIVES

Compared with studies on the genital tract of female rodents, research on mammary gland involvement after perinatal exposure to DES and other sex hormones has been relatively limited. In general, existent data point to possible increases in tumor and dysplasia risks resulting from hormone treatments during development. Longterm effects may involve the mammary tissues directly and also the endocrine glands regulating breast growth and function. However, some of the data are contradictory. In particular, high neonatal doses of sex steroids and DES in mice may have longterm effects which suggest inhibition of responses (and estrogen receptor levels) and inhibition of mammotropic hormone secretion. Exposure to estrogen relatively early in fetal life may also inhibit mammary gland development [cf. 31-33]. Much more experimental investigation is needed, using a wide range of hormone doses given at different times, prenatally and neonatally. Although there have as yet been no reports on increased breast disease in DES daughters, and information indicating abnormal endocrine function is minimal (as indeed is the number of clinical investigations needed to determine this issue), studies with rodent models strongly support the desirability of an increased concern with clinical possibilities involving persistent changes in breast sensitivity and in hormonal balance.

SUMMARY

The effects of early exposure to estrogens on the mammary glands of experimental rodents are reviewed. These effects include hyperplastic and dysplastic changes, as well as neoplastic changes in the MTV-expressed mouse. Increased sensitivity to hormones and to carcinogens occurs in the adult. Exposure to high dose levels or exposure in early fetal life may lead to inhibited mammary development in both females and males, including reduced estrogen receptor levels. Effects may be direct upon the mammary gland or indirect, mediated by alterations in levels of mammotropic hormones.

ACKNOWLEDGMENTS

Research from our laboratory has been supported by Grant No. CA05388 awarded by the National Institutes of Health, DHHS. We are indebted to Aniko Mos for micro-technical assistance and to Susie Castillo for manuscript preparation.

REFERENCES

1. H.A. Bern and F.J. Talamantes, Jr. in: The Developmental Effects of Diethylstilbestrol (DES) in Pregnancy, A.L. Herbst and H.A. Bern, eds. (Thieme-Stratton, New York 1981) pp. 129-147.
2. T. Mori, H. Nagasawa, and H.A. Bern, J. Environ. Pathol. Toxicol. 3, 191-206 (1979).
3. M.R. Warner, Cell Tiss. Kinetics 9, 429-438 (1976).
4. Y. Tomooka and H.A. Bern, J. Natl. Cancer Inst. 69, 1347-1352 (1982).
5. H.A. Bern, K.T. Mills, and L.A. Jones, Proc. Soc. Exp. Biol. Med. 172, 239-242 (1983).
6. J.M. Strum, Virchows Arch. Cell Pathol. 42, 227-233 (1983).
7. T. Mori, H.A. Bern, K.T. Mills, and P.N. Young, J. Natl. Cancer Inst. 57, 1057-1062 (1976).
8. L.A. Jones and H.A. Bern, Cancer Res. 37, 67-75 (1977).
9. L.A. Jones and H.A. Bern, Cancer Res. 39, 2560-2567 (1979).
10. M.R. Warner and R.L. Warner, J. Natl. Cancer Inst. 55, 289-298 (1975).
11. M.R. Warner and R.L. Warner, In Vitro 13, 477-483 (1977).
12. M.R. Warner, J. Endocrinol. 77, 1-10 (1978).
13. M.R. Warner, L. Yau, and J.M. Rosen, Endocrinology 106, 823-832 (1980).
14. C.J. Shellabarger and V.A. Soo, Cancer Res. 33, 1567-1569 (1973).
15. H. Nagasawa, R. Yanai, M. Shodono, T. Nakamura, and Y. Tanabe, Cancer Res. 34, 2643-2646 (1974).
16. H. Yoshida and R. Fukunishi, Gann 69, 627-632 (1978).
17. E.S. Boylan and R. Calhoon, J. Toxicol. Environ. Health 5, 1059-1071 (1979).
18. E.S. Boylan and R.E. Calhoon, J. Natl. Cancer Inst. 66, 649-652 (1981).
19. E.S. Boylan and R.E. Calhoon, Cancer Res. 43, 4879-4884 (1983).
20. T.C. Rothschild, R.E. Calhoon, and E.S. Boylan, Proc. Amer. Assoc. Cancer Res. 76th Annual Meeting, Abstract no. 770 (1985).
21. M. Rustia and P. Shubik, Cancer Res. 39, 4636-4644 (1979).
22. H. Nagasawa, T. Mori, R. Yanai, H.A. Bern, and K.T. Mills, Cancer Res. 38, 942-945 (1978).
23. S. Kawashima, H.A. Bern, L.A. Jones, and K.T. Mills, Endocrinol. Japan. 25, 341-348 (1978).
24. T. Kalland, J.-G. Forsberg, and Y.N. Sinha, Endocrine Res. Comm. 7, 157-166 (1980).
25. R.A. Huseby and S. Thurlow, Am. J. Obstet. Gynecol. 144, 939-949 (1982).
26. J. Lopez, L. Ogren, and F. Talamantes, Life Sci. 34, 2303-2312 (1984).

27. M. Edery, M. McGrath, L. Larson, and S. Nandi, Endocrinology 115, 1691-1697 (1984).
28. G. Verhoeven, G. Vandoren, W. Heyns, E.R. Kuhn, J.P. Janssens, D. Teuwen, P. Goddeeris, E. Lesaffre, and P. DeMoor, J. Endocrinol. 95, 357-368 (1982).
29. P.H. Heidemann, J.L. Wittliff, R.E. Calhoon, and E.S. Boylan, J. Toxicol. Environ. Health 78, 667-686 (1981).
30. Y. Tomooka, H.A. Bern, and S. Nandi, Cancer Letters 20, 255-261 (1983).
31. C. Jean and P. Delost, J. Physiologie (Paris) 56, 377 (1964).
32. K. Hoshino and M.T. Connolly, Anat. Rec. 157, 262 (1967).
33. C. Jean, Arch. Sci. Physiol. 25, 145-185 (1971).

DISCUSSION

MCLACHLAN: Is the mitotic activity in the mammary gland of neonatal mice reduced immediately following estrogen treatment?

BERN: I cannot say anything about mitotic rate per se, but Dr. Y. Tomooka has found less ductal branching in glands of mice treated with estrogen for 5 days and examined on the 6th day, and we assume this reflects decreased cell proliferation.

BOYLAN: Regarding the question of mitotic activity: Bergman and Boylan (Proceedings of Endocrine Society, 1982) show reduced ^{3}H-thymidine/uridine labeling in neonatal rat mammary gland after neonatal DES exposure.

TUCHMANN-DUPLESSIS: Did you have a group of animals treated with agents which determine prolactin release, like phenothiazines?

BERN: No. However, mice treated as neonates for 5 days with prolactin show no changes in any genital, mammary or pituitary feature examined. It would be necessary to sustain the prolactin release, and this kind of experiment would be well worthwhile doing.

JONES: What was the effect with progesterone and what did the question mark mean? We have shown that neonatally progesterone-treated mice do cycle. However, they do develop cervicovaginal lesions as well as tumors. There is no reduction in the ability to be impregnated nor in the number of the offspring.

BERN: Equivocal; hence, the question mark indicated uncertainty.

OVARIAN STRUCTURE AND FUNCTION IN NEONATALLY ESTROGEN TREATED FEMALE MICE

JOHN-GUNNAR FORSBERG, ARTUR TENENBAUM, CHRISTINA RYDBERG, AND CHRISTINA SERNVI

Department of Anatomy, University of Lund, Biskopsgatan 7, S-223 62 LUND, Sweden

ABSTRACT

Neonatal female mice of the NMRI strain were treated with daily doses of 10^{-6} to 5µg diethyl-stilbestrol (DES) for the first five days after birth. A dose of 10^{-1}µg DES, or higher, resulted in significantly reduced uterine wet weight at 28 days, and this response was ovary-independent. Except for the occurrence of multi-oocyte follicles, DES exposed and control ovaries developed in a similar way in the prepubertal period. After puberty, females treated neonatally with 10^{-4}µg, or higher daily doses of DES, had ovaries lacking corpora lutea but with follicles and hypertrophy of the interstitial tissue. Homogenates of DES exposed ovaries metabolized ^{3}H-pregnenolone into a pattern of ^{3}H-steroid metabolites which was different from that in control homogenates and characterized by high levels of ^{3}H-progesterone and increased levels of ^{3}H-androstenedione while the levels of ^{3}H-17α-hydroxyprogesterone, 20α-dihydroprogesterone and ^{3}H-testosterone were low. This pattern was similar in 8-week-old and 12-month-old ovaries. Treatment with human chorionic gonadotropin or LH-RH reversed the abnormal pattern to that typical for homogenates of control ovaries. In spite of the striking difference in ^{3}H-progesterone extracted from control and DES homogenates, the plasma level and ovarian content of progesterone (RIA) were similar in control and DES treated females.

INTRODUCTION

By treating female mice with estrogen during the first five

days after birth, permanent and life-long changes are induced in different organ systems.The normal cycling vaginal epithelium is changed into a permanent cornified epithelium which,depending on dose and mouse strain used, may be of an ovary-dependent or ovary-independent type [1,2]. The latter is caused by a direct estrogen effect on the vaginal cells [1]. In animals more than one year old, the latter epithelium may develop into a hyperplastic type with cancer - like lesions [1]. Neonatally estrogen treated (estrogenized) and later ovariectomized females demonstrate a deviating response to a later challenge with estrogen. The histochemically demonstrable activity of alkaline phosphatases in the vaginal epithelium is decreased as is also the mitotic activity [1,3,4]. Just the opposite response is true for non-estrogenized females. The proliferative behaviour of the uterine epithelium is also different from that in controls [4]. The uterotropic response to estrogen is decreased at weaning in rats but not later when hormonal feed-back mechanisms are functional [5]. The altered and reduced estrogen response in adult estrogenized females may be related to a lower concentration of cytoplasmic estrogen receptor and altered function of new receptor protein [6,7].

Contrary to these results, an increased production of a specific cell product was described after a challenge to estradiol in adult ovariectomized and estrogenized females [8]. This difference to control females was ascribed to both systemic hormonal factors as well as to factors within the cervicovaginal region.

Ovaries from estrogenized mice are characterized by absence of corpora lutea, presence of follicles in various stages of development and hyperplasia - hypertrophy of the interstitial tissue [2,9-11]. The ovarian changes are generally considered secondary to estrogen effects in the hypothalamic - pituitary control system, resulting in no cyclic LH surges [12,13]. Estrogens have a sex organizational effect in the hypothalamic region which, in rats, is morphologically apparent in the sexually dimorphic nucleus of the preoptic area [13,14]. In estrogenized rats, the mechanism responsible for LH-RH release is permanently altered and thus also the cyclic release of LH from the pituitary gland. There are still measurable and tonic levels of LH in plasma [15]. The serum level of LH in

estrogenized rats has been described as normal [16] or similar
to the level in controls at proestrus [17]; FSH was intermediate
between diestrus and proestrus levels [17]. Thus the pituitary
gland is not silent with respect to gonadotropin release.

Prolactin interferes with ovarian steroid synthesis [18,19].
No effect was seen on plasma prolactin in one study of
estrogenized mice [20] while in another the level was as in
proestrus/estrus control females and significantly higher than
in diestrus/metestrus [21]. Bromocriptine reduced the
increased prolactin level in estrogenized rats but did not
result in recovery of cyclic LH release [17,22].

The aberrant gonadotropin pattern in estrogenized females
could be of primary importance for gonadal dysfunction but the
possibility of an additional direct estrogen – induced
disturbance should not be over-looked. When ovaries from
control mice were grafted on ovariectomized females, a cyclic
estrus pattern occurred in 71% of the females grafted and this
percentage decreased with increasing age of donor females.
Ovaries from estrogenized females resulted in 42-48% of the
hosts resuming vaginal cyclicity and this percentage did not
change with increasing age [11]. These experiments demonstrate
the possibility of a direct ovarian estrogen effect.

The serum level of estradiol in adult estrogenized female
rats was significantly lower than in controls at proestrus but
significantly higher than at diestrus [23]. The female
offspring (8-month-old) from pregnant mice treated with
diethylstilbestrol (DES) on days 9 through 16 of gestation had
plasma levels of total estrogen not different from those in
controls [24].

In conclusion, treatment of neonatal female rats and mice
with estrogen results in effects in the hypothalamic area, and
in turn, in a loss of cyclic LH surges. However, LH,FSH, and
prolactin can be measured in the circulation and some studies
indicate circulatory levels of estrogen within the normal
control range.

Critical phases in the development of the hypothalamic –
pituitary control system, which in rodents can be demonstrated
in the perinatal period, in the human fetus are probably
occurring in the period between 11 and 17.5 weeks of fetal
age [25]. However, it is not justified to postulate identical

mechanisms in this development between rodents and man, nor to
anticipate a similar response to exogenous estrogens. Only
little information exists on the hormonal pattern in women
exposed to DES in fetal life. The serum values for LH,FSH,
total estrogens,progesterone, and testosterone were reported
to be within normal limits in patients having problems to
achieve pregnancy [26]. Increased testosterone levels were
found in the postovulatory and perimenstrual phases of the
menstrual cycle [27]. So far, no information is available on
prolactin. Some studies indicate that in utero DES exposed
women have menstrual irregularities [28-30] but no conclusions
can be drawn about causal factors.

In this paper will be discussed structural, functional, and
synthetic aspects on the prepubertal and postpubertal ovary
from neonatally DES treated female mice. An increased in vitro
testosterone production (RIA) on a per ovary basis has earlier
been described after fetal exposure to DES [31].

GENERAL ASPECTS ON EFFECTS OF NEONATAL ESTROGEN TREATMENT IN FEMALE NMRI MICE

In 1969, we reported results from a histological study of the
upper part of the vagina and uterine cervix from adult mice
treated with daily doses of 5µg estradiol-17β for the first
five days after birth [10]. Instead of the normal squamous
epithelium we found more or less widespread regions with a
columnar epithelium. Apparently, the normal transformation of
the fetal columnar epithelium into a squamous epithelium had
not taken place in these regions. After puberty, the hetero-
topic columnar epithelium (HCE) formed glandular-like
down-growths into the stroma , resulting in a state of adenosis,
particularly in the uterine cervix [10]. The developmental
mechanisms for HCE and adenosis have been discussed [32].

Neonatal treatment with DES resulted in the same epithelial
aberrations but in this case the adenosis progressed into
changes morphologically similar to well-differentiated
adenocarcinoma [33], which so far has not been observed after
estradiol treatment [33]. The pathological changes induced by
DES in the mouse uterine cervix have been compared to those
seen in the human cervix after fetal exposure to DES [34].

The mouse HCE could be a quite benign epithelium upon which

different factors could act to result in malignancy or the HCE
could contain dormant malignant cells, resulting from a direct
DES attack in the neonatal treatment period. In the former case,
it remains to find the factor(s) responsible for malignant
degeneration; in the latter case, the factors responsible for
growth initiation of malignant cells are of interest. The same
problems are relevant also for the relation between human
adenosis and DES associated clear-cell adenocarcinoma.Recently
atypical adenosis was described in DES exposed patients and
thus, as in the mouse, adenosis was linked to the carcinoma[35].

Among factors of importance for progression of HCE into
adenosis and later malignancy are virus, immune competence and
hormonal environment. In mice, the neonatal DES treatment
results in permanent immune disturbances and a reduced activity
of Natural Killer (NK) cells [36,37]. The reduced NK activity
is parallell to an increased sensitivity to chemical carcinogen
[38]. The failure of progression of HCE into adenosis after
ovariectomy indicates that this progression is ovary-dependent
[10,33]. Because of this, we started experiments to look for
ovarian function in neonatally DES treated NMRI mice.

A definite answer to the complicated question about the
importance of hormonal factors for the HCE progression cannot
be given at the present time. More information is needed on
plasma binding, peripheral conversion, metabolism and hormonal
kinetic,etc. In fact, we have not yet a clear picture of
estrogens because of problems to define what we are actually
studying in some experiments. Thus,the present paper should
be considered a progress report

THE PREPUBERTAL OVARY
Morphological studies

Follicular development and antrum formation in ovaries trom
immature mice is dependent on gonadotropins [39,40]. A DES
effect on gonadotropin secretion and release in the prepubertal
period might be reflected in ovarian development.

Ovaries were removed from female mice on days 6,8,12,21, 28,
and 35 and prepared for routine histological study. "DES
ovaries" were from females treated with a daily dose of 5μg
DES in olive oil for five days after birth; control ovaries
were from females treated with olive oil only. Ovaries from at

least 3 females were studied at each stage

At 6 days after birth, both DES and control ovaries were characterized by a broad cortical zone of immature follicles; in the center of the ovaries were scattered growing follicles surrounded by a single layer of follicular cells. The follicles were separated by stromal cells of a fibroblast-like type. Bi-layered follicles were seen at 8 days in control ovaries and at 12 days in DES ovaries. The most characteristic trait of the latter was the appearance of numerous bi-layered follicles containing 2 - 3 or even more oocytes. A distinct layer of theca cells surrounded the follicles. Large multi-layered follicles were seen in 21-day control ovaries and in some follicles disintegration among the follicular cells indicated a beginning antrum formation. The disintegration process was less pronounced in 21-day DES ovaries than in controls.Numerous follicles in DES ovaries contained multiple oocytes, in some follicles as much as six oocytes could be identified. At 28 days, antrum follicles occurred in both control and DES ovaries; the characteristic trait of follicles in DES ovaries was still the multi-oocyte phenomenon. Degenerating follicles in various stages of development occurred in both control and DES ovaries and albeit no quantitative study was done, the over-all impression was that the degeneration process was similar in both types of ovaries.

At 35 days, numerous cells with the morphology of interstitial cells were prominent on tissue sections from both control and DES ovaries. Cells with this morphology could be traced back to the 21-day stage. With special techniques (electron microscopy,histochemistry), they have been described from 10 - 12-day-old ovaries [41]. The interstitial cells have been classified as "primary", arising from stromal cells, or "secondary", arising from the theca of atretic follicles [41]. In our material from 28- and 35-day-old females, the interstitial cells were linked to atretic follicles but also localized to perivascular regions.

Except the occurrence of numerous multi-oocyte follicles in DES ovaries and a possible slight developmental retardation (later appearance of bi-layered follicles, later antrum formation), the DES ovaries and control ovaries were similar at the different stages studied. It can therefore be concluded

that factors regulating ovarian development,at least up to and
including 35 days after birth,are acting in a similar way in
control and DES females. The mechanism behind the appearance of
multi-oocyte follicles is unknown.

Ovarian_influence_on_uterine_growth

In FIG.1 is shown the uterine weight in control female mice
injected with olive oil for the first five days after birth.
Apparently there are two periods of accelerated weight increase,
one from day 8 to 12, and a second one from day 21 to 28.After
ovariectomy on day 1,there is a pronounced weight reduction
in 28-day-old females which indicates that at least the
increase from day 21 to day 28 is ovary-dependent. Then it was
of interest to study if the prepubertal DES exposed ovary could
support a normal uterine weight increase.

Beginning on the day of birth (day 1), female NMRI mice were
treated with daily subcutaneous injections of 10^{-4} to 5µg DES
in olive oil for five days. In some experiments, 5 or 20µg
doses of estradiol-17β were used. Females were killed on days
6, 8, 12, 21, and 28 and the uterine wet weight and body-weight
recorded. All data were analysed statistically using linear
regression analysis (uterine wet weight on body-weight). The
results are summarized in FIG.1.

The highest and lowest DES doses used (5 and 10^{-4}µg)
resulted in a slight but statistically significant increase in
uterine weight in the interval 6 - 12 days.A much more
pronounced stimulation was obtained wuth the 10^{-2}µg dose. At
12 days, the mean weights of the control group, the 10^{-2}µg
group and the 5µg group were close to each other. Contrary to
this,at 21 days the uterine weight of females treated with
10^{-2},10^{-1}, 1, and 5µg was significantly lower than in controls.
One week later (28 days), this reduction was still significant
for the 10^{-1},1 and 5 µg doses but not for 10^{-2}µg. The
weight reduction showed a definite dose-response dependency.
In fact, the daily 5µg dose reduced   the weight to a
significantly lower value than that representative for females
ovariectomized on day 1. A dose of 5µg estradiol-17β had no
weight reducing effect while that obtained with 20µg
estradiol was similar to that with 1µg DES.

The prepubertal mouse ovary develops competence to respond

334

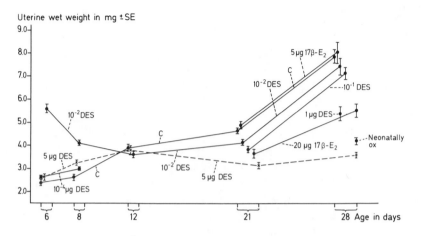

FIG.1. Uterine wet weight at different ages after
treatment with various doses of DES or estradiol-17β
for 5 days after birth. C controls. Neonatally ox
females ovariectomized on day 1 and killed on day 28.
17β -E$_2$ estradiol-17β. Every point represents the mean
from 50 females,except the group treated with 10^{-2}μg DES
and killed on day 12 (n=25).

to gonadotropins between day 2 and 7 after birth and _is_ then
competent to secrete different steroids, including
estradiol-17β, at least under in vitro conditions [42]. Serum
concentrations of LH begin to increase at about 5 days after
birth and increase successively to a maximal value on day 19
only later to return to the low levels seen in the neonatal
period [42 - 45]. The situation is about the same for serum
FSH but the peak appears somewhat earlier, on day 10-11 [43,44].
In rats, plasma estradiol-17β and FSH show a similar pattern
between 5 and 35 days and a feedback mechanism was operative
[46]. The possibility now exists, that the reduced uterine
weight in 28-day-old female mice after 10^{-1} to 5μg DES doses
neonatally, is the result of a DES interference with the
pituitary - ovarian axis. To test this, 25 - 27-day-old
females were treated with estradiol-17β.

Females treated with daily doses of 5μg DES in the neonatal
period were later injected with 1 μg estradiol-17β on days

25 - 27 and killed 24 hours after the last injection. In control females, this treatment resulted in about a 4.9-fold weight increase; in DES females, the weight increase was about 4.2-fold and in females ovariectomized on day 1 the increase was 7.7-fold (FIG.2). The latter result indicates that the low initial uterine weight of the DES females is not a factor per se responsible for the less dramatic weight response as compared with the ovariectomized females. Then, the less response in the DES females could be due to factors within the uterus, such as defects in receptor mechanisms [6,7] or the small uterus could be under the influence of an abnormal ovarian steroid secretion. To differentiate between these possibilities, 5µg DES females (n=33) were ovariectomized on day 21 and treated with 1µg estradiol-17β on days 25 - 27. The uterine weight of these females on day 28 was not different (regression analysis) from that in non-ovariectomized 5µg DES females treated with estradiol-17β ($\bar{y}$ = 15.0 vs. 14.9 mg). The failure of uterine weight increase from day 21 to day 28 in 5µg DES females is thus ovary-independent and the slight response to exogenous estrogens compared with neonatally ovariectomized females is not a result of an ovarian hormone influence.

A further argument for the latter conclusion is based on the fact that ovaries from females treated neonatally with 10^{-4} to 5µg DES have the same morphology and synthetic pattern in the postpubertal period (see below) but only 10^{-1} to 5µg resulted in effects on uterine weight at 28 days.

The conclusion from these studies on the prepubertal ovary is that neonatal DES exposure is compatible with normal development (except appearance of multi-oocyte follicles) and support of uterine growth.

THE POSTPUBERTAL OVARY

Morphological studies

Ovaries from 8-week-old female NMRI mice, treated with daily doses of 10^{-5}µg for the first five days after birth were similar to those from control females [47]. A ten-fold higher daily DES dose (10^{-4}µg) resulted in all ovaries lacking corpora lutea [47]. Cross-sections from these ovaries were dominated by follicles and the interstitial tissue, the latter arranged in nodular or cord-like formations. The interstitial cells had

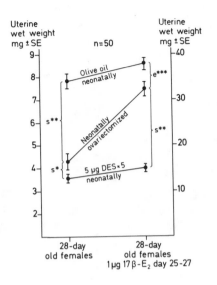

FIG.2. Effect of estradiol-17β on uterine weight in
28-day old females after different types of treatment
in the neonatal period. Results were compared with
regression analysis. Significance levels: [*] 0.05>p>0.01;
[**]0.01>p>0.001; [***] p<0.001. e = elevation; s = slope.
Every point represents the mean of 50 females.

a larger cytoplasmic – nuclear ratio than the same cells from
control ovaries.

The histological picture characteristic for ovaries from
females treated with 10^{-4}μg DES was also seen in ovaries from
females treated with higher DES doses, up to and including 5μg
per day. At all dose levels, the ovaries contained follicles in
various stages of development. The multi-oocyte follicles,
which formed such a prominent trait in prepubertal DES exposed
ovaries were also found at 8 weeks but only occasionally did
they have more than two oocytes. Ovaries from females exposed
to the 5μg dose had about a 30% lower weight than those from
controls [47]. Ovarian cysts were seén ih about 25% of the
ovaries studied [47].

The histological picture as described here for ovaries from
neonatally DES treated females at doses higher than and

including 10^{-4}µg DES is similar to that reported earlier after
neonatal estrogen treatment [2,9 - 11], but in this study we
have been able to establish a threshold dose for DES. Ovaries
from the female offspring of pregnant CD-1 mice treated with
100µg DES per kg body-weight on days 9 through 16 of
gestation, and killed at 4 weeks or later in life,had vacuolated
interstitial cells, stained with oil-red-O which could point to
a high steroidogenic activity [31]. At 6 months, the ovaries
contained corpora lutea [48], which has never been observed in
our material from neonatally treated females. The incidence of
ovaries with cysts is about the same (25%) in 8-week-old
prenatally or neonatally treated females [47,48]. Extensive
inflammatory changes were a prominent trait of prenatally
exposed ovaries [48] at 8 weeks, but not in those exposed
neonatally.

With increasing age of the neonatally DES exposed females,
the number of follicles decreased. At 9 months, most of the
ovarian cross-section was formed by interstitial tissue.
Interspersed in this were groups or scattered large cells with
an eosinophilic cytoplasm. Usually, these cells are referred to
as ceroid containing cells. A similar age-related reduction
in oocytes and follicles has also been reported from studies of
prenatally exposed ovaries [48].

When ovaries from 4-week-old, neonatally DES treated (5µg)
females were grafted under the kidney capsule of inbred control
females (ovariectomized) of the same age, numerous corpora
lutea were seen when the grafted ovaries were sectioned 8 weeks
later [47].In the reverse type of experiments (control ovaries
on DES females), the control ovaries adopted the typical DES
appearance. These experiments demonstrate that the morphological
traits characteristic for DES exposed ovaries are reversible
and controlled by systemic factors in the females. Of obvious
interest in this connection are gonadotropins. Thus 8-10-week-
old DES (5µg)females were injected with 50 IU of human chorionic
gonadotropin (hCG) and the ovaries sectioned 24, 48, 72, and
96 hours after the injection. At 24 hours, the vascularization
was increased and at 48 hours scattered corpora lutea were
seen. Because some of the corpora lutea structures had remnants
of what seemed to be degenerating oocytes, the possibility
exists that the corpora lutea structures were formed by

338

luteinisation of the follicles without ovulation. Corpora
lutea were also seen in DES exposed ovaries (5µg DES) after
treating the females with LH-RH (des-Gly^{10},[im-Bzl-D-His^6]-LH-
RH ethylamide, Sigma Chemical Co.; 2µg twice daily for 3 days,
females killed 24 hours after the last injection).

Fertility test

None of the neonatally DES treated females (test doses: 10^{-2}
to 5µg) has ever become pregnant in repeated fertility tests.

Prenatal exposure to DES (0.01 - 100 g DES per kg body-
-weight on days 9 through 16 of gestation) resulted in a
dose-dependent decrease in reproductive capacity of the female
offspring, with high frequency of total sterility at the
highest dose level [24].Even at the highest DES dose used in
these experiments, some of the ovaries had corpora lutea.
Superovulation after PMSG-hCG treatment resulted in degenerating
ova [24].

Ovarian steroid synthesis

Ovaries from 8-week-old, neonatally DES treated females or
control females, were homogenized in Parker medium 199 and the
homogenate incubated in the presence of co-factors and
^{3}H-pregnenolone for 60 min at 37°C in an atmosphere of 95% air
and 5% CO_2. After incubation,the steroids were extracted in
ethyl acetate and then separated in a two-dimensional thin
layer chromatography system (TLC). The identity of the different
^{3}H-steroids recovered from the TLC areas were verified in
recrystallization experiments [47]. After initial kinetic
studies (effect of incubation time, homogenate concentration,
^{3}H-pregnenolone concentration) an optimal incubation system
was defined as homogenate representing one ovary in 2 ml medium
in the presence of 440,000 dpm ^{3}H-pregnenolone [47].The recovery
of radioactivity from TLC areas representing ^{3}H-17α-hydroxy-
pregnenolone, ^{3}H-dehydroepiandrosterone,^{3}H-estrone,^{3}H-estradiol-
17β, and ^{3}H-estriol was low (<8%) while a high-activity group
included ^{3}H-progesterone (^{3}H-P), ^{3}H-17α-hydroxyprogesterone
(^{3}H-17OH-P), ^{3}H-androstenedione (^{3}H-A), and ^{3}H-testosterone
(^{3}H-T). Recrystallization experiments showed that the area
tentatively taken to represent ^{3}H-17OH-P in fact contained a
mixture of this steroid and ^{3}H-20α-dihydroprogesterone (^{3}H-20-P)

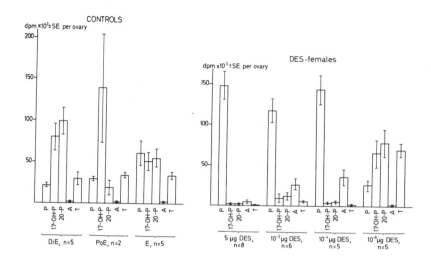

FIG.3.The pattern of ^{3}H-steroids (high-activity group)
formed in homogenates of ovaries from females in different
phases of the estrus cycle and from females treated with
various doses of DES in the neonatal period. All values for
radioactivity calculated as 100% recovery. Separation on
TLC and identity verification after recrystallization.
DiE diestrus; PoE proestrus; E estrus; P ^{3}H-progesterone;
17-OH-P ^{3}H-17α-hydroxyprogesterone; 20-P ^{3}H-20α-dihydro-
progesterone; A ^{3}H-androstenedione; T ^{3}H-testosterone.
(Reproduced with permisson from J.Reprod.Fert.[47])

had to be taken into account.In the following only results from
the high-activity group will be discussed. A maximum of 18%
radioactivity was recovered from the TLC area representing
^{3}H-pregnenolone.

The typical pattern of ^{3}H-steroids present in the homogenates
after 60 min incubation is shown in FIG.3. Homogenates of
control ovaries were characterized by high levels of ^{3}H-17OH-P
relative to ^{3}H-P in diestrus and proestrus but similar levels
in estrus. Moderate levels of ^{3}H-T but very low ones
representing ^{3}H-A were typical for all three cyclus phases
studied. This pattern was in strong contrast to that found in
homogenates of neonatally DES exposed ovaries,from females
treated with 10^{-4} to 5µg DES.The lowest dose, 10^{-6}µg DES,

resulted in a pattern similar to that in controls.

Homogenates of ovaries exposed to 10^{-4} µg or higher DES doses had essentially the same pattern of ^{3}H-steroids and this was characterized by high levels of ^{3}H-P and,in comparison to this, the levels of the remaining ^{3}H-steroids studied were very low (FIG. 3). Not only was there a shift from relative dominance of ^{3}H-17OH-P over ^{3}H-P,as typical for controls, to a ^{3}H-P dominance in DES homogenates, but also a shift from ^{3}H-T dominance relative to ^{3}H-A (controls) to a higher level of ^{3}H-A relative to ^{3}H-T in DES homogenates.The ^{3}H-A dominance over ^{3}H-T tended to increase with lower DES doses [47].

The results demonstrated in FIG. 3 are calculated on a per ovary basis. Because the weight of the DES ovaries was about 30% lower than that of control ovaries, the difference in ^{3}H-steroid pattern between control and DES homogenates is not changed after weight correction.

In the morphological studies discussed above, daily neonatal doses of 10^{-4} µg DES resulted in a typical "DES ovarian structure with absence of corpora lutea and hypertrophy of the interstitial cells. This dose, but not a 100-fold lower, resulted in ^{3}H-P dominance and thus there is a parallellism between morphology and synthetic activity.

When the studies on synthetic activity were repeated on ovarian material from 1-year-old females,the same pattern as observed at 8 weeks emerged.

In all our experiments, only minute amounts of ^{3}H-estrogens have been recovered after incubation with ^{3}H-pregnenolone. If anything, ^{3}H-estrone dominated in the minute ^{3}H-estrogen pool. To further study the aromatization capacity, homogenates from control and DES exposed (5µg DES)ovaries were incubated in presence of 440,000 dpm ^{3}H-androstenedione and co-factors. After extraction of ^{3}H-steroids, they were separated on column chromatography (Sephadex LH-20, benzene/methanol 85:15). The radioactivity in the frations tentatively taken to represent ^{3}H-estrone and ^{3}H-estradiol was too low to allow any further characterization. Material from the fractions tentatively taken to represent ^{3}H-androstenedione and ^{3}H-testosterone were further separated in a TLC system (first run:chloroform/methanol 98:2, second run bensene/ethyl acetate 13:1). The ^{3}H-andro-stenedione fractions proved to be homogenous for this steroid

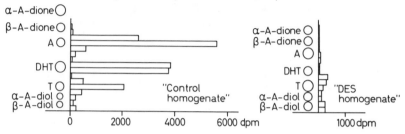

FIG.4. TLC separation of ³H-steroids in the
"³H-testosterone" fractions after Sephadex LH-20
chromatography. Homogenates incubated in
³H-androstenedione.

while those tentatively taken to represent ³H-testosterone
were a mixture of different steroids (FIG.4). Beside an
over-spill of ³H-androstenedione into the ³H-testosterone
fractions, significant amounts of radioactivity could be
recovered from the TLC areas representing 5α-dihydrotestosterone
and testosterone when control homogenates were analysed. With
DES homogenates, only very low amounts of radioactivity were
recovered from the same areas. Again, these experiments
demonstrate a difference in metabolic activity between control
homogenates and DES homogenates. These results also support
those from incubations using ³H-pregnenolone as precursor,which
pointed to a pronounced inhibition of ³H-T formation in DES
homogenates. The question about aromatization capacity in the
homogenates is still open and has not been solved in these
experiments.

After grafting of DES exposed ovaries (5µg DES) from 4-week-
-old females to the kidney of ovariectomized controls of the
same age, the synthetic pattern changed to that typical for
controls [47]. When control ovaries were grafted on DES hosts,
the pattern changed to that typical for DES ovaries.

The DES-typical pattern of steroid synthesis was also

shifted into a normal type when 8-week-old DES females (5µg DES)
were treated with hCG (0.5 - 50 hCG per day for 3 days, females
killed 24 hours after last injection) or LH-RH (des-Gly^{10}[im-
-Bzl-D-His^6]-LH-RH ethylamid, Sigma; 2µg twice daily for 3 days,
females killed 24 hours after last injection). Both hCG and
LH-RH resulted in a relative depression of the high ^{3}H-P value
in DES females and increased values for ^{3}H-17OH-P and ^{3}H-2O-P.
It can be concluded, that the pattern of ^{3}H-steroid
synthesis, as far as described in this paper, is different in
homogenates from control and DES exposed ovaries. The abnormal
pattern is reversible and can shift into a normal one under
different experimental conditions: grafting experiments,
treatment with hCG and LH-RH. On the contrary, the DES pattern
was not influenced by estradiol-17β or 5α-dihydrotestosterone
(DES females injected with 5µg of each steroid for 4 days and
killed 24 hours after last injection).Nor had the prolactin
release inhibitor CB-154 (2-bromo-α-ergocryptine mesylate,
50µg twice a day for 7 days, females killed 24 hours after last
injection) any effect.

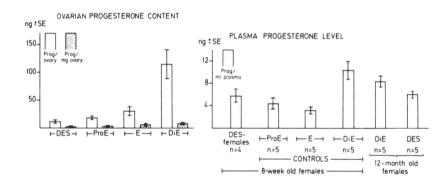

FIG.5. Results from RIA studies on ovarian
progesterone content and plasma levels of
progesterone. The same females were used for
ovarian and plasma analyses.

Studies on ovarian progesterone content and plasma levels of
progesterone

Because of the pronounced difference in ^{3}H-P recovered after

incubation of control and DES homogenates it was of interest
to study the ovarian progesterone content and plasma
progesterone levels in the same females, using RIA technique
[49]. The ovarian progesterone content was found to be similar
in DES exposed (5µg DES) and in control ovaries from females
in proestrus and estrus, but significantly lower than in
diestrus ovaries (FIG.5). This was true when the values were
calculated both on a weight basis and a per ovary basis. The
plasma levels of progesterone were in the same range in DES
treated females and in control diestrus females, but higher
than in proestrus or estrus females (FIG.5). Finally, the
plasma level was similar in 8-week-old and 12-month-old DES
females.

CONCLUSION

   In the prepubertal period, control ovaries and neonatally
DES exposed ovaries do not differ in any major structural
(except occurrence of multi-oocyte follicles) or functional
(support of uterine growth) respects, as far as evident from
these studies.
   Adult DES females have ovaries characterized by hypertrophy
of interstitial tissue and absence of corpora lutea. After
incubation of homogenates of DES ovaries in the presence of
^{3}H-pregnenolone, high levels of ^{3}H-progesterone and increased
levels of ^{3}H-androstenedione were recovered,while the radioactivity representing ^{3}H-17α-hydroxyprogesterone, 20α-dihydro-
progesterone and ^{3}H-testosterone was very low compared with
controls. In spite of the high in vitro ^{3}H-progesterone level,
the ovarian content and plasma level of progesterone were as
in controls.
   The pattern of ^{3}H-steroid synthetic activity,as found in
homogenates of DES ovaries in these studies,is different from
results from studies of ovarian steroid production (RIA) after
hypophysectomy in rats [50 - 52]. Androgenized female rats,
which lack corpora lutea, had non-detectable levels of
progesterone and 20α-dihydroprogesterone after hypophysectomy
[50]. Because of the results from experiments involving hCG
and LH-RH, and against the background of earlier studies
discussed in Introduction, it seems reasonable to postulate a
low and tonic level of LH in neonatally DES treated female mice

as a factor of importance for the pattern of tritiated
steroids recovered from homogenates. The general impression is
that of a reduced activity of 17α-hydroxylase,17β-ol-dehydro-
genase, and 20α-dehydrogenase. Another possibility is, possibly
associated with the reduced enzyme activities, that low LH
levels in vivo result in a rapid uncoupling of LH regulated
steroid synthesis in vitro and an autonomous Δ^5-3β-ol-dehydro-
genase activity [53]. Only further studies can give a complete
picture of the control mechanisms.

Acknowledgement

The results presented in this paper are based on studies
supported by grants from the Swedish Cancer Society (project
1870-B85-03XC).

REFERENCES

1. N.Takasugi,T.Kimura, and T.Mori, in: The Post-Natal
   Development of Phenotype, S.Kazda and V.H.Denenberg,
   eds. (Academia,Prague 1970) pp.229-249.
2. T.Kimura,S.L.Basu, and S.Nandi, J.exp.Zool. 165,
   71(1967).
3. T.Mori, Proc.Japan Academy 44,516(1968).
4. T.Mori, J.Endocr.(London) 64,133(1975).
5. L.J.Lerner, A.Vitale, and C.Oldani, in: Research on
   Steroids, vol.7, A.Vermeulen, A.Klopper,F.Sciarra,
   P.Jungblut, and L.J.Lerner,eds. (North Holland Press,
   Amsterdam 1977) pp.77-94.
6. G.Shyamala,T.Mori, and H.A.Bern, J.Endocr.(London)
   63,275(1974).
7. M.Aihara,T.Kimura, and J.Kato, Endocrinology 107,224(1980).
8. T.Kalland,S.-O.Døskeland, and J.-G.Forsberg, Endocrinology
   99,1548(1976).
9. N.Takasugi, and H.A.Bern, J.natl.Cancer Inst. 33,855(1964).
10. J.-G.Forsberg, Br.J.exp.Patol. 50,187(1969).
11. T.Mori, J.exp.Zool. 207,451(1979).
12. R.A.Gorski,R.E.Harlan, and L.W.Christensen, J.Toxicol.
    Environm. Health 3,97(1977).
13. R.A.Gorski, in: Sexual Differentiation:Basic and Clinical
    Aspects, M.Serio,M.Motta,M.Zanisi, and L.Martini,eds.
    (Raven Press, New York 1984) pp.65-77.
14. K.-D.Döhler,A.Coquelin, F.Davis, M.Hines,J.E.Shryne,
    Brain Res. 302,291(1984).
15. N.Goomer, R.N.Saxena, and A.R.Sheth, J.Reprod.Fert.
    50,239(1977).
16. E.Aguilar, C.Fernández Galaz, M.D.Vaticón, A.Tejero, and
    A.Oriol, J.Endocr.(London) 97,319(1983).
17. H.Nagasawa, R.Yanai, S.Kikuyama, and J.Mori, J.Endocr.
    (London) 59,599(1973).

18. J.H.Dorrington,H.L.McKiracher, A.K.Chan, and R.E.Gore-
    -Langton, J.steroid Biochem. 19,17(1983).
19. G.F.Erickson, and D.A.Magoffin, J.steroid Biochem. 19,
    113(1983).
20. T.Kalland,J.-G.Forsberg, and Y.N.Sinha, Endocr. Res.
    Commun. 7,157(1980).
21. H.Nagasawa,T.Mori,R.Yanai,H.A.Bern, and K.T.Mills,
    Cancer Res. 38,942(1978).
22. E.R.Kühn, E.J.Nouwen,L.Nieuwborg, W.Heyns, and F.Bertiau,
    J.Endocr.(London) 85,319(1980).
23. H.Nagasawa,R.Yanai, M.Shodono, T.Nakamura, and Y.Tanabe,
    Cancer Res. 34,2643(1974).
24. J.A.McLachlan,R.R.Newbold, H.C.Shah, M.D.Hogan, and
    R.L.Dixon, Fertil.Steril. 38,364(1982).
25. J.S.D.Winter, C.Faiman, and F.Reyes, in: Mechanisms of
    Sex Differentiation in Animals and Man, C.R.Austin, and
    R.G.Edwards, eds. (Academic Press, New York 1981)
    pp.205-253.
26. M.Bibbo, W.B.Gill, F.Azizi,R.Blough, V.S.Fang,R.L.Rosen-
    field,G.F.B. Schumacher, K.Sleeper, M.G.Sonek, and
    G.L.Wied, Obstet.Gynecol. 49,1(1977).
27. C.H.Wu, C.E.Mangan, M.M.Burtnett, and G.Mikhail,
    Obstet.Gynecol.55,157(1980).
28. L.Cousins, W.Karp., C.Lacey, W.E.Lucas, Obstet.Gynecol.
    56,70(1980).
29. A.L.Herbst, M.M.Hubby, F.Azizi, and M.M.Makii,
    Am.J.Obstet.Gynecol. 141,1019(1981).
30. M.R.Peress, C.C.Tsai, R.S. Mathur, H.O.Williamson,
    Am.J.Obstet.Gynecol. 144,135(1982).
31. A.F.Haney, R.R.Newbold, and J.A.McLachlan, Biol.Reprod.
    30,471(1984).
32. J.-G.Forsberg, Natl.Cancer Inst.Monogr. 51,41(1979).
33. J.-G.Forsberg, and T.Kalland, Cancer Res. 41,721(1981).
34. J.-G.Forsberg, Biol.Res.in Pregnancy 2,168(1981).
35. S.J.Robboy,R.H.Young, W.R.Welch, G.Y.Truslow,J.Prat,
    A.L.Herbst, and R.E.Scully, Cancer 54,869(1984).
36. T.Kalland, Banbury Report 11,217(1982).
37. T.Kalland, Immunopharmacology 7,127(1984).
38. T.Kalland, and J.-G.Forsberg, Cancer Res. 41,5134(1981).
39. T.W.Purandare, S.R.Munshi, and S.S.Rao, Biol.Reprod.
    15,311(1976).
40. S.Lintern-Moore, Biol.Reprod. 17,635(1977).
41. S.L. Quattropani, Anat.Rec. 177,569(1973).
42. J.E.Fortune, and J.J.Eppig, Endocrinology 105,760(1979).
43. J.Dullaart, J.Kent, and M.Ryle, J.Reprod.Fert.
    43,189(1975).
44. S.D.Michael, O.Taguchi, and Y.Nishizuka, Biol.Reprod.
    22,342(1980).
45. S.D.Michael, S.B.Kaplan, B.T.Macmillan, J.Reprod.Fert.
    59,217(1980).
46. H.M.A. Meijs-Roelofs, J.Th.J. Uilenbroek, F.H. de Jong,
    and R.Welschen, J.Endocr. (London) 59,205(1973).
47. A.Tenenbaum, and J.-G.Forsberg, J.Reprod.Fert.
    (1985) in press.
48. R.R.Newbold, B.C.Bullocj, and J.A.McLachlan, Biol.Reprod.
    28,735(1983).
49. A.Tenenbaum, C.Sernvi, and J.-G.Forsberg, Biol.Res. in
    Pregnancy (1985) in press.
50. R.J.C. van Straalen, F.G.Leemborg, J.T.M. Vreeburg, and
    G.H.Zeilmaker, Acta Endocrinol.(Kbh) 98,437(1981).

51. K.Taya, and G.S. Greewald, Endocrinology 110,390(1982).
52. I.Kim, and G.S.Greenwald, Biol.Reprod. 30,824(1984).
53. K.Taya, and G.S.Greewald, Biol.Reprod. 25,683(1981).

DISCUSSION

BOVING: Could polyovular follicles be regarded as a failure of separation by ovarian stroma? It seems mechanically easier to visualize than oocytes proliferating within one follicle.

FORSBERG: It could be a result of failure of separation, but then the next question is: "Why?" A possible cause could be changes in the cell membrane of the follicular cells.

JONES: We have seen an increased number of follicles before 2 months of age in neonatally progesterone-treated Balb/c mice (Jones and Bern, Cancer Res., 37, 67, 1977). However, between 2 months to 6 months of age the ovaries of these animals undergo super ovulation. Have you looked at the ovaries of your treated animals at 2, 4, 6, etc., months?

FORSBERG: In the postpubertal period, we have only studied 8-week-old and 9-month-old ovaries, as far as it relates to the experiment described here. We have not studied super ovulation, but we have treated females with HCG. In these experiments, we obtained structures similar to corpora lutea but with degenerating oocytes. Thus, in this system, we don't think the follicles are able to ovulate.

Critical Evaluation of the Role of Environmental Estrogens

in Premature Sexual Development

PREMATURE THELARCHE AND ESTROGEN INTOXICATION

MARIA I. NEW, M.D.
Department of Pediatrics, New York Hospital - Cornell Medical Center,
New York, NY 10021

INTRODUCTION

We are here to address the problem of exogenous estrogen exposure, and its relationship to the incidence of premature thelarche among Puerto Rican infants and children. As Chairman of the session on the Critical Evaluation of the Role of Environmental Estrogens in Premature Sexual Development, I have undertaken a survey of the literature (Table I), which is by no means exhaustive, but which provides a representative sample of the types of exogenous estrogen exposure described to date.

SUMMARY

As this review of the literature indicates, there have been few documented epidemics of premature thelarche. The literature contains case reports of estrogen intoxication via consumption of ointments, vitamins, and medicines; possible food contamination; and accidental estrogen exposure by ingestion of stilbestrol pills and creams, absorption of stilbestrol ointment, and inhalation of stilbestrol dust. As can be seen in Table II, the reports from Puerto Rico indicate a much higher prevalence than ever reported before. The significance of this dramatically high frequency must be evaluated carefully. Is this an epidemic or is it normal? Is it an environmental intoxication? Is there a genetic or familial susceptibility? Factors that must enter the investigation are indicated in Table III. Uniform assessment of the signs of sexual development is imperative if we are to establish accurately an incidence of precocious thelarche. With advanced technology, the source and nature of a potential environmental toxin may be detected. However, pigmentation of genitalia, a uniform symptom of estrogen intoxication in past reports, is not prominent in the Puerto Rican cases. Thus the possibility of an estrogen intoxicant seems unlikely. The contribution of phytoestrogens, mycotoxins and lignans may be important in the evaluation of the effect of nutrition on sexual development. It does not seem likely that such dietary factors would suddenly increase the prevalence of precocious development. Therefore, genetic factors should be given special attention in the investigation of the cases in Puerto Rico.

TABLE I. Select review of the literature on estrogen intoxication.

Report; Location	Cases (Age, sex)	Time to appear / disappear	Symptoms	Hormone levels	Estrogen source and outcome
Dunn, 1940 [1]; Philadelphia, USA	6 y, F	6 w /	Breast enlargement: 2.5 cm diam, 1 cm thick	NA	Rx for gonorrheal vaginitis: stilbestrol solution (1 mg/cc, 3 drops/d x 6 w)
Hesselvik, 1952 [2]; Uppsala, Sweden	10 m, M	5 m / 6 m	Breasts enlarged: 2 cm diameter, 5 mm thick breasts; pigment increase in areolae, penis, scrotum; pubic hair; rectal exam nl; BA nl	No urinary estrogenous substance; 17-KS 0.9 mg/d	Mother used stilbestrol ointment before breast feeding (0.1% diethylstilbene; 300 g used in 5 m)
	5 m, M	At 0.3 g/d x 1 m, no effect; then at 0.7 g/d x 2 w, breasts enlarged; in 2 m, 10 mm diam	(Autopsy after 3.5 m Rx): breast enlargement; histology of breasts: proliferation of efferent ducts, no acini; Pigment of areolae, linea alba; pubic hair; pituitary, adrenals and testes nl	NA	Experiment in child with myelomeningocele: 0.3 g/d topical stilbestrol ointment
Prouty, 1952 [3]; Wisconsin, USA	4 y, M	Breasts "several weeks" > mother started job; pigment over 5 m / 3 w	2 cm diameter breasts; linea alba, areolae, scrotum pigmented; axillary and pubic hair; testes nl size; adrenals nl; BA nl	17-KS 6.6 mg/d; gonadotropin < 1 rat unit	Breasts began after mother packaging 15 mg stilbestrol tabs, came home without changing clothes; about 2 m later, packaging machine brought home
	10 y, F (sib)	/ 2 w, menses stopped, pigment decreased over 4-5 m	Pigmented areolae; menses	NA	"

Report; location	Cases (Age, sex)	Time to appear / disappear	Symptoms	Hormone levels	Estrogen source and outcome
Cook et al, 1953 [4]; Boston, USA	4 y, F	? 4 m / ? 2 m	Breast enlargement; dark pigmented areolae; slight pubic hair; vaginal bleeding; vaginal smear estrogenized; at laparotomy, uterus and fallopian tubes large, ovaries nl; biopsy of ovaries: nl with no follicular activity; BA nl	Urinary estrogens <1 ng; 17-KS 0.37 mg/d; 11-oxo-steroids 0.1 mg/d; FSH < 6.5 U	Mother took stilbestuol until 4 m before breasts; estrogen ingestion not proven
	7 y, F	4 w / 2 m all symptoms gone and urinary gonadotropins nl	Breast enlargement; pigmentation of areolae and linea alba; vaginal bleeding; vaginal smear estrogenized; uterus and cervix enlarged	Urinary gonaadotropins 3.3 mouse units	Stilbestrol, 2 mg/d mistakenly given for vitamin C by M.D. father
Hertz, 1958 [5]; National Institutes of Health, USA	5 y, M	40 d / 6 w	Breast enlargement; pubic hair; enlargement of penis	NA	Vitamins taken for 40 d, equivalent of 150 mg estrone
	7 y, F (sib)	40 d / 6 w	Breasts 1 cm; no acini; pigmented areolae; fine pubic hair; enlarged labia; vagina moist; hair upper lip; uterus nl size	NA	"
	8 y, M	90 d / 6 w	Breast enlargement	NA	Vitamins containing estrogens
	10 y, M (sib)	40 d / 6 w	Breast enlargement	NA	"

NOTE: Inhibitory effect of dietary glutathione on melanin formation is neutralized by estrone, and therefore pigmentation is prominent in the above cases of estrogen intoxication.

Report; location	Cases (Age, sex)	Time to appear / disappear	Symptoms	Hormone levels	Estrogen source and outcome
Weber et al, 1963 [6]; San Francisco, USA	4 F, 1-8 y	7-44 d / 3 m: vaginal estrogenization gone in 10 d; breasts in 3 m; pubic hair still present > 3 m	Breast development after 1 mg ingested over 11 d, but no breasts with 0.8 mg over 7 d; pigmented areolae and linea alba; pubic hair; vaginal bleeding; vaginal discharge, 10 d; BA nl	17-KS 0.4, 1.8 mg/d; FSH 2.5 mouse units; urinary estrogens 10 "g/d in 1 child, others none	INH Rx of tuberculosis contained diethylstilbestrol due to contaminated tablet machine; 0.8-4 mg total dose (0.012-0.09 mg/d x 7-44 d)
	3 M, 5-10 y	"	Breast enlargement; pigmented areolae and linea alba; pubic hair; BA nl	17-KS 0.1, 0.2 mg/d; urinary estrogens < 3 "g/d	"
Silver & Sami, 1964 [7]; Colorado, USA	Review of cases of 16 F: 87.5% before 2 y; 68% before 1 y; 38% in first month	Breasts persisted up to 7 y	Bilateral breast enlargement in 15/16, unilateral in 1/16; height and weight nl; BA nl; negative family history	17-KS and urinary gonadotropins nl; urine desquamated cells + for estrogen in 15/16 vs. 7/86 controls	1 mother received progestational agent during pregnancy
Ramos and Bower, 1969 [8]; Connecticut, USA	3 y, F	6 m / 3 m	Breast enlargement; deeply pigmented areolae; sparse pubic hair; vaginal bleeding; vaginal cytology +; uterus nl; moist vagina; >2 SD above height age; BA nl	Urinary estrogens 4 "g/dl	Grandmother's facial cream containing 10,000 U/oz estrogen; child took about 2500 U
Beas et al, 1969 [9]; Santiago, Chile	4 M, 4-8 m; 3 F, 4 m-2 y	2-18 m / by 4 y all nl	Breast enlargement; pigmentation of areolae, genitals and linea alba; pubic hair; in F, vaginal discharge and bleeding, vaginal smear +; BA ni	Urinary gonadotropins, 17-KS and pregnatriol nl	Ointment for diaper rash contained estrogen

Report; location	Cases (Age, sex)	Time to appear / disappear	Symptoms	Hormone levels	Estrogen source and outcome
Hemsell et al., 1977 [10]; Dallas, USA	11 y, M		Breasts T IV; slightly pigmented areolae; axillary hair; sparse pubic hair (T III); tall; testes nl; BA 15 y	NA	Increased aromatase in breasts
Andler and Zachmann, 1979 [11]; Essen, W. Germany	17 y M testicular feminization, castrated at 3 y		Breast development; no pubic hair	NA	Due to aromatized adrenal androgen
Scaglioni et al, 1978 [12]; Fara et al, 1979 [13]; Milano, Italy		/ 2-8 m	Enlarged breasts (0.5-3 cm diameter; moderately pigmented areolae noted in only 3 girls and 1 boy; fine pubic hair; moist vagina; siblings in other schools not affected	FSH, LH, prolactin nl; 17-β-estradiol slightly elevated	Meat suspected but unable to be tested; subsequent meat from same supplier had no estrogen
Kimball, 1981 [14]; Bahrain, Lebanon	1 M, 2 y; 7 F, 1.5-6.5 y		Breast enlargement; pigmented linea alba in 2/8	Nl serum estrogens and chorionic gonadotropin levels	6/7 drank from cow given oestinyl injection, but unaffected sib drank from same cow; estrogen intoxication not proven; affected less likely to eat red meat than controls (0/7 vs 6/9)

School outbreak:

Age, Sex	% Affected	Controls
3-5 y F	22% (8/37)	6%
6-10 y M	58% (58/100)	8%
6-7 y F	67% (45/67)	5%
11-14 y M	23% (15/66)	35%

Report; location	Cases (Age, sex)	Time to appear / disappear	Symptoms	Hormone levels	Estrogen source and outcome
Saenz et al, 1982 [15,16]; Puerto Rico (70% from city of San Juan)	62 F 1972-77, 256 F 1978-; 81, 198 6-24 m, 57 2-4 y; 40 4-6 y; 27 6-7 y	87% had involution in 3 m after diet change	Premature thelarche; sonograms in 60 showed ovarian cysts in 41; only 5 had ovarian cysts, increased E_2 and accelerated BA; 45% of pts with ovarian cysts had + family history; BA increased in 26	Tested 75 for E_2, FSH and LH: FSH and LH nl; 15 had increased urinary E_2, of these 10 had ovarian cysts	97% had breast tissue appear when weaned to local whole milk; older pts ate more local whole milk, poultry and beef; suggests estrogen consumption (veterinary stilbestrol and zeranol available without prescription) plus ? genetic predisposition
Comas, 1982 [17]; Puerto Rico	229 8 y or younger seen in 10 y		121 with precocious puberty (118 F, 3 M): increased BA, gonadotropin or prolactin levels; 121 with premature thelarche; BA increased in 54; 6/10 had ovarian cysts	86 had increased gonadotropins; increased FSH and/or LH in 145; increased estrogens in 156	2 exposed to estrogen in cream or pill; dietary contamination suspected but not proven (1 set of twins with same diet and home: 1 has marked breasts other unaffected)
Pasquino et al 1982 [18]; Rome, Italy	3 F: 7 y, 17 m, 9 m	/ 3-5 m	Breasts T II; pigmented areolae and genitals; no pubic hair; vaginal bleeding; vaginal smear +; BA nl	Serum E_2 nl; serum gonadotropins after LHRH injection very low	Believe it was food but not proven
Bongiovanni, 1983 [19]	(COMMENT)				Some meat and poultry had + cytosol receptor assay for estrogens; note that since publicity, incidence of condition has decreased, and average weight of poultry in local markets has decreased

Report; location	Cases (Age, sex)	Time to appear / disappear	Symptoms	Hormone levels	Estrogen source and outcome
Frazer de Llado et al, 1983 [20]; South Puerto Rico	100 F cases (1 case/60 F births		Premature thelarche	No increase in E_2 or E_1 compared to controls	Same diet as controls
Saenz, 1984 [21]; Puerto Rico				Zearalenone isolated in serum of some patients	

Abbreviations: M, male; F, female; m, month; y, year; nl, normal; BA, bone age; 17-KS, 17-ketosteroids; NA, not reported; T, Tanner stage of development

TABLE II. Number of children reported with precocious breast development attributed to potential or certain estrogen intoxication.

Before Puerto Rico Report (1952-1982)

Boys	Girls	Includes epidemics in Bahrain, Chile, Rome and
94	70	Milan, Italy [2-11,13,14,18,24,25]

Puerto Rico Experience

Saenz et al, 1982   322 cases (256 between 1978-81) [15,16,21]

Comas, 1982   272 cases of precocious puberty, 121 precocious
                       thelarche only (70 cases between 1978-82) [17]

Frazer et al, 1983   100 cases of precocious thelarche in 1982 [20]

TABLE III. Aspects of estrogen intoxication in children.

---

1. Boys as well as girls affected?
2. Age of onset?
3. Family members or classmates affected?
4. Are ethnic groups in different places affected?
5. Are diverse ethnic groups in the same place affected?
6. Polymorphism of clinical syndrome (uniform case assessment).
7. Rate of appearance and disappearance of manifestation.
8. Ultimately is puberty normal? Is age of puberty normal?
9. Are there late complications in adulthood?
10. Source of intoxicant?
11. Nature of intoxicant?
12. Does intervention stop the epidemic?

REFERENCES

1. C.W. Dunn, J.A.M.A. 115, 2263-2264 (1940).
2. L. Hesselvik, Acta Pediatr. 41, 177-185 (1952).
3. M. Prouty, Pediatr. 9, 55-57 (1952).
4. C.D. Cook, J.W. McArthur, and W. Berenberg, New England J. Med. 248, 671-674 (1953).
5. R. Hertz, Pediatr. 21, 203-206 (1958).
6. W.W. Weber, M. Grossman, J.V. Thom, J. Sax, J.J. Chan, and M.P. Duffy, New England J. Med. 268, 411-414 (1963).
7. H.K. Silver and D. Sami, Pediatr. 34, 107-111 (1964).
8. A.S. Ramos and B.F. Bower, J.A.M.A. 207, 368-369 (1969).
9. F. Beas, L. Vargas, R.P. Spada, and N. Merchak, J. Pediatr. 75, 127-130 (1969).
10. D.L. Hemsell, C.D. Edman, J.F. Marks, P.K. Siiteri, and P.C. MacDonald, J. Clin. Investigation 60, 455-464 (1977).
11. W. Andler and M. Zachmann, J. Pediatr. 94, 304-305 (1979).
12. S. Scaglioni, C. DiPietro, A. Bigatello, and G. Chiumello, Lancet 1, 551-552 (1978).
13. G.M. Fara, G. Del Corvo, S. Bernuzzi, A. Bigatello, C. DiPietro, S. Scaglioni, and G. Chiumello, Lancet 2, 295-297 (1979).
14. A.M. Kimball, R. Hamadeh, R.A.H. Mahmood, S. Khalfan, A. Muhsin, F. Ghabrial, H.K. Armenian, Lancet 1, 671-672 (1981).

15. C.A. Saenz, M.A. Toro-Sola, L. Conde, and N.P. Bayonet-Rivera, Bol. Assoc. Med. P. R. 74, 16-18 (1982).
16. C.A. Saenz de Rodriguez and M.A. Toro-Sola, Lancet 1, 1300 (1982).
17. A.P. Comas, Lancet 1, 1299-1300 (1982).
18. A.M. Pasquino, R. Balducci, M.L. Manca Bitti, G.L. Spandoni, and B. Boscherini, Arch. Dis. Child. 57, 954-956 (1982).
19. A.M. Bongiovanni, J. Pediatr. 103, 245-246 (1983).
20. T. Frazer de Llado, C. Sanchez, G. Bird, and D. Mayes, Pediatr. Res. 162A (1983).
21. C.A. Saenz de Rodriguez, New England J. Med. 310, 1741-1742 (1984).
22. G.A. Bannayan and S.I. Hajdu, Am. J. Clin. Pathology 57, 431-437 (1972).
23. P.A. Lee, J. Pediatr. 86, 212-215 (1975).
24. A. Caufriez, R. Wolter, M. Govaerts, M. L'Hermite, and C. Robyn, J. Pediatr. 91, 751-753 (1977).
25. J.L. Mills, P.D. Stolley, J. Davies, and T. Moshang, Jr., Am. J. Dis. Child. 135, 743-745 (1981).
26. R. Schoental, Lancet 1, 537 (1983).

358

PREMATURE SEXUAL DEVELOPMENT IN PUERTO RICO: BACKGROUND AND CURRENT STATUS

Lillian Haddock, M.D.,[*] Gloria Lebron, M.S.,[**] Ruth
Martínez, Ph.D.,[**] Jose F. Cordero, M.D., M.P.H.,[***] Lambertina W.
Freni-Titulaer, M.D., M.S.P.H.,[***] Francisco Carrion, M.D.,[*] Carlos
Cintron, M.D.,[*] Lillian Gonzalez, M.D.[*]

[*]School of Medicine and [**]Graduate School of Public Health, University of
Puerto Rico, Medical Sciences Campus, San Juan, Puerto Rico 00936
[***]Center for Environmental Health, Centers for Disease Control, Atlanta,
Georgia 30333

INTRODUCTION

In this paper we describe three aspects of the investigation on the

reported increase of premature thelarche cases seen by pediatric

endocrinologists in Puerto Rico: an investigation on the magnitude of the

problem, the search for etiologic factors, and some clinical data on the

patients with the condition.

BACKGROUND

In February 1982, Sáenz and coworkers [1] published a series of 322

cases of premature thelarche (PT) seen between 1971 and January 1982, 80%

of which were seen in the last 5 years. Among recent cases, 41 of 60 in

which pelvic sonograms had been performed were reported to have ovarian

cysts. The authors stated: "It was clearly observed in 97% of the cases

that the appearance of abnormal breast tissue was probably related to the

weaning of a formula to a local whole milk in the infant group. At a

later age, a dietary history of a greater consumption of local whole

milk, poultry and beef was referred by the parents." The Secretary of

Health of Puerto Rico then asked the Centers for Disease Control (CDC) to

conduct an investigation.

The CDC began its investigation in February 1982. CDC personnel

visited the island's pediatric endocrinologists and learned that the

physicians had seen more cases of PT in recent years. Samples of meat

including beef and chicken, and milk were obtained from the market and sent to the Food and Drug Administration (FDA) for testing. Of the chicken samples tested two were positive for estrogenic activity by the immature mouse uterine weight bioassay. This finding increased community concern about the possibility of estrogen contamination as a source of the reported increase of premature thelarche.

In August 1982, the Secretary of Health requested that the Chancellor of the Medical Sciences Campus appoint a Commission to investigate the increasing reporting of PT and early sexual development (ESD) in female infants and young girls.

The immediate goals of the Commission were to assess the magnitude of the problem and to develop a questionnaire to be used in an epidemiologic study of a representative sample of the cases. In September 1982, a special clinic was started in the Pediatric University Hospital for the followup of patients with premature thelarche and early sexual development.

MAGNITUDE OF THE PROBLEM

A survey was conducted among 304 pediatricians and 46 adult and pediatric endocrinologists to obtain information on the incidence of PT and ESD. Responses were received from 58 of 304 pediatricians contacted. A total of 174 patients with PT and 38 with PT and other signs of ESD were reported by 35 respondents. The remaining 23 pediatricians reported not seeing any patients with PT. Of the 174 patients with PT, 150 (86%) had been referred to pediatric endocrinologists and of the 38 with other signs of ESD, 31 had been referred.

Among the endocrinologists contacted, responses were obtained from all adult endocrinologists and 8 of the 11 pediatric endocrinologists. The 35 adult endocrinologists had seen a total of 23 cases, 10 of which had been seen in the early 70's. One adult endocrinologist was following

five cases in her practice; the others referred their cases to the
pediatric endocrinologists.

The eight pediatric endocrinologists reported 905 cases with PT and
38 cases with PT and other signs of ESD. These 38 patients had either
pubic or axillary hair or both. Sáenz informed the Commission about
various cases of pseudoprecocious puberty seen in her practice. Perez
Comas reported 121 cases of what he called true precocious puberty on the
basis of single elevated serum levels of follicle stimulating hormone
(FSH), luteinizing hormone (LH), or both [2]. In 48 of these subjects he
reported an increased bone age. In the same publication he reported 30
cases of premature adrenarche.

From the survey 1,137 cases of PT were estimated to have occurred
between 1971 and 1982. Table I shows the distribution of these cases by
age of onset. The group with onset of PT between 0.5 to 1.9 years
comprises 762 (67%) of the total and includes 467 cases (41%) that had
thelarche at birth which was maintained after 6 months.

TABLE I. Premature thelarche in Puerto Rico, by year of onset, 1971-1982

Onset of thelarche (years)	Number of cases	Percentage
0.5 - 1.9	762	67.0
2.0 - 3.9	140	12.3
4.0 - 5.9	116	10.2
6.0 - 6.9	91	8.0
7.0 - 7.9	28	2.5
Total	1,137	100

To obtain information about the incidence of PT and true precocious
puberty (TPP) in other countries, a questionnaire was sent to members of
the chapters of the International Endocrine Society. Responses were
received from institutions in 12 countries [3-17]. Completed
questionnaires were received from 7 institutions. Table II shows data on

the number of cases of PT and TPP provided by these respondents. The National Institute of Pediatrics of Budapest, Hungary, reported that of 3,143 patients seen in a hospital setting from 1978 to 1982, 46 (1.46%) had PT and 11 (0.34%) had TPP, a ratio of PT to TPP of 4.5. The ratio of PT to TPP cases seen in the other reporting children's hospitals were in Japan, 2.5; in Cuba, 2.3; in Cardiff, England, 2.5; in Heidelberg, 1.0; and in Switzerland, 0.6. All the respondents wrote that the reported PT cases were the number of patients seen by pediatricians and that no incidence data were available. None of the respondents were aware of outbreaks in their areas that could be associated with estrogen contamination of food products.

From informal conversations with pediatric endocrinologists in the continental United States and Latin America, no increase in referrals of PT or ESD was reported. No population studies on the prevalence or incidence of PT and ESD were found in the literature.

In September 1984, the CDC and the University of Puerto Rico Medical Sciences Campus sponsored a scientific meeting to discuss all the available data and studies that had been conducted so far in the investigation of the problem. At that meeting five pediatric endocrinologists reported patients with various types of early sexual development seen in their private and/or institutional practices. These included PT (1,542 cases), premature adrenarche (242 cases, including 32 males), pseudoprecocious puberty (158 cases), precocious puberty (124 cases), and prepubertal gynecomastia (49 cases).

SEARCH FOR POSSIBLE ETIOLOGIC FACTORS

In February 1982, CDC conducted a pilot case-control study among 20 cases and 20 controls to search for obvious sources of estrogens. In this study, the only factor found to be associated with PT was a maternal history of ovarian cysts.

TABLE II. International experience on premature thelarche and true precocious puberty, 1978-1982.

	Premature Thelarche Age group		True Precocious Puberty Age group	
	<2 yrs.	≥2 yrs.	<4 yrs.	≥4 yrs.
1. Kanagua Children Medical Center Yokohama City, Japan	37	17	11	11
2. National Institute of Endocrinology Fajardo Hospital, Havana, Cuba	10	15	11 (5 yrs.)	--
3. National Institute of Pediatrics Budapest, Hungary (3,143 children in Hospital setting)	13	33	5	6
4. Department of Child Health National School of Medicine, Cardiff, England	2	8	--	4
5. Division of Pediatric Endocrinology University of Heidelberg Children's Hospital, Heidelberg, Germany	7	10	9 (<6 yrs.)	9 (6-8 yrs.)
6. Kinderspital, Department of Endocrinology Zurich, Switzerland	14	10	12 (<5 yrs.)	32 (>5 yrs.)
7. The Middlesex Hospital London, England (1982 only)	3	6	5	7

In April 1982, samples of fresh milk, poultry from two local
production companies, and frozen chicken, beef, liver, and pork were
collected by the Puerto Rico Department of Health and were sent to the
FDA for analysis. A mouse bioassay using uterine weight as an indicator
of estrogenic activity was used as a screening test for these samples. A
preliminary report of the analysis showed that two chicken samples were
presumptively positive. One of these samples was from a local poultry
farm, and the other was from a company on the mainland United States.
Subsequent chemical analyses of the two presumptively positive samples
for estradiol, estrone, DES, and zearalanol were negative.

The preliminary report sent to the Secretary of Health was published
in the media, and the possible use of estrogen as an anabolic product in
the raising of poultry in Puerto Rico and on the mainland was widely
reported in the local and national newspapers.

There were allegations that anabolic products were used illegally in
raising cattle and poultry in Puerto Rico. Farmers, veterinarians, and
representatives of the beef and poultry producers in Puerto Rico denied
that these products were used. Beef consumed in Puerto Rico comes mainly
from the continental United States and from Central and South American
countries. Less than 20% of the beef and 27% of the poultry consumed in
Puerto Rico is locally produced. Representatives of the U. S. Department
of Agriculture (USDA) assured the Commission that the strictest measures
are taken in the inspection of meat imported from other countries.
Random samples are inspected regularly, but hormonal assays are not
usually performed. Between October 1982 and February 1983, the USDA
analyzed 64 additional samples of beef, 20 of beef livers, 63 of chicken
livers, and 11 of egg products, using the mouse uterine weight bioassay
[18]. Chemical analyses (mass spectrometry) of three presumptively
positive samples, two of beef and one of chicken liver, did not show the
presence of either estradiol, estrone, DES, or zearalanol.

ACTIVITIES OF THE COMMISSION

In March 1983, CDC sponsored a meeting to discuss the problem of PT

in Puerto Rico. A group representing the Commission and its consultants

presented the findings of the survey and discussed the research proposal

and the questionnaire prepared for the epidemiological study.

Representatives of the USDA, FDA, and National Institutes of Health (NIH)

participated in this meeting. All participants agreed that although some

uncertainty existed about whether there was a real increase of PT in

Puerto Rico, they thought that an investigation should be conducted.

The participants proposed the following recommendations: (1) conduct

a survey of households of PT cases and controls, (2) conduct a

case-control study of PT, (3) establish a surveillance of PT, and (4)

develop a follow-up program of PT cases to assess the natural history of

the condition. All recommendations, except the third, were fully

implemented.

HOUSEHOLD SURVEY

In April 1983, the Commission, in collaboration with the CDC,

conducted a survey of 14 households, 8 of recent PT cases and 6 of

controls. This survey was conducted with three objectives: (1) to

ascertain a source of estrogen or estrogenic activity that might explain

the condition, (2) to raise hypotheses on potential environmental

etiologies of PT, and (3) to collect biological samples to search for the

presence of estrogens, including estrogenic pesticides and zearalenones.

These samples included household water, food, blood from parents, and

urine from mothers and from the case and control children. In the search

for specific pesticides with known estrogenic activity, the U.S.

Geological Survey analyzed samples of household water for methoxychlor,

Kepone, and DDT and its metabolites. Laboratory analyses of the food and

biological samples collected in the household survey did not identify or confirm any estrogen or estrogenic chemicals in any of the samples. The serum levels of methoxychlor and Kepone from parents of PT cases and controls were below detection limits. The levels of DDT and DDE metabolites were not significantly different from levels found in whites in the United States as reported in the second National Health and Nutrition Examination Survey (HANES) study [19].

SURVEY OF PREMATURE THELARCHE CASES

The Commission, for two reasons, decided to include in a survey for a case-control study only patients who were initially diagnosed as having PT by a pediatric endocrinologist. First, the Commission's preliminary survey showed that over 90% of the cases reported had an initial diagnosis of PT. Second, the pathogenesis and pathophysiology of other forms of ESD, such as premature adrenarche, is considered to be different from that of PT [20]. If the patients later developed other signs of early sexual development, they were not excluded from the study.

Case Definition

A case was defined as a girl between the ages of 6 months and 8 years who had palpable breast tissue of at least 1.5 cm in diameter and who did not have other evidence of early sexual development at the time of the diagnosis.

Sample Selection

In the sample for the case-control study, we included only cases diagnosed in the years 1978-1982, because 80% of the cases reported by the pediatric endocrinologists were diagnosed during that period.

A questionnaire was sent to the pediatric endocrinologists to obtain more specific data about their cases diagnosed between 1978-82. It asked for the name of the patient, the address, the telephone number, the date of birth, the age at the time the thelarche was first noticed, and the

366

date of the first visit to the pediatric endocrinologist. Two pediatric
endocrinologists with the largest practices were visited to obtain this
information from their records. Seven of the remaining nine pediatric
endocrinologists provided the information to the Commission by mail.

TABLE III. Premature thelarche by age of onset and year of diagnosis

Age of onset (Years)	Year of diagnosis 1978	1979	1980	1981	1982	Total	Percent
0.5 - 1.9	24	34	65	73	191	387	70
2.0 - 3.9	3	5	10	4	12	34	6
4.0 - 5.9	4	3	6	11	35	59	11
6.0 - 6.9	2	3	5	8	23	41	7
7.0 - 7.9	1	3	5	3	19	31	6
Total	34	48	91	99	280	552	100
Percent	6.0	8.7	16.5	17.9	50.7	100	

Table III shows the number of cases seen by year and by age group. The
age group corresponds to the age at which thelarche was first noticed, and the
year corresponds to the year in which the case was diagnosed.

The group less than 2 years old comprised 70% of the cases. Fifty percent
of the cases were diagnosed in 1982. From the 552 cases, 130 were selected
for the case-control study.

Table IV gives the rate of PT by year of diagnosis. These rates should be
considered minimum estimates, since they include only those patients who were
diagnosed by participating endocrinologists.

The preliminary results of the case-control study were presented at a
September 1984 meeting, and the recommendations of the consultants were
considered in the subsequent analysis.

The analysis was conducted for 120 cases; 10 were excluded for diverse
reasons. The distribution of the 552 cases and the 120 cases in the final
sample is given by year of diagnosis and year of onset of thelarche as shown
in Table V.

Although 50% of the cases were first diagnosed by a pediatric

TABLE IV. Premature thelarche, number of cases and rate by year of diagnosis, Puerto Rico

Year	Number	Rate*
1978	34	1.2
1979	48	1.7
1980	91	3.2
1981	99	3.7
1982	280	10.4
Total	552	4.0

*Rate per 10,000 girls less than 8 years old. The denominators were estimated from data on the population by year and distribution by age and sex in the Annual Report of Vital Statistics, Puerto Rico Department of Health (1981).

endocrinologist in 1982, the actual onset of PT according to the mother does not show this sharp increase. The mothers of the PT patients took anywhere from 1 month to 2 1/2 years before they sought medical attention for their children. Because the problem was extensively covered in the media, the public's increased awareness and the mothers' increasing concern may partly explain the increase in cases diagnosed in 1982.

CLINICAL DATA

Some clinical followup was available for selected groups of patients. In a case-control study questions were asked about subsequent development of other signs of ESD. We also asked whether the breast enlargement had disappeared, and if this was the case, when it was first noted to have disappeared.

All patients that pediatric endocrinologists saw with breast enlargement as the only sign of early sexual development were eligible for this study. If other signs of early sexual development developed later, however, these cases were not excluded. Of the 85 patients with onset before the age of 2 years, 8 developed other signs of early sexual development before age 8 years and between the time of diagnosis and the time of interview; 7 developed pubic hair, and 1 developed vaginal bleeding. The interval in months

368

Table V. Number of cases by year of diagnosis and year of onset of thelarche

Year	New cases diagnosed by pediatric endocrinologist		Sample used in analysis			
	Number	(%)	Diagnosis by PE *	(%)	Onset of PT**	(%)
1978	34	(6)	5	(4)	19	(16)
1979	48	(9)	10	(8)	19	(16)
1980	91	(16)	20	(17)	27	(22)
1981	99	(18)	23	(19)	30	(25)
1982	280	(51)	62	(52)	25	(21)
TOTAL	552	(100)	120	(100)	120	(100)

* As reported by pediatric endocrinologist
** According to the mother

between onset and interview was comparable for the group that developed pubic hair or vaginal bleeding and for the group that did not. The mean interval was 33 months, with a range of 17-64 months for those with other symptoms, and 33 months, with a range of 6-81 months for those without other symptoms.

Of the 35 patients with onset at age 2 or over, 14 subsequently developed pubic hair before the age of 8 years, one of whom also developed vaginal bleeding starting at the age of 4 1/2 years. Four of the patients with pubic hair had menarche at ages 8 2/12, 8 4/12, 9 2/12, and 9 3/12 years. The respective ages at the time of interview were 9 6/12, 10 10/12, 10 6/12, and 9 10/12 years. One patient had only vaginal bleeding which developed at age 6 years. Of these cases with onset at age 2 or over, the group that developed other signs of ESD had a longer interval between onset and interview than the group that did not develop other signs. The mean interval for those with other signs was 41 months, with a range of 13-58 months. For those without other symptoms the mean interval was 26 months, with a range of 8-65 months. This difference is statistically significant ($p = 0.009$).

Table VI shows the mean age and range in months of PT cases by age group and occurrence of other signs of ESD.

369

Table VI. Mean age in months and range of PT cases by age group and occurrence of other signs of early sexual development.

Age Group (months)	Time	PT only Number	Mean	Range	PT and other signs Number	Mean	Range
0-23	Onset	77	6.5	0-21	8	4.1	0-12
	Interview	77	39.5	14-88	8	37.8	22-76
24-95	Onset	20	66.0	36-90	15	65.2	24-94
	Interview	20	92.0	65-130	15	106.0	68-131

Clinical and Institutional Practices of Pediatric Endocrinologists

The Commission conducted a follow-up of PT patients for whom a record was available at the Pediatric University Hospital. A total of 136 were identified from 1966 to 1977; 31 subjects could be contacted. In 18 or 58% the thelarche disappeared after 8 to 68 months, with an average of 28 months (Table VII).

Table VII. Evolution of thelarche for a group of patients with onset between 1966 and 1977

COURSE	BIRTH	<2 yr.	≥2 yr	TOTAL
Disappeared	2	13	3	18
Decreased	1	1	1	3
Maintained	3	1	1	5
Increased	2	1	2	5
TOTAL	8	16	7	31

Fifteen of these girls had had their menarche already (Table VIII). One of these had true precocious puberty; four developed pubic hair before age 8, but their linear growth and bone age were normal. The remaining 10 did not develop any other secondary sexual characteristics before age 8. The mean age at menarche of these girls, excluding the TPP

370

case, was 11.2 years and that of their mothers, 12.4 years. Of the 16

girls who have not had the menarche, 2 have developed pubic hair. Their

height is normal for age. Thus, 6 of 30 cases or 20% developed pubic

hair before age 8, but have shown a normal linear growth. The number of

cases with a family history of ovarian cysts was similar in both groups.

Table VIII. Premature thelarche of a group of patients with onset
between 1966 and 1977

	Post-menarche	Pre-menarche
Number of Subjects	15	16
Age at Evaluation	9.8 – 21.6 yrs.	7.9 – 12.8 yrs.
Age at Time of Menarche	8 – 14 yrs	N/A
Mean Age at Menarche	11.2	N/A
Mothers' Age at Time of Menarche	11 – 14 yrs.	10 – 17
Mean Mothers' Age at Time of Menarche	12.4 yrs.	13.0
No. of Patients with Other Secondary Sex Characteristics Before Age 8	4	2
Number with Normal Height	14	N/A
Ovarian Cysts in Females of the Family	6	8

In September 1982 a clinic for the followup of cases with thelarche

and ESD was started in the Pediatric University Hospital. Before

starting this clinic, an average of eight new patients with PT were seen

yearly in the Pediatric Endocrine Clinic from 1975 to 1981. Once the

Commission was formed to investigate the problem and the public became

more aware of the condition, the number of patients referred to the

special clinic increased dramatically. Between September 1982 and

December 1984, 206 patients were referred with the diagnosis of PT. We

have studied the natural history of the condition in 135 patients

followed for at least 6 months. Of these 135 patients, 7 have developed

pubic hair, of whom 3 have accelerated bone age. The latter 3 were

considered cases of TPP. These patients had onset of thelarche at ages

4 9/12, 6 6/12, and 7 4/12 years, and pubic hair appeared 16, 12, and 13
months later. Of the four patients who developed pubic hair but in whom
the bone age was normal, one developed thelarche at age 6 months and the
remaining developed thelarche between ages 5 and 6 6/12 years. Pubic
hair appeared in the former at age 7 8/12 years, 86 months later, and in
the remaining 3, between 13 and 28 months later.

Stimulation tests using gonadotropin releasing hormone (GnRH) were
performed in these cases and in an additional patient who developed
breast enlargement at age 7 4/12 years. The LH response was prepubertal
in one of the patients who had pubic hair and normal bone age. Her age
at the time of the test was 7 6/12 years. The remaining seven patients
showed a pubertal LH response. The maximal increase of LH from baseline
levels ranged from 25 to 90 mIu/ml. The ages at the time of the test of
the latter group ranged from 7 5/12 to 10 years. One of the three girls
with TPP had her menarche at 9 3/12 years; the remaining 7 had not had
their menarche.

Table IX shows the course of the breast enlargement in the remaining
127 cases. Thelarche disappeared in 31 subjects (24%) after 3 to 48
months, with an average of 21 months for the whole group; the thelarche
disappeared after an average of 19 months for the group with breast size
<2.5 cm and after an average of 26 months for the group with breast size
of ≥2.5 cm. The present age range of this group is between 1 1/2 to
7 6/12 years.

The group that has maintained the breast enlargement makes up the
largest number of cases, with 50 of the 75 patients having breast sizes
larger than 2.5 cm.

In none of the patients did we find evidence of exposure to overt
estrogenic sources, such as estrogenic creams, or accidental exposure to
any estrogen-containing compound.

Pelvic sonography was performed in 64 cases, of which 31 (48%) were
normal. The most common finding was the presence of fluid-containing

areas in the presence of a normal infantile uterus. The range in size of the fluid-filled structures was from 0.5 cm to 2 cm in the group of patients with onset of PT before age 2, and 0.8 cm to 3 cm in the older patients. Larger ovaries and an inverted uterine ratio was seen in the patients who developed pubic hair and accelerated bone age. A normal population of girls has not been studied. The findings of positive sonograms have to be considered in the light of the power of the new technology for detecting subtle changes in the growth and development of the female reproductive organs.

Between September 1982 and December 1984, 15 patients with premature adrenarche have been followed in the Pediatric Endocrine Clinic. The rates of referral for this condition have remained stable during the past 10 years.

In May 1984, Ariza and coworkers [21] studied the onset of menarche in a group of 524 Puerto Rican girls and a group of 75 girls from the United States, Cuba, and Latin America residing in Puerto Rico. Their ages ranged from 8 to 17 years. The mean age at menarche of the Puerto Rican girls was 12.2 years, and that of the other group was 12.3 years. The median age was 12.1 years in both groups. The values followed a normal distribution curve. In the group of Puerto Rican girls, 5.5% had their menarche before age 10 compared with 1.3% in the other group. The sample size, however, was too small for this difference to be statistically significant.

RECOMMENDATIONS OF THE MEDICAL SCIENCES CAMPUS COMMISSION

On the basis of the findings of the investigation, the Commission rendered a report to the Secretary of Health in December 1984 with a series of recommendations for further investigation of the problem. This report is available upon request [22].

Table IX. Natural history of thelarche, Pediatric University Hospital, Sept. 1982 to Dec. 1984

COURSE	AGE OF ONSET			TOTAL	SIZE IN CM.	
	Birth	<2 yrs.	≥2 yrs.		<2.5 cm.	≥2.5 cm.
Disappeared	7	19	5	31 (24%)	22	9
Reappeared	--	3	–	3 (2%)	3	--
Disappeared in one breast and variable changes in the other	3	2	–	5 (4%)	2	3
Decreased and maintained	8	28	–	36 (28%)	9	27
Maintained	10	27	2	39 (31%)	16	23
Increased	4	8	1	13 (10%)	9	4
TOTAL	32 (25%)	87 (69%)	8 (6%)	127	60	67

| Present age (range, average and standard deviation) | 1.2 yrs. x = 2.4 yrs. S.D. = 11 mos. | 11 mo. - 7.7 yrs. x = 2.3 yrs. S.D. = 13.2 mos. | 5.8 - 8 yrs. x = 6.5 yrs. S.D. = 10.6 mos. | | | |

Currently, the staff of the special clinic of the Pediatric University Hospital is closely following cases of PT and ESD to assess the natural history of the condition, giving particular attention to the possible change from an isosexual to a heterosexual type of disorders. A complete endocrinological evaluation will be performed in a selected group of patients. A study of the growth and development of a sample of 8,000 children in Puerto Rico and additional clinical and basic research studies are in the planning stage.

ACKNOWLEDGEMENTS

We acknowledge the assistance of many individuals to the Medical Sciences Campus Commission and the Centers for Disease Control in this project. Their assistance is kindly appreciated. In Puerto Rico, we thank Dr. Norman Maldonado, Chancellor of the University of Puerto Rico Medical Sciences Campus; members of the Commission, Dr. Carlos Vicéns, Dr. Francisco Aguiló, Dr. Carl Gemzell, and Dr. Pedro Sostre; the pediatric endocrinologists in Puerto Rico who provided the Commission access to their patients for this study; from the University of Puerto Rico, Graduate School of Public Health, Dr. Jaime Ariza, Dr. Carlos Muñoz, Maggie Alegría, M.S., Mildred Vera, M.S., and the 16 students of the Graduate Program of Public Health who performed the interviews in the case-control study; Dr. Manuel Soldevila and Dr. Wilma Rodríguez who served as consultants to the Commission.

In Atlanta we acknowledge the assistance of Dr. Godfrey P. Oakley and Dr. J. David Erickson who reviewed the manuscript and provided very useful suggestions.

REFERENCES

1. C.A. Sáenz, M.A. Toro Sola, L. Conde, and N.P. Bayonet Rivera,
    Bol. Asoc. Med. P. R. 74, 16-19, (1982).
2. A. Pérez Comas, Bol. Asoc. Med. P. R. 74, 245-251, (1982).
3. C. A. Brooke, personal communication from the Middlesex Hospital,
    London, England, 1982.
4. S.K. Jivami, personal communication from the Blackburn District
    Lancashire, England, 1983.
5. D.C.L. Savage, personal communication from the Pediatric Endocrine
    Unit, Royal Hospital for Sick Children, Bristol, England, 1983.
6. I. A. Hughes, personal communication from Welsh National School of
    Medicine, Department of Child Health, Health Park, Cardiff, England, 1983.
7. P. J. Sinail, personal communication from the Royal Aberdeen
    Children's Hospital, Aberdeen, Scotland, 1983.
8. J. Maenpaa, personal communication from Aurora Children's
    Hospital, Helsinki, Finland, 1982.
9. M. Zachman, personal communication from the Department of
    Endocrinology, Kinderspital, Zurich, Switzerland, 1982.
10. R. Wasikowa, personal communication from Academia Medyczna,
    Institut Peditrii, District Wroclaw, Poland, 1983.
11. V. Schreiher, personal communication, Czechoslovakia Endocrine
    Society, Prague, Czechoslovakia, 1982.
12 O. Matio de Acosta, personal communication from Instituto Nacional
    de Endocrinología Vedado-Hospital Fajardo, Havana, Cuba, 1983.
13. B. Halasz, personal communication from Hungarian Society of
    Endocrinology, National Institute of Pediatrics, Budapest, Hungary,
    1983.
14. D. J. Carson, personal communication from Department of Child Health,
    Institute of Clinical Science, Belfast, Ireland, 1983.
15. L. Matajc, personal communication from University Clinic of
    Pediatrics, Ljubljana, Vrazov, Yugoslavia, 1983.
16. S. Suiva, personal communication from Kanagua's Children Medical
    Center, Kyoto, Japan, 1983.
17. D. D. Schoenberg, personal communication from Division of Pediatric
    Endocrinology, University of Heidelberg Children's Hospital, Heidelberg,
    Germany, 1983.
18. E. A. Montgomery, personal communication, 1984.
19. National Center for Health Statistics, HANES Study Section, personal
    communication to Dr. H. Hannon, 1984.
20. L.N. Parker, W.O. Odell, Am. J. Physiol. 236, E616-E620, (1979).
21. J. Ariza, personal communication, 1984
22. Commission on Premature Thelarche, Final report, 1985.

DISCUSSION

SIITERI: How much chicken does a child less than age 2 consume in Puerto Rico?

HADDOCK: Chicken starts to be included in the diet at about 9 months. It is difficult to state how much they consume for usually they chew the meat but do not ingest it.

MCLACHLAN: Since the majority of the cases of premature thelarche are under the age of two, this raises the possibility for prenatal exposure to an estrogen source. If one makes the hypothesis that this is the case, then the experiment has already been done. I can't imagine any environmental exposure to estrogens at levels comparable to the therapeutic treatment of pregnant women with diethylstilbestrol. If the offspring of these pregnancies did not have premature thelarche, this mechanism seems less likely.

HADDOCK: We have recommended that a group of such patients be identified so as to study the development of these conditions (premature thelarche and early sexual development) in their siblings and in that of subsequent generations. I think Dr. Edward O'Neill, a member of the new Commission on Premature Thelarche, could do this study in Puerto Rico. Other interested groups could do it in the United States and abroad.

MILLS: I would like to respond to the question, "Is prenatal hormone exposure responsible for premature thelarche?" We examined this issue in our Philadelphia case-control study. Six of the mothers of cases (of 46) received sex hormone treatment during the pregnancy that produced the case. Only two of the control mothers (N=47) received such treatment. The difference was not significant (p=.13). But this illustrates the need for a controlled study since hormone treatment in this time period was not uncommon.

SIITERI: Transplacental passage of exogenous estrogen is an unlikely mechanism for premature sexual development in view of 50-100 mg/day of endogenous placental estrogen production unless the estrogen is very unusual and retained in tissue for months or years. If it is endogenous, it likely derives from peripheral aromatization of adrenal androgens (androstenedione in particular) which is suggested by evidence for advanced adrenarche. We reported a case of prepubertal gynecomastia due to massive peripheral aromatization which was not evident until adrenal androgen precursor was available.

BERN: The issue to be considered may derive from the experiments performed on mice; namely, whether a prenatal exposure to estrogen which does not result in perceptible breast changes at birth, followed by a postnatal exposure to estrogen, which also by itself would not result in significant changes, could underlie the premature thelarche observed. Does the early exposure so change the sensitivity of the breast tissue as to allow response to the second stimulus? The same argument would apply to internal changes in the genital tract (see Ostrander et al., JNCI, 1985, in press).

ADLERCREUTZ: Many baby foods contain soy and nobody knows how much phytoestrogens is transferred to children in this way. Baby foods contain other beans as protein supplements and also chicken, which could be possible sources of estrogens. Cow milk contains rather much equol in unconjugated form, and the baby can get some exposure to phytoestrogens during lactation if the mother consumes soy products. On the other hand,

Japanese people consume a lot of soy products and they do not have, as far as I know, any problems of this kind. Therefore, I do not believe that phytoestrogens can cause these symptoms, but that does not mean that I am not interested in investigating phytoestrogen action in these subjects.

NAFTOLIN: The work done in Puerto Rico has exposed an area of ignorance and may have indicated a special problem for Puerto Ricans. However, the evidence of endemic or epidemic precocious activation of sex hormone responsive tissues remains unconvincing. Prior to extensive biochemical testing of a selected population, general prospective and cross-sectional incidence studies are indicated. Identified cases found during this study should then be studied/treated according to their individual findings.

HADDOCK: The Commission has recommended to the Secretary of Health that prevalence and incidence studies be done in Puerto Rico regarding premature thelarche, early sexual development (to include premature adrenarche and precocious puberty), and prepuberal gynecomastia. The Centers for Disease Control has also recommended that the prevalence and incidence of premature thelarche and early sexual development be done in a Puerto Rican population in the United States and other ethnic group (Anglo-Saxon). I, therefore, agree with you.

BOVING: Have you done vaginal cytology in these girls? If so, was there maturation that could be interpreted as estrogenic effect? I think that would indicate that there is an estrogen in the system.

HADDOCK: Yes, we do vaginal smears in the cases. The vaginal smears done in 83 cases showed mild to moderate etrogenic effect in 8 patients whose ages ranged from 10 months to 6-1/2 years. Of the four patients with thelarche and pubic hair, the vaginal smear was done in 3 and showed mild estrogenic effects, vaginal smear was not available in the other.

KIRKLAND: The response (to GnRH) of the LH levels in children with premature thelarche is comparable (25-90 mIu/ml peak values) to older children (pubertal) and adults. If one assumes an exogenous source of an "estrogenic compound" to be responsible for premature thelarche in Puerto Rico, but with no other signs of puberty, how does one hypothesize an explanation with the known concept of the hypothalamic-pituitary-gonadal axis?

HADDOCK: The patients in which GnRH stimulation tests gave maximal LH increases ranging from 25 to 90 mIu/ml were 6 girls who had thelarche and pubic hair and one with thelarche only. Three of the girls were classified as having precocious puberty because the bone age was advanced in two and accelerated linear growth was seen in the other. The remaining 3 of that group had pubic hair, thelarche and normal bone age. The ages of these girls at the time of the test ranged from seven and 5/12 years to 10 years. The LH response was pubertal in all. We have classified three of them as true precocious puberty on the basis of their LH response to GnRH and the observed acclerated bone age and growth. We have not postulated an exogenous source in these cases. In 6 patients with thelarche, in whom GnRH stimulating tests were performed, the maximal LH response was like that seen in prepuberal girls (maximal increase of LH less than 10 mIu/ml. The ages of these girls at the time of the test ranged from two and 2/12 to three and 3/12 years. Basal values of LH and FSH were normal in these two set of patients. Serum estradiol 17β was elevated in two of the cases with precocious puberty (80 pg/ml and 200 pg/ml) and normal in the rest of the patients. We are doing GnRH stimulation tests in all the patients that have a breast size larger than 2.5 cm and in those that develop other signs of early sexual development. Repeated testing in the same patients will be done so as to determine whether their response is sustained or not. The type of LH response may help us predict the course of the condition. In this respect, we are following the recommendation of Dr. Robert Kelch.

BERN: Have you measured serum prolactin levels?

HADDOCK: Yes, serum prolactin (PRL) has been measured in 83 subjects and showed slight to moderate elevation in 14 patients (PRL>22 ng/ml). The values ranged from 24 to 63 ng/ml. Basal LH was normal in all, and there was a slight elevation of FSH in 2. In 10 of 11 patients on whom the test was repeated, in two occasions the serum prolactin decreased to normal values. At the time of the second test, the thelarche had disappeared in 1 case, had decreased in 5, and remained of the same size in 4. A statistical analysis done of this using the Pearson product moment correlation coefficient and the Spearman rank correlation relating the size of the breast to the serum prolactin levels and the change in size to the change of prolactin did not show any significant correlation.

KUPFER: A possible reason for the lack of detectable levels of methoxychlor in blood could be due to rapid metabolism of methoxychlor to demethylated products. Therefore, one should look for the mono- and bisphenolic derivatives of methoxychlor. In addition, the uterine cytosol assay for binding to estrogen receptor is inadequate since it will miss detecting proestrogens in samples (e.g., methoxychlor). In our assay, methoxychlor is a proestrogen and does not bind to the estrogen receptor.

SETCHELL: Is there a correlation between incidence of this condition and social class?

HADDOCK: No, we have found premature thelarche and early sexual development in girls from all social classes.

SETCHELL: What is the incidence of premature thelarche in Puerto Ricans who have emigrated and now reside in other countries between 1978-1984?

HADDOCK: We do not know. This is the type of study that we want Dr. Maria New to conduct in New York.

SETCHELL: Have liver function tests been carried out, because estrogens will influence liver function tests and may provide an indication of exogenous estrogen?

HADDOCK: All the patients get SMA12 examinations which include: serum bilirubin, serum cholesterol, SGOT and LDH, total proteins and A/G ratio. We have not found any abnormalities in these tests in our patients.

BOURDONY: Concerning the possibility of altered liver function in children with premature sexual development if an exogenous estrogenic substance is considered as etiologic, of the 50 cases I have studied, more than 50% had mild elevation of transaminases. This finding is being pursued further and more specific studies of liver function may reflect the effect of an ingestion of estrogenic substance in the organism.

ELLIS: Have you noted any new or different clinical conditions in your new cases of premature thelarche or sexual development. New cases would be those observed in 1984, for example.

HADDOCK: As presented, of 8 patients seen initially with thelarche, 3 have developed true precocious puberty and 5 early puberty. We have not seen cases with prepuberal gynecomastia. We are seeing an average of 7 cases of premature adrenarche per year.

MCLACHLAN: I have two fundamental questions: (1) Do you think there is an epidemic; and (2) Do you think it derives from an exogenous source?

HADDOCK: I don't know. I cannot say there is an epidemic of premature sexual development for there are no prevalence or incidence data in Puerto Rico or in any other place in the world. All books state that premature thelarche is common, but no data is available to verify this anecdotal observation. Furthermore, we have not been able to prove that the condition is due to an exogenous source. The state-of-the-art of the technology (mass spectometry, HPLC, estrogen receptor assay) has limited our investigation. The analyses of food and sera have lacked reproducibility. Poultry contamination with estrogens has been postulated by Dr. Saenz; yet in our patient population that develop thelarche before age 2, 55% had not eaten chicken before developing the breast enlargement and 25% had the breast enlargement at birth which was maintained after 6 months of age; the latter represent another unexposed group (to chicken food or any other type of food).

380

PREMATURE THELARCHE IN PUERTO RICO: DESIGN OF A CASE-CONTROL STUDY

Jose F. Cordero, M.D., M.P.H,* Lillian Haddock, M.D.,**
Gloria Lebron, M.S.,*** Ruth Martinez, Ph.D.,*** Lambertina W.
Freni-Titulaer, M.D., M.S.P.H.,* James L. Mills, M.D., M.S.****

*Birth Defects Branch, Center for Environmental Health, Centers for
Disease Control, Public Health Service, U. S. Department of Health and
Human Services, Atlanta, GA 30333; **School of Medicine and ***Graduate
School of Public Health, University of Puerto Rico, San Juan,
Puerto Rico 00936; ****Epidemiology and Biometry Program, National
Institute of Child Health and Human Development, National Institutes of
Health, Bethesda, MD 20205

INTRODUCTION

Premature thelarche (PT) is usually defined as breast enlargement in

girls less that 8 years old who do not have other evidence of early sexual

development (ESD). A 1982 report of an increase in the number of PT cases

seen by pediatric endocrinologists in Puerto Rico led to an investigation

of possible environmental sources of estrogens. The large variety of

estrogens in the environment, deriving from many diverse sources, required

that an extensive epidemiologic and laboratory investigation be

developed. We describe the development of a case-control study to search

for possible environmental causes of the reported increase.

BACKGROUND

There are several types of ESD: premature thelarche, premature

adrenarche, precocious puberty, and prepubertal gynecomastia. Premature

thelarche is the presence of breast enlargement without other signs of

ESD. Premature adrenarche refers to the development of pubic and/or

axillary hair before the age of 8 years. This condition usually results

from an increase in the adrenal androgen secretion and is not related to

the gonadal secretion of sex hormones. Precocious puberty refers to early

development of puberty, including breast enlargement, increased bone age,

elevation of gonadotropins, and the presence of pubic and/or axillary

hair. Prepubertal gynecomastia refers to the development of breast enlargement in males before the age of 8 years. Each of these types of ESD may result from a different pathophysiologic mechanism.

In February 1982, Saenz and coworkers reported an increase in the number of patients with PT seen in their practices from 1979 through 1981 when compared with the previous years [1-2]. Ovarian cysts were reported in 41 of 60 patients who had pelvic sonography. In a study of 272 cases of ESD, Perez-Comas reported an increase in PT for the years 1978 through 1980 [3]. In addition, he reported an isolated increase of precocious puberty for 1980. Many of these cases, however, may represent PT, since the diagnosis was based in most cases on elevated follicle-stimulating hormone and luteinizing hormone levels in random serum samples [4]. Other pediatric endocrinologists normally consider such cases as PT if there is no evidence of sexual development other than breast enlargement.

In August 1982, the Commission on Premature Thelarche was created in Puerto Rico to study the reported increase of PT and its possible causes. Cases were defined on the basis of presence of breast enlargement without other evidence of ESD at the time of the initial diagnosis. Other types of ESD were not included, since they may have different etiologies and no significant increase in their reporting was observed.

The Commission surveyed all 11 pediatric endocrinologists in Puerto Rico to ascertain cases of PT diagnosed between 1978 and 1982 [5]. Responses were obtained from 9 of them. A total of 552 cases were ascertained for that period. A threefold increase in the rate of PT was seen in 1981 when compared with 1978. In about 70% of the cases, onset was before age 2. No geographic clustering was found; the cases were reported from virtually all municipalities. All socioeconomic strata were represented among the reported cases. These findings were considered in designing a case-control study to search for the possible causes of the reported increase of PT in Puerto Rico.

ETIOLOGIC CONSIDERATIONS

Little is known about the etiology of PT [6]. Both human and animal data implicate estrogens or substances with estrogenic activity as causes of breast enlargement. Several commercial estrogens have been found to cause breast enlargement in humans; among them are diethylstilbestrol (DES) [7], ethynyl estradiol, and mestranol [8].

A number of substances with no apparent chemical similarity to steroidal estrogens have been shown to have estrogenic effects in animals and or humans. Among them are some DDT metabolites, Kepone, methoxychlor, and some mycotoxins [9]. A derivative of the mycotoxin zearalanone, zearalanol, is used as a growth promoter in cattle and sheep.

Breast enlargement has also been reported among prisoners of war with chronic malnutrition after they were given a normal diet [10].

Previous Outbreaks

Outbreaks of abnormal breast development following estrogen contamination of several types of foods, drugs, and air have been reported. An outbreak of breast enlargement among children in a kibbutz in Israel was attributed to the ingestion of chicken necks containing residues of DES pellets [7]. Kimball and coworkers reported a cluster of one boy and seven girls with breast enlargement in Bahrain, which was traced to consumption of milk from a cow that had received monthly injections containing oestronyl [11]. Hertz reported two siblings with bilateral breast enlargement that was traced to vitamin pills contaminated with DES; the vitamin tablets were manufactured in the same uncleaned equipment used to make DES tablets [7]. Contamination of isonicotinic acid hydrazide (INH) with DES was reported as the cause of an outbreak of breast enlargement in a tuberculosis ward in the United States; three boys and three girls were affected [12]. Breast enlargement was reported in four sons of workers in a pharmaceutical plant in Poland that produced DES. The outbreak was attributed to DES dust brought into the home on the parents' clothes [13]. Several cases of gynecomastia from use of creams and lotions with estrogenic activity have been reported. An example is the report by Edidin and Levitsky of a 5-year-old boy who developed gynecomastia after using a hair cream [14]. Menstrual irregularities and gynecomastia have been reported in workers of an oral contraceptive manufacturing plant in Puerto Rico. Air sampling revealed contamination with the active ingredients [8]. An outbreak involving 120 boys and girls with breast enlargement in a school in Italy was traced to the consumption of meat, although the relationship could not be confirmed by laboratory tests [15].

Given the number of diverse substances with estrogenic activity and the many potential sources of estrogens, many hypotheses had to be considered in the design of the case-control study.

STUDY OBJECTIVE

The primary objective of this study was to evaluate various hypotheses potentially related to the etiology of the increase of PT cases reported in Puerto Rico. Some of these hypotheses were derived from previous reports, others came from local community concerns in Puerto Rico, and some emerged from a household survey and from a pilot study. A prominent hypothesis considered in the study design was the possible association between meat consumption and PT. This was derived from the reports of contamination of foodstuffs in previous outbreaks and from strong community concern about the meat supply possibly being contaminated with estrogens. Several physicians had postulated that contamination of beef, poultry, and milk with exogenous estrogens may have been the cause of the problem.

STUDY DESIGN

The basic design of this study is a matched-pairs case-control design. The selection of subjects on the basis of the presence or absence of PT defines it as a case-control study. The selection of one control subject for each case on the basis of certain characteristics of that case defines the matched-pairs design. An alternative method for selecting of controls would be to select them from the general population without any attempt to match them with the cases.

Definitions

Case definition A case was defined as a girl between the ages of 6 months and 8 years who had palpable breast tissue of at least 1.5 cm in diameter at the time of the diagnosis and who at that time did not have evidence of other signs of ESD. All cases included had onset of the condition between 1978 and 1982.

Control definition A control was defined as a girl who never had breast enlargement after the age of 6 months and who was of similar age as the case with whom she was matched.

Age definition Age of onset was defined as the age in months when breast enlargement was first noted. For controls, the same age as that for the matched case was used to determine exposure status before onset of PT. For the pairs where the case had continuous breast enlargement from birth, three months was considered the age of onset for the purpose of defining exposure.

Selection of Subjects

Selection of cases The sample for the study derived from the 552 cases of PT diagnosed between 1978 and 1982 that were reported to the Commission, in a 1982 survey, by 9 of the 11 pediatric endocrinologists practicing in Puerto Rico. The Commission contacted all the parents by letter to request permission to interview them and to review the medical records, if necessary. A signed consent form was received from 397 (72%). The cases whose parents responded were not significantly different from the 552 cases with regard to year of diagnosis, age of onset, pediatric endocrinologist, and municipality of residence. Of the 397 cases, a stratified systematic sample of 130 (33%) patients was selected. The stratifying variables were pediatric endocrinologist, age of onset, year of diagnosis, and municipality of residence. Thus, the sample of interviewed cases was representative of the cases whose parents agreed to participate in the study.

Selection of controls Each case was pair-matched with a control. Mothers of cases were asked to name a friend or an acquaintance with a female child of the same age as the girl with PT. When the mother was unable to do so, a control was selected from the case's source of pediatric care: for girls with a private pediatrician, he or she was contacted to select a control; when the case received her pediatric care from a local health clinic, controls were selected from the Maternal Infant Care (MIC) program clinic that serves the Northeast Health District.

If at the time of first contact the parent of the potential control was uncertain about the presence of PT, or if the parent thought that the girl had enlarged breasts, the child was examined by the interviewer for the presence of palpable breast tissue. If palpable breast tissue was present, another child was selected as a control. To verify the absence of PT in the past, interviewers asked control parents if they had observed breast enlargement in the girl at any time between the ages of 6 months and 8 years. We assumed that the controls did not have any other form of ESD. Although the control parents were not asked specifically about other forms of ESD, the rarity of this condition and the absence of reference to it in the responses to the open-ended question about the control's medical problems make it unlikely that this condition was present.

Matching criteria Two criteria were used for matching on age. For cases who were less than 2 years old at the onset of PT, the control had to be at least 6 months of age and within 6 months of the case's age. For cases 2 years of age or older at the onset of PT, the control had to be at least 2 years old and within a year of the case's age. The younger cases were matched more closely on age to control for the rapid changes in feeding patterns and other exposures that occur in infancy.

Interview Procedures

A standardized home interview of the subject's mother, which lasted about 90 minutes, was used for collecting exposure data. To minimize bias in collecting exposure data, we divided the interview into two parts administered by different female interviewers. The first interviewer asked about family history of PT and, for the cases, the natural history of the condition, the diagnosis of ovarian cysts in the child, and the presence of other signs of ESD. When the first part of the interview was completed, the mother was instructed not to reveal to the second interviewer the status of her child as a case or control. The second interviewer asked about the subject's consumption of various food items and water, her medical history (excluding PT), therapy for treatment of illnesses, occupational histories of all household members, the mother's reproductive history, prenatal exposures, and history on use of insecticides, herbicides, and exterminator services in and around the house.

Exposure Definitions

Food items   The rationales for evaluating food items—particularly milk, beef, pork, chicken, eggs, and grains—are similar. All these commodities could be contaminated with estrogens. If this occurred, consuming these items could induce PT. Some grain products such as corn and rice may play host to Fusarium rosea, a fungus that produces the mycotoxin zearalanone, which has estrogenic activity [16]. In the interview the types of foods consumed by the subject—fresh, frozen, baby food, and the commercial brand, if available—were obtained. For each type of food the age in months when it was first consumed, the usual frequency of consumption, and whether the food was consumed at the time of the interview were noted. For milk consumption the age at which each type of milk was discontinued was also obtained. For all other categories of food it was assumed that once they were introduced, their consumption would continue.

Drugs PT may have been caused by exposure to estrogen-containing pills, creams, or ointments. It seems unlikely that parents would have deliberately given a child oral contraceptives. However, toddlers may have ingested oral contraceptives accidentally. Mothers may have used their own estrogen-containing creams on their daughters. We asked whether the mother used oral contraceptives after the subject's birth. If this was the case, the brand, date when started, and the duration of use were ascertained. We also asked whether the subject's mother used facial, skin, and vaginal creams. For each cream used, the brand name was obtained and the composition was reviewed to determine the presence of estrogens.

Occupation of household members Several reports have described the development of breast enlargement among children of workers in DES plants. Puerto Rico manufactures about 95% of the oral contraceptives consumed in the United States [17]. We obtained an occupational history for each adult household member, starting from 1 year before the birth of the subject. If any household member worked at a pharmaceutical plant producing sex hormones in the 3 months period before the onset of PT, or equivalent reference age for the control, the subject was considered exposed.

Pesticides Some pesticides such as DDT, methoxychlor, and Kepone are known to have estrogenic activity. We asked about pesticide use in the household and the use of exterminating services.

Maternal history of ovarian cysts In a pilot study of PT in Puerto Rico, an association was found between PT and a maternal history of ovarian cysts. In most instances this diagnosis is based on clinical findings. We asked the mother of each subject if a physician had ever

388

told her that she had ovarian cysts. If so, we asked if surgery was ever performed, and if so, what was the postsurgical diagnosis as described by the physician. We also asked if any family member had been diagnosed as having ovarian cysts. If this was so, we asked what the relationship with the index child was.

Prenatal factors and exposures We asked the mother about the events surrounding the pregnancy of the subject child. History of threatened abortion, X ray exposures, sonograms, smoking, and alcohol use during pregnancy were covered. We also asked about infertility problems. A threatened abortion was only considered as such in those instances where a physician had made the diagnosis.

Familial factors Because of the association between PT and maternal history of ovarian cysts noted above, history of ovarian tumors, breast cysts, diabetes, thyroid disease, and other endocrine disorders in the family were obtained. If there was a positive history, we asked how the affected person was related to the subject.

Water source Drinking water may be another source of potential estrogen contamination, for instance, through contamination with waste products from the chemical industry. We considered the water source for a possible association with PT in categories of tap water, deep well, bottled, or other.

STATISTICAL METHODS

In the analysis of a matched-pairs study a similar pattern is followed for each hypothesis. The odds ratio (OR) provides a summary measure of the magnitude of the association between the exposure of interest and PT. A simple 2 x 2 table provides the data from which the OR is computed without consideration of, or adjustment for the effects of other variables. It has the following layout:

```
                           Control's
                        Exposure Status
                          +       -

        Case's          +    a       b
    Exposure Status
                        -    c       d
```

The cells labelled "b" and "c" represent discordant pairs. The pairs where the case was exposed and the control was not fall into the "b" cell. The pairs where the case was not exposed and the control was go into the "c" cell. The OR is computed as the ratio of the number of pairs that are discordant for the exposure, b/c. Data from the cells labelled "a" and "d" are not used because they provide no information for or against the hypothesis. The 95% confidence limits will be estimated with an exact method based on the probability distribution of the binomial as described by Clopper and Pearson [18]. Associations with a p-value of 0.05 for a 2-tailed test are considered to be statistically significant. One-sided tests would be more appropriate, if the only associations tested were between PT and products possibly contaminated with estrogens. As such, contamination cannot protect subjects from developing PT. However, many of the factors studied are possible correlates of exposures to such substances, and therefore the associations could be either positive or negative.

Categories where the number of discordant pairs is fewer than 6 are not analyzed, since statistical significance at alpha = 0.05 (2-tailed) cannot be attained with such small numbers.

Since many hypotheses are considered, many tests of statistical significance will be performed. With alpha set at 0.05, one can expect that roughly 5% of independent tests will be significant by chance alone. One way of remedying this is to apply the Bonferroni method [19]. With this method one divides the p-value considered to be statistically significant by the number of comparisons made and adjusts the confidence

390

intervals accordingly. We will not use this method for three reasons. First, the fact that some findings are due to chance does not necessarily detract from the finding of any particular instance of statistical significance. Second, this is the first case-control study of PT in Puerto Rico, which should be considered as hypothesis generating, and therefore all possible associations should be reported. Third, the sample size of this study is such that moderately strong associations can be detectable at the 5% significance level, but it is too small to for such associations to be detected at significance levels of 1%, 0.5%, or even smaller.

Effect Modification and Confounding

Effect modification   Effect modification is also referred to as interaction. It occurs when the magnitude of the exposure-disease association (i.e., the magnitude of the OR) varies among subgroups of the cases. For example, consider the age of onset of PT as a potential effect modifier. If the OR were 4.0 for cases whose age of onset was less than 2 years old, and if the OR were 1.5, for cases whose age of onset was 2 years or older, we would say that there could be effect modification by age of onset. In practical terms, this means that the effect of the exposure would not be the same for both age groups. The only factor considered as a potential effect modifier before the analysis is age of onset. Separate analyses will be performed for the two age categories.

Confounding   The relationship between an exposure and a disease may be confounded by extraneous variables. A confounder is defined as a factor independently associated with the exposure and the condition under study. For example, maternal age may be a confounding factor in a study of spermicide failure and chromosomal defects since older women are more likely to be users of spermicides and have a higher risk of having children with chromosome abnormalities. These confounders could have the effect of either diminishing or increasing the magnitude of the

exposure-disease relationship.

When the potential confounders are not known a priori, it is necessary

to search for them in the analysis. One method of searching for

confounders is to perform separate analyses for subjects with and without

a possible confounding factor. This is often called a stratified

analysis. If the odds ratios found for these subgroups (strata) are

different from those obtained when all strata are combined, it is assumed

that confounding is present, and this factor must be a controlled for in

the analysis. In matched studies, this simple approach is often not

feasible because the case-control pairs have to remain together, leading

to at least four strata for each possible confounding factor. Therefore,

an analysis can often not be performed because the number of discordant

pairs in each stratum is too small.

A statistical technique that can be used in such situations is

conditional logistic regression. With this procedure, the effect of

several exposures and confounders can be studied simultaneously, and OR's

can be estimated that are adjusted for all variables present in the

model [20]. The program that will be used in the analysis of this study

is PROC PHGLM, a procedure in the Statistical Analysis System (SAS) [21]

that was designed to fit a proportional linear hazard model to the data

but that can also be used for conditional logistic regression of matched

pairs in a case-control study [22].

Multivariate models will be fitted for both age groups, as well as for

all ages combined. All variables with OR's of at least 2 or at most 0.5

in the univariate analyses will be included in the initial models, as well

as variables that show statistically significant associations.

Subsequently, those variables that are the least significant will be

removed one at a time in a stepwise fashion, until the models contain only

those variables that are significant at the 5% level. In the analyses for

both age groups combined, all exposures found to be associated in the univariate analyses and interaction terms for these exposures with age of onset will be included.

Breast size may reflect the level of exposure: girls with the smaller breast sizes may represent the lower exposure group; this group may also represent background cases, not related to the reported increase, and only identified because of increased awareness. Including these cases may dilute a statistical association. To determine whether possible associations are diluted because cases with only limited breast enlargement were included, we will perform separate multivariate analyses on the subset of cases in which the diameter of the largest breast is at least 2.5 cm, a size that represents clearly visible breast enlargement to the untrained observer.

DISCUSSION

The primary objective of this study was to test specific hypotheses on the possible etiology of PT. We chose the case-control design, since there were many hypotheses to be tested, it was relatively inexpensive, and it could provide answers in a reasonable period of time. The alternative, a prospective study of children exposed to certain products would have been very costly and time consuming and would have required a sample size of over 10,000 girls.

Controls were selected from daughters of friends and acquaintances of mothers of the cases. In addition to matching for age, we selected controls that tended to match the geographical area and socioeconomic status of the cases. This could lead to overmatching for variables that are associated with residence and socioeconomic status. The effect of the overmatching would be to decrease the power of the study. An advantage of matching is that it may help to control for unknown or unmeasurable confounding variables that would otherwise bias the estimated odds ratios. An additional advantage of matching in this study is that it simplifies defining exposure in the control group. We considered the

3-month period before the onset of PT as the exposure window. In the situation of an unmatched sample, defining exposure in the controls might have been quite difficult.

Alternatively, we could have selected children from the general population, using a frequency matching with regard to age of onset of the cases. The advantage of not matching would be that the controls might be more representative of the general population than the controls selected for this study, especially with regard to socioeconomic status. Since PT cases are distributed throughout the island, a localized factor is probably not the cause of the reported increase.

This study was conducted amid a great deal of publicity. There were public allegations of possible estrogen contamination of milk products, and meat, especially fresh chicken. The interviewers were aware of this publicity. Since some of the questions raised in the media were related to questions being asked in the interview, this might have introduced a serious bias if the interviewer probed more for exposures in the cases than in the controls. That is why the interviews in this study were conducted in a blinded fashion.

In a case-control study, exposures are ascertained in a retrospective fashion. The accuracy of the response depends on the accuracy of the interviewed subject's recall. This is particularly a concern in the responses to food items. As time elapses, remembering what foods were consumed and when is more difficult [23]. In the interview we asked the age in months when the food was introduced. The mother may not have remembered the correct age when the food was started. However, there are no specific reasons why the mothers of cases would remember more or less than the mothers of controls, except for a possible selective recall by the mothers of cases for consumption of fresh milk and fresh chicken. If there is poor recall occurring more or less randomly, the result will be to reduce the likelihood of finding a true association.

Most of the exposures that were considered in this study reflect vehicles or sources of estrogens and not the estrogenic substance per se. If certain products are contaminated with estrogenic substances sometimes, but not always, some associations might not be detectable. Although comparing consumption of possibly contaminated food products by calendar time might be preferable in this situation, we decided that the age at which products were consumed would be better for comparison, especially in pairs where the control was younger than the case and might not have had an equal opportunity for exposure in the calendar time of interest.

In the analyses of occupational exposure we assume that if the parents or other household members were exposed, then the subjects were also exposed. That might not be true in all instances. Probably, exposure to these substances varied with the worker's tasks; some workers may have received negligible exposures, whereas others may have been heavily exposed. Exposed workers may have introduced variable amounts of estrogen-containing dust into the home environment.

SUMMARY

In recent years, the number of PT cases seen by pediatric endocrinologists in Puerto Rico has increased. The condition is relatively rare. After considerable publicity in 1982, the number of newly diagnosed cases in that year was 1 in every 1,000 girls under the age of 8 years [5]. Therefore, the only feasible approach to find possible etiologic factors was a case-control study. To our knowledge, only one other case-control study of PT has been performed [6]. This study was based on 46 cases and 47 controls. Two possible associations were found with PT: breast feeding and treatment of the mother with sex hormones during pregnancy. Both associations were not statistically significant, possibly because of the limited sample size.

In this study, a large number of hypotheses will be tested. They include associations between PT and environmental and familial factors. Given the large number of statistical tests, we expect that a few statistically significant associations will be found by chance alone. Each statistically significant finding will be judged on its own merits. The interpretation of associations will include considerations of the accuracy and completeness of the data from which the association is derived, the biologic plausibility of the association in the light of other animal and human data, and the magnitude of the association.

REFERENCES

1. C.A. Saenz, M.A. Toro-Sola, L. Conde, et al, Bol. Asoc. Med. P. R. 74, 16-19 (1982).
2. C.A. Saenz de Rodriguez and M.A. Toro-Sola, Lancet I, 1300, (1982).
3. A. Perez-Comas, Lancet I, 1299-1300, (1982).
4. A. Perez-Comas, Bol. Asoc. Med. P. R. 74, 245-251 (1982).
5. L. Haddock, G. Lebron, R. Martinez, et al, in: Estrogens in the Environment: Influences in Development, J.A. McLachlan, ed. (Elsevier/Holland, 1985).
6. J.L. Mills, P.D. Stolley and J. Davis, Am. J. Dis. Child. 135, 743-745 (1981).
7. Hertz, R. in: Estrogens in the Environment, J.A. McLachlan, ed. (Elsevier/North Holland, 1979) pp. 347-352.
8. J.M. Harrington, G.F. Stein, R.O. Rivera, et al, Arch. Environ. Health 33, 12-14, (1978).
9. G. Klatskin, W.T. Salter and F.D. Humm, Am. J. Med. Sci. 213, 19-30, (1949).
10. J.A. Katzenellbogen, B.S. Katzenellbogen, T. Tattee, et al in: Estrogens in the Environment, J.A. McLachlan, ed. (Elsevier/ North Holland, New York, 1979) pp. 33-51.
11. A.M. Kimball, R. Hamadeh, R.A.H. Mahmood, et al, Lancet I, 671-672 (1981).
12. W.W. Weber, M. Grossman, J.V. Thom, et al, N. Engl. J. Med. 268, 411-414, (1963).
13. A. Budzinka, R. Wasikowa and J. Zajac, Polish Med. J. 6, 1249-1256 (1967).
14. D. Edidin and L. Levitsky, Am. J. Dis. Child. 136, 587-588 (1984).
15. G.M. Fara, G. Del Corvo, S. Bernuzzi, et al, Lancet II, 295-297 (1979).
16. S.V. Pathre and C.J. Mirocha in: Estrogens in the Environment, J.A. McLachlan, ed. (Elsevier/North-Holland, New York, 1979), pp. 265-278.
17. Food and Drug Administration, personal communication, 1982.
18. C.J. Clopper and E.S. Pearson, Biometrika 26, 404-413 (1934).
19. J. Neter, W. Wasserman and M.H. Kutner, Applied Linear Statistical Models (Richard D. Irwin Inc., Homewood, Illinois, 1985), pp. 583-584.
20. D.G. Kleinbaum, L.L. Kupper and H. Morgenstern, Epidemiologic Research (Lifetime Learning Publications, Belmont, California, 1982).
21. SAS Institute Inc., SUGI Supplemental Library User's Guide, (SAS Institute, Cary, North Carolina, 1983).
22. N.E. Breslow, N.E. Day, K.T. Halvorsen, et al, Am. J. Epidemiol. 108, 299-307 (1978).
23. F.E. Van Leeuwen, H.C.W. De Vet, R.B. Hayes, et al, Am. J. Epidemiol. 118, 752-758 (1983).

DISCUSSION

SETCHELL: I have developed a considerable interest in phytoestrogens since the discovery for the first time of equol in human urine and following our demonstration of the effects of soya in adults. There seems to be a general pessimism about the possible role of phytoestrogens in oestrogenic effects in man, and I would like to point out several things. Firstly, there has been an exponential increase in the use of soya based food products over the last five years, and I keep thinking of the effects which occurred in sheep ingesting isoflavones in clover. While I accept that in the case of sheep the levels of phytoestrogen ingestion far exceed that in man, I have an open mind about whether phytoestrogens may be important in these cases. However, what I showed in my presentation was that relatively large quantities of equol are absorbed and excreted in adults following soya ingestion. The second point I would like to stress is that not all people are able to produce equol given the challenge of soya since it requires the active bacterial enzymes in the gastrointestinal tract to convert the phytoestrogen precursors to equol. Bacterial flora and activity will vary between individuals and populations, and this is reflected, for example, in the different profiles of fecal metabolites which can be measured. It is conceivable that this may explain why some of the described effects are not seen in all infants. Finally, one could speculate that the clinical features may be explained by a combination of the suggestion of Dr. John McLachlan, that prenatal sensitization of the tissue by earlier use of DES 10-15 years previously could be coupled with the ingestion of low levels of phytoestrogens sufficient to stimulate tissue growth. I think we cannot yet exclude a role for phytoestrogens.

MCLACHLAN: Perhaps the question I asked Dr. Haddock would be more appropriately asked to you, a practicing epidemiologist. Do you think there is an epidemic of premature sexual development in Puerto Rico?

CORDERO: To determine that an epidemic exists, several criteria should be fulfilled. First, one needs to know the baseline incidence of the condition of the population. Second, one must show that the incidence of the condition is significantly increased. We do not know of any population-based data on the incidence of premature thelarche (PT). The reported incidence of PT is based on cases seen by pediatric endocrinologists. Some of the data presented by Dr. Haddock suggests a change in pattern of referrals to pediatric endocrinologists. There is one prevalence study of breast enlargement in children. Fara and coworkers studied a population of girls of 3 to 8 years old to serve as controls for another group in which an outbreak of breast enlargement had been reported. In about 5% of the control subjects, palpable breast tissue was found. The highest the incidence rate of PT in Puerto Rico was 1% that was seen by pediatric endocrinologists in Puerto Rico in 1982. A population study of the prevalence of PT in girls residing in Puerto Rico, a comparison group of Puerto Rican girls residing in mainland United States and, perhaps, a group of non-Hispanic girls may provide the final answer.

O'NEILL: Is there a problem in regard to premature thelarche or not? The magnitude of the problem whether epidemic in nature or not is irrelevant.

CORDERO: As far as the people of Puerto Rico are concerned, there is a problem. The pasture of the local and federal government has been to assume there is a problem. That is why the Centers for Diseases Control have collaborated with the Commission on Premature Thelarche in undertaking the studies described here today.

JONES: Puerto Rico is a major center for the production of birth control pills. How are the precursor products and waste products disposed of? It is possible that contaminants from these plants have been incorporated into the food chain. Therefore, these studies need to use controls outside of Puerto Rico. It may be that all were once exposed to low levels of contaminants for an extended period of time. However, differences in incidence of disorders may be due to a variety of secondary factors.

CORDERO: The waste treatment facilities in the municipalities where the oral contraceptive plants are located cannot handle the levels of effluents from these plants. Most of the waste products are collected and taken to the sea in barges where they are dropped. If low levels of estrogen contaminated many products in the food chain, this study would not be able to detect an association.

NEWBOLD: Are there any changes observed in other species? It seems the Caribbean primate colony in Puerto Rico may provide a good model to look for estrogenic effects.

CORDERO: I agree.

NAFTOLIN: What about the siblings of the identified cases--was there premature thelarche in them and was it concurrent? Also, what about other family members in the "control" population--was there premature thelarche in them?

CORDERO: Premature thelarche had never been present in family members of 16 cases and of 17 controls. Whether these were mothers, aunts or siblings has not been analyzed; information whether PT was concurrent is not available.

NAFTOLIN: If we apply the same percentage of misdiagnosis of maternal ovarian cysts to both the control and case population (40% or 3/7), I believe that the statistical significance of differences between groups for this variable would no longer be present--is that correct, i.e., that maternal history of ovarian cysts is not a marker of either control or case populations?

CORDERO: There were 23 cases of whom the mother of the case had ovarian cysts and the mother of the control not, and 6 controls where the mother had ovarian cysts and the mother of the case subject not. Three out of eight mothers, who had had surgery, or 38% had a diagnosis other than ovarian cysts. If we apply this percentage "overdiagnosis" to the ratio 23 over 6, it becomes 14 over 4. This results in an ratio of 3.5, which is not statistically different from one. However, women who require surgery for "ovarian cysts" cannot be considered a representative sample of all women who were ever told they had ovarian cysts. Therefore, we do not believe that this "adjustment" of the data should be done.

398

ESTROGENS IN FOOD PRODUCTS AS DETERMINED BY CYTOSOL RECEPTOR ASSAY

Alfred M. Bongiovanni, M.D., Department of Pediatrics, Pennsylvania
Hospital, School of Medicine, University of Pennsylvania

In the fall of 1978 I was living in Ponce and was beginning my

second year as the Dean of the medical school there. Dr. Adolfo Perez-

Comas was on that faculty and was teaching human genetics to our students.

We have never worked directly together but I had known of him as an

endocrinologist and clinician of excellent reputation. One day in late

1978 he stopped into my office to tell me of the peculiar increase in the

incidence of premature breast development in little girls in the region

around Mayaguez. I do not recall the exact month when he was first

suspicious. This was my first acquaintance with the problem and it was

later that I learned of the happenings in the region around San Juan

through Dr. Carmen Saenz with whom I had worked some years ago. I found

the matter sufficiently interesting to communicate with Dr. James Mills

who was already working in the epidemiology branch of the National

Instututes of Child Health where he works still. This correspondence is

a matter of record. Nothing came of it and within a year I learned from

Dr. Carmen Saenz that she had a large number of cases. I visited her

office in 1982, examined a number of her excellent records and concluded

that a truly unduly large number of children with early sexual develop-

ment were being seen in a single practice. I should also tell you that

I had known Dr. Saenz for some years and that she had worked with me a

long time ago at the University of Pennsylvania. In the spring of 1982

we received a number of specimens of meat and milk from Dr. Saenz which

were shipped frozen to my laboratory. The studies I am about to describe

were limited because of budgetary constraints as well as the small staff

of my laboratory. Therefore, what I am about to present I have regarded

as tentative. But I felt that the results, such as we encountered, were

sufficient to merit investigation by agencies equipped to undertake such a matter. In deciding to look for estrogens in the meat and milk products which we examined, we were at first bewildered by the very large number of estrogens described in the literature both natural and synthetic so that I concluded there was little point to employing highly specific techniques such as radioimmunoassay. Such an exploration would have required perhaps a hundred or more separate assays. In turning to bioassay with which I have had considerable experience I was obliged to reject the notion of whole animal assays because of lack of funds and because in the last ten years we have had no special facilities for housing whole animals in the laboratory. On this basis and since we were involved in some cytosol receptor studies with Dr. Robert Brent of Jefferson Medical College we decided to go that route.

The cytosol preparations were made from the uteri of immature rabbits which were stored at minus 100 degrees until processed. Tissues were homogenized in tris buffer pH 7.4 containing 1 mM EDTA, 1 mM Diathiotreitol and 5 mM Sodium Molybdate. The supernate after centrifugation at 100,000 g for 1 hour had a protein concentration of 4.5 - 7 mg./ml. Binding activity for estradiol was determined by incubation of 0.2 ml. cytosol and 1 ng. of radioactive estradiol tritiated at 2, 4, 6, 7 with a specific activity of 100 mCi per uM. Binding activity of the cytosol varied between 100 - 320 fmol estradiol per mg. of protein. Incubation was for two hours at 4 degrees and the unbound isotope was separated by use of a dextran-charcoal suspension. An aliquot of the supernate was counted by liquid scintillation at 30% efficiency in a model 6890 Searle Delta counter.

We examined specimens of meat and milk which were prepared in three different ways. First we decided to measure what we considered total estrogens by submitting the specimens to rigorous acid hydrolysis without any prior extraction. Except for the milk, the other specimens were homogenized in a Waring blender in aqueous phosphate buffer, pH 7.2, for 30 minutes. This was then heated to 100 degrees C. for two hours with 10% HCl, 0.1 M KCl and 0.002 M bisulfide. This mixture was then brought to pH 12 with 10% NaOH and extracted three times with an equal volume of ethyl ether which was then discarded. This was then brought to pH 1 with concentrated HCl and extracted three times with an equal volume of methylene chloride. The methylene chloride was washed five times with one-third volume of water and evaporated.

We then attempted to separate the conjugated from the free estrogens in the following manner employing fresh specimens of the food products. On this occasion they were homogenized in the Waring blender as above with two volumes of a mixture of 50% each ethyl ether and methylene chloride. This was filtered through gauze and dried. The residue was partitioned between aqueous buffer pH 7.2 and ethyl ether. The latter was dried and analyzed and was regarded as the free. The former was hydrolyzed and treated as in the previous paragraph. In all of these studies approximately 100 gram portions of the meats were employed for each specimen.

In four specimens of milk from Puerto Rico and three specimens from Philadelphia we found the equivalent of 10 - 15 ng. per kg. estradiol. Estradiol was employed in all experiments as the standard. We employed specimens of chicken obtained from supermarkets in the Philadelphia area as controls. In the beginning two specimens revealed low levels in muscle of the birds. In early experiments we found between 3 - 49 ng. per kg. as free and there was nothing in the conjugate. However, one local chicken contained 532 ng. per kg. when measured as the total but only 20 as the conjugate and 100 as the free when partitioned as described. Chickens from Puerto Rico revealed 470 - 2537 ng. per kg. as total estrogens. And in one instance there was 7750 ng. per kg. measured as the free when partitioned as described above.

We attempted to separate the organs of the frozen specimens which was difficult. In the skin, neck and liver we were able to detect 3.1 - 26.0 ng. per kg. with smaller amounts as conjugates. Therefore, the examination of the separated tissues revealed quantities lower than those detected in the muscle as described in the previous paragraph.

In an attempt to identify the particular estrogen in a few specimens showing high levels by cytosol receptor we performed gas liquid chromatography. We prepared standards for only three estrogens. These were zeranol, diethylsilbestrol (DES) and estradiol. We did not have available nor did we include any metabolites of the substances. The zeranol employed as a standard was from a commercial source obtained by Dr. Carmen Saenz in Puerto Rico at a farmer supply store. We were able to characterize each of these very well as three different derivatives. Acetates, bistrimethylsilylacetamids and trimethylchlorosilanes. We do not currently have mass spectroscopy so that for identification we insisted that any compound would need to confirm to the standards examined on GLC in all three derivatives and not any single one. The equipment was a capillary SE-54 column and Hewlett-Packard model 5840A gas chromatograph.

Although several peaks were present in all specimens we were unable to identify them and they did not coincide with our standards with one exception. One specimen showed a strong signal at the retention time for estradiol acetate but this was not confirmed with the other two derivatives and therefore we were unwilling to accept this. In another specimen there appeared to be large amounts of zeranol as determined with two separate derivatives. However, further examination of the acetate at different attenuations had this peak resolve into three spearate ones none of which were acceptable. The nature of our methods and equipment were such that with the employment of GLC we would not have achieved a sensitivity less than 10 ng. per kg. of specimen. Although we did

402

experiment with two other derivatives capable of giving strong signals
there was so much "noise" that we were unable to draw any conclusions.

We tested several estrogen like substances in our cytosol system in
order to compare their reactivity with estradiol. Each substance was
tested at numerous levels but these will be briefly summarized as follows.
Diethyl stilbestrol in an amount of 500 pg. was equivalent to 25 of
estradiol. In the case of estrone 1000 was equivalent to 10 of estradiol and 16-hydroxy estrone did not react at all even at very high
concentrations. With estriol 1000 pg. was equivalent to 20 of estradiol.
In the case of zeranol 500 was equivalent to 54 of estradiol and 1000
equivalent to 84. It can be seen from these results that if zeranol
were the culprit there is far more present in some of the specimens than
indicated in the results where the standard was always estradiol.

We studied several specimens of beef and pork but the levels were
generally moderate and in the lower range found in some of the chickens.

In conclusion, preliminary investigations of specimens of food from
Puerto Rico employing the cytosol receptor assay suggested the presence
of large quantities of estrogens. This was also true of certain specimens
obtained in the greater Philadelphia area. Our work was very carefully
conducted and we believe these results call for further investigation.
We do not agree that whole animal assays are superior and that the uterine
weight method is highly sensitive and reproducible. It is clearly not
strictly reproducible by contemporary concepts of such a notion.
Different people dissect differently and there are variations in the
stripping of extraneous tissue from the uteri. We highly recommend the
cytosol system for large scale screening. However, the resources of
government will be needed to define the problem in precise terms in
Puerto Rico and bring about its prevention. It is also suggested that

some degree of surveillance is required in the continental United States as well.

EFFECTS OF ENVIRONMENT HORMONAL CONTAMINATION IN PUERTO RICO

Carmen Sáenz de Rodríguez,MD, Director Pediatric Department, De Diego
Hospital, San Juan, Puerto Rico
Alfred M. Bongiovanni, MD, Professor University of Pennsylvania,
Philadelphia, Pennsylvania
Lillian Conde de Borrego, MD, Director Ultrasound Department, De Diego
Hospital, San Juan, Puerto Rico

ABSTRACT
     In the last three years the incidence of premature sexual
development and reactive hypoglycemia has increased alarmingly
in Puerto Rico. Both conditions may be related to environmental
hormone contamination, specifically estrogens.
     Several samples which were analyzed by Cytosol receptor
assay revealed significant levels of an estradiol equivalent
substance in some of the food tested. The early sexual
development and reactive hypoglycemia may be caused by
exogenous estrogen contamination in the food ingested by the
children and their mothers, as well as some other sources of
contamination in the environment in Puerto Rico.

INTRODUCTION
     Premature sexual development among Puerto Rican children has been
reported previously in Puerto Rico by several investigators. [1,2,3,4,5 &
6]. Reactive hypoglycemia has not been associated before to environmental
hormone contamination by estrogen. The high prevalence of both conditions
may be indicative of estrogen contamination in the island.

Patients, Material & Methods
     We have seen 914 patients with early sexual development during the last
9 years, 80% of them from 1982-85. The incidence of premature thelarche,
premature pubarche, precocious pseudopuberty, prepuberal gynecomastia and
vaginal bleeding in this group is shown in Table #1. During the same
period of time, 319 cases of reactive hypoglycemia in children were
observed. The patients with this condition presented the following
symptoms: dizzy spells, headaches, blurred vision, abdominal pain,
tachycardia, paleness and diaphoresis. Some of them had chest pain and
vomiting, 14 patients had syncope.

Endocrine Studies
     Serum total estrogens, FSH LH, and urinary gonadotrophins were
determined by radioimmune assay; total estrogens by MacAnally and Hausmann
method [7,8]. Seventeen K's determination was done by the Zimmerman method.
Bone age was determined by Greulich and Pyle Atlas [9]. Vaginal smears
were stained with Shorr's solution.
     The pelvic sonograms were done with a Gray Scale B scanner [Rohe and
Picker]. A 3.5 and 5.0 NH2 transducer was used. Patients under 24
months were sedated using Chloral Hydrate (50 mgs/Kg). The urinary
bladder was satisfactorily filled in most of the cases. The volume of
the ovaries was calculated using the formula of Sample [10] which is as
follows:

$$\text{Ovarian volume (cc)} = \frac{\text{Height x depth x length}}{2}$$

     An enlarged prepuberal ovary was considered when the volume exceeded
1.2 cubic centimeters. A puberal uterus was classified when the uterine
body was more prominent than uterine cervix.

Cytosol Receptor Assay

The Cytosol assay was conducted by using immature rabbit uterus according to the method of Moncharmont et al. [11] Gas liquid chromatography was employed as described by Bongiovanni [12] using the combined methoxyamine-trimethylsymidazole, 0 - bistrimethysiltlacetamide, trimethylchorosilane derivative as described. The Hewlett-Packard Model 5840A gas chromatograph equipment was used.

The Cytosol receptor assays are expressed as estradiol equivalents. The standard curves were constructed with this estrogen as the standard. In all cases the test was repeated with an excess of DES introduced into the assay and in all specimens the results were reduced to zero.

Results

Classification of patients with premature sexual development is shown in Table 1. The age group of this condition and reactive hypoglycemia is depicted in Table 2.

Endocrine tests performed in the patients with premature sexual development are outlined in Table 3. Those with reactive hypoglycemia are in Table 4. Among the girls with early sexual development, 130 had significant cornification of the vaginal cells. Advancement of the epiphyseal maturation was found in 73 patients in which a wrist bone age was performed. Serum insulin levels were elevated in a small group of patients with reactive hypoglycemia. Blood sugar levels ranged between 25 to 55 mg/dl. at the 2nd. and 3rd. hour of the GTT in the patients with reactive hypoglycemia.

Pelvic sonogram results are summarized in Table 5.

A control group of 40 girls demonstrated that in half of the patients under 3 years of age, the ovaries were not visualized. In the rest of the control group, 1 patient had a cyst of .3 cm. at the age of 9 years, associated with a puberal uterus. Girls from 9 months to 11 years did not have ovarian cysts above .3 cm. Excluded from the control group was a 6 year old girl, who had a cyst of 1.5 cm. and developed premature thelarche 3 months after these findings.

Results of Cytosol receptor assay on several food specimens are shown on Table 6. We were unable to identify any estradiol, zeranol or DES in any specimen by use of GLC.

After withdrawal of suspected food contaminants, involution of the breast tissue was observed within 2 to 6 months in 48% of the patients. The ovarian cysts decreased or disappeared significantly in the same period of time.

Patients with reactive hypoglycemia were started on a diet excluding refined sugars and significant remission of their symptoms was noticed in 3 weeks. Two patients needed Proglicem (Diazoxide) for control of their symptoms.

DISCUSSION

We consider that the early sexual development observed in these children is related to exogenous contamination of estrogens because:
1) Endogenous endocrine disorders were excluded
2) High levels of estrogen like substances were found by cytosol receptor assay in some food specimens
3) A genetic predisposition is not considered a causative factor because several ethnic groups have been affected in Puerto Rico
4) Estrogenic effect on vaginal smears were detected in 50% of post menopausal women in several local hospitals
5) The importation of hormones for veterinary use to the island was directly proportional to the increase incidence of these conditions

6) Exclusions diets (of suspected food contaminants) resulted in remission of symptoms or marked improvement in 48% of the cases

7) Related conditions as reactive hypoglycemia increased during the same period of time. Islet cell hyperplasia and increased levels of insulin have been reported in animals exposed to growth promotants since 1970. [13,14,15] We postulate that these growth promotants may be related to the reactive hypoglycemia observed in our patients. Gonadal steroids and related compounds have been reported to stimulate islet cell to increase secretion and growth. These effects may be seen in the absence of pituitary and adrenal glands, so they are not mediated through these glands [16]

8) Pharmaceutical companies in Puerto Rico have an extraordinary production of estrogenic compounds and other drugs which produce breast enlargement such as cimetidine and digitalis. The geographic distribution of patients do not correlate with the location of these pharmaceutical companies, but the contamination of waste products from them has not been thoroughly investigated.

9) Infant girls not directly exposed to this contaminants may be affected because their mothers were exposed during gestation. Experimental work with laboratory animals proves that intrauterine or neonatal exposure to several estrogens may lead to long lasting endocrine disturbances in the offspring, [17] The adverse effects of all these hormones have been shown in experimental animals so the long term effects in our population is of concern.

Conclusion

The increased prevalence of premature sexual development and related conditions as prepuberal gynecomastia, postmenopausal bleeding and reactive hypoglycemia strongly suggest the presence of a severe exogenous hormone contamination in Puerto Rico.

REFERENCES

1. Pérez-Comas, A. Precocious Sexual Development in Puerto Rico, Lancet 1:1299, (1982).
2. Bongiovanni, Alfred M. An Epidemic of Premature Thelarche in Puerto Rico, J. of Pediatrics 103:245, (1983).
3. Sáenz de Rodríguez, C.A.; Bongiovanni, A.M. An Outbreak of Premature Thelarche in Puerto Rico (Abstract), Ped. Res. 17:171A, (1983).
4. Sáenz de Rodríguez, C.A.; Toro Solá, M.A.; Conde, L; Bayonet, N. Premature Thelarche and Ovarian Cyst Probably Secondary to Estrogen Contamination, Bol. Asoc. Med. P.R. 74:16, (1982).
5. Sáenz de Rodríguez, C.A.; Toro Solá, M.A. Anabolic Steroids in Meat and Premature Thelarche, Lancet 1:1300, (1982).
6. Sáenz de Rodríguez, C.A; Bongiovanni, A.M. An Epidemic of Precocious Development in Puerto Rican Children, Journal of Pediatrics, In press for publication.
7. Commercial Kits from R.J.L. Radioimmuno Assay System Laboratories and Clinetics Corporation, California
8. MacAnally, J.S., Hausmann, E.R. The Determination of Urinary Estrogen by Fluorescence, J. Lab. & Clinic Med. 44-647, (1954).
9. Greulich and Pyle Atlas, Stanford University Press, Second Edition, (1983).

TABLE I - Classification of Patients with early Sexual Development
(January 1976 - February 1985) 914

CONDITION	NUMBER OF PATIENTS
Premature Thelarche	551
Precocious Pseudopuberty	188
Premature Adrenarche	130
Females	105
Males	25
Prepuberal Gynecomastia	45
Vaginal Bleeding	35

TABLE 2 - Age of Patients with Premature Thelarche and Precocious
Pseudopuberty

b - 24 months	350
25 - 36 "	73
37 - 90 "	326

Age of Patients with Reactive Hypoglycemia

1 - 3 years	41
4 - 6 "	67
7 - 9 "	81
10 - 12 "	69
13 - 15 "	41
16 - 18 "	20

TABLE 3 -

ENDOCRINE TESTS	NORMAL PREPUBERAL VALUES	# OF TESTS	ELEVATED VALUES
FSH	0-8 MIU/ML	352	11
LH	0-7 MIU/ML	352	8

TOTAL ESTROGENS			
Serum	Below 40 picograms		131
Urine	Below 5 micrograms		
17 ks	0-4 mg/day	144	None
DEAS	0.1-0.6 mcgr./ml.	14	None
Serum	0.1-2.2 ng./ml.	22	None

TABLE 4 -

Insuline Levels	46
Normal	13
Elevated	28
Low	5

TABLE 5 - Pelvic Sonograms (295)

	Percent
Ovarian cysts (greater than 1.4 cm.)	49.9%
Enlarged ovaries (above 1cc.)	56%
Enlarged uterus	35%
Pubertal Type Uterus	38%
Multicystic ovaries	5.3%

408

TABLE 6 - Cytosol Receptor Assay (as ng. Estradiol/kg)

P. R. Milk #1	14
P. R. Milk #2	10
P. R. Milk #3	14
P. R. Milk #4	10
P. R. Milk #5	10
Phila. Milk #1	15
P. R. Chicken #1	2500
P. R. Chicken #2	470
Phila. Chicken #1	532
Phila. Chicken #2	30
P. R. Pork #1	89
P. R. Babilla	89
Phila Pork #1	161
Phila Beef #1	850

10. Sample W.F.; Lippe B.M.; Giepes M.T. Gray Scale Ultrasonography of the Normal Female Pelvis, Radiology 125 477-483, (1977).
11. Moncharmont B. Parikh I; Pica, G.A.; Cuatrecases, P. Effect of Sodium Molybdate on Cystosolic Estrogen Receptor, J. Steroid Biochem 16:361-368, (1982).
12. Bongiovanni, A.M. Urinary Steroidal Pattern of Infants with Congenital Adrenal Hyperplasia, J. Steroid Biochem 13:809-811, (1980).
13. Allen Trenkle, Plasma Levels of Growth Hormone, Insulin and Plasma Protein-Bound Iodine in Finishing Cattle, Journal of Animal Science Vol. 31, (1970).
14. Borger, M.L.; Sink, J.D.; Wilson, L.L. Zeranol and Dietary Protein Level Effects on DNA, RNA and Protein Composition of Three Muscles and the Relationship to Serum Insulin and GH Levels of Steers, Journal of Animal Science Vol. 36 No. 4, (1973).
15. Borger, M.L.; Wilson, L.L.; Sink, J.D. Zeranol and Dietary Protein Level Effects on Live Performance, Carcass Merit, Certain Endocrine Factors and Blood Metabolite Levels of Steers, Journal of Animal Science Vol. 36, No. 4, (1973).
16. Haist, R.E. Effect of Steroids on the Pancreas. In Dorfman, Ralph I. (Ed.) Methods in Hormone Research, Vol. IV, Part B, Academic Press, N.Y. Page 193 (1965).
17. Susumu K.; Isutom S. Neonatal Exposure to Zearalenone Causes Persistent Anovulatory Estrus in Rats, Arch Taxicol, 50:279-286, (1982).

DISCUSSION

FRENI-TITULAER: Based on the result of earlier and of recent sonograms in your patients, you implied that something that was in the environment before has disappeared now. How do you explain that you do not see fewer cases of premature sexual development now?

SAENZ: According to my records and the experience of all other pediatric endocrinologists as well as sonographists, there has been a radical change in the pelvic sonogram findings of these patients. I continue to see cases of premature sexual development, yet, my only explanation could be that some compounds that were added to animal feed have been discontinued in their use. There is a long list of accepted drugs available in Puerto Rico for animal husbandry. Chorionic gonadotropin may have been added and withdrawn, but other types of estrogen may be still in use.

CORDERO: One of the concerns about premature thelarche in Puerto Rico relates to the number of new cases being seen by year. From your table on number of new cases by year, you showed about the same number of cases for 1982-1984. What period of time did you include for 1985: January, February, and part of March? Then you have had a stable number of cases from 1982 through 1985.

SAENZ: You refer to these cases as premature thelarche. The numbers that
I gave you included: premature thelarche, premature pubarche, prepuberal
gynecomastia, and precocious pseudopuberty.

    1982 : 184
    1983 : 207
    1984 : 204
    1985 : 49

The difference is that in the year 1982, most of the cases were premature
thelarche, but from the year 1983 on, 38% of the cases were classified as
premature pubarche or pseudopuberty. So, it does not show a stable number
of premature thelarche as you claim.

NEW: In the appearance of the breasts in the cases of precocious thelarche, pubertal and prepubertal gynecomastia presented by Dr. Saenz, I am
impressed with the absence of pigmentation such as that reported in
patients with documented estrogen intoxication. We must conclude that the
present phenomenon is a high frequency of precocious thelarche of the
usual type.

SAENZ: First you must define what you mean by precocious thelarche of the
"usual type." Many of the patients without pigmentation came to me many
months after they were diagnosed by the pediatrician. The infants that
had thelarche by the effect of their exposure in utero were seen at least
six months after birth. I did not expect to see pigmentation after such a
long lapse of time. Other patients that came at a later age (2 to 7 yrs)
did present pigmentation, as well as the boys with prepuberal gynecomastia. The cases of premature thelarche that I presented had ovarian
cysts over 1.4 cm in 49% of the cases; enlarged ovaries in 56%; pubertal
type uterus in 38%. You only saw four cases of premature thelarche in
1984. This was accepted by you. By definition, we define premature thelarche as the appearance of breast tissue before age 8 in the female,
without sonographic changes nor accelerated bone age as many of these
patients did.

JORDAN: Dr. New, I am rather intrigued by your observation that the
areola of the breast is not pigmented in the Puerto Rican cases although
other confirmed reports of estrogen poisoning are pigmented. May I
suggest that other pharmacologic agents could be involved to cause the
thelarche in children. We should consider that other environmental agents
or pharmaceutical products could be the culprit rather than focus entirely
upon estrogens.

KIRKLAND: What are the biochemical criteria that you used for making a
diagnosis of reactive hypoglycemia?

SAENZ: Reactive hypoglycemia was defined when the patient had a drop in
blood sugar below 55 mg/dl at the second or third hour in the glucose
tolerance test. In some cases, this was accompanied by a rise in insulin.
These patients were referred by their pediatricians with symptoms of
hypoglycemia; that is, paleness, dizziness, abdominal pain, diaphoresis,
headaches, blurred vision. In a small group of patients where insulin
levels were determined, 60% had hyperinsulinism.

BOURDONY: With regard to Dr. Saenz's statement that she seems to be seeing an increased frequency of cases with reactive hypoglycemia, the percent of cases admitted to the Pediatric Endocrinology Clinic of the San Juan City Hospital from the Pediatric Endocrinology Screening Clinic was as follows:

Hypoglycemia Cases Admitted/ Total Cases Referred for Hypoglycemia		Percentage of Cases Admitted for Hypoglycemia
1979	1/17	5.9
1980	4/22	18.2
1981	7/26	26.9
1982	5/38	13.2
1983	12/48	25
1984	10/51	19.6
Total	39/202	15.8

Of 34 cases followed for hypoglycemia of any etiology only 3 cases have shown any signs of premature sexual development.

SAENZ: Other pediatric endocrinologists, Dr. Adolfo Pérez Comas, Dr. Angel Solla, as well as many pediatricians claim that they are seeing more hypoglycemia since 1982. The cases that you refer to were not studied with insulin levels; and, therefore, the question whether there was hyperinsulinism remains unanswered. Of 914 cases followed from 1976 to 1985 with premature sexual development, 12% present carbohydrate intolerance. In your series of 34 cases with hypoglycemia of unknown etiology, 3 (10%) have shown signs of premature sexual development.

PASQUALINI: Do you have some correlation of the cases of premature development with the estrogen concentration and production in the maternal compartment during pregnancy?

SAENZ: No, I don't. The cases were referred to me when the baby was at least 6 months of age. However, there is ample evidence in the literature of the effects of hormones on the offspring by the exposure of the mother (K. Susumu and S. Isutom, Arch. Toxicol. 50, 279, 1982).

Published 1985 by Elsevier Science Publishing Co., Inc.
Estrogens in the Environment, John A. McLachlan, Editor

412

ENDOCRINOLOGY OF PREMATURE THELARCHE

JAMES L. MILLS
Epidemiology and Biometry Branch
National Institute of Child Health and Human Development
National Institutes of Health, Bethesda, Maryland 20205

INTRODUCTION

Premature thelarche has proved to be a frustrating problem for

epidemiologist and endocrinologist alike. The epidemiologist still cannot

say what the expected rate of premature thelarche is in any large

population. It has not even been determined whether it is a common or an

uncommon condition. Since it is uncertain how common premature thelarche

is, it is impossible to determine when a large number of cases is identified

whether or not they constitute an epidemic.

Life is no easier for the endocrinologist. Many laboratory studies

have produced few conclusive results. Although most experts agree that

hormones are in some way responsible for premature thelarche, the etiology

remains unknown in the majority of cases. It is only where premature

thelarche has followed accidental contamination by estrogenic compounds that

the cause is considered established.

WHAT IS PREMATURE THELARCHE?

The generally agreed upon definition of premature thelarche is breast

development in a girl occurring prior to age eight. There should be no

other signs of puberty: no growth spurt, no advancement of bone age, no

pubic hair or menses. Breast tissue in the neonatal period is the result of

prenatal hormone exposure and is not considered premature thelarche.

Endocrinologists generally use Tanner's system to classify breast

growth. His five categories, shown in Table 1 [1], describe the stages of

breast development from pre-pubertal (stage 1) to adult (stage 5). Most

girls with premature thelarche develop to stage two or stage three [2].

As noted, there are no data on how common premature thelarche is in any large population. Several clinical studies have provided information on the prevalence of breast enlargement in hospital populations. A breast study conducted at Victoria Royal Children's Hospital, Australia [3] found that 18 of 94 girls between nine weeks and 30 months of age had more than one centimeter of palpable breast tissue. Nelson [4] reported that among 68 surviving low birth weight infants ($\leq$ 1000 grams), six developed breast nodules (20 to 40 mm) after six months of age. It should be noted that this is a very unusual group of babies. Besides being very low birth weight (mean 786 grams), several showed evidence of central nervous system abnormalities. A very small number of normal full-term infants was examined periodically by McKiernan and Hull [5]. As expected, breast tissue was palpable in most of the term infants at birth. By ten months of age only seven subjects were still available for study. All three of the girls still had palpable breast nodules [6]. These very limited studies suggest that premature thelarche may be a fairly common condition; however, the small number of subjects in each and the ways by which they were identified make it impossible to draw firm conclusions.

TABLE 1. STAGES OF BREAST DEVELOPMENT[a]

Stage 1. The infantile stage which persists from the immediate postnatal period until the onset of puberty.
Stage 2. The "bud" stage. The breast and papilla are elevated as a small mound, and the diameter of the areola is increased. The development of this appearance is the first indication of pubertal development of the breast.
Stage 3. The breast and areola are further enlarged and present an appearance rather like that of a small adult mammary gland with a continuous rounded contour.
Stage 4. The areola and papilla are further enlarged and form a secondary mound projecting above the corpus of the breast.
Stage 5. The typical adult stage with a smooth rounded contour, the secondary mound present in stage 4 having disappeared.

[a]From Marshall [1]

Somewhat more is known about the age of onset of premature thelarche and its outcome than is known about its incidence. The information comes from referral populations which may not be typical. For example, persistent cases are probably more likely to be referred. Nonetheless, the findings from different centers are quite consistent.

Virtually all studies agree that most cases occur within the first two years of life [7, 8, 9, 10, 11]. Mills et al. [7] reported that of 40 cases with known time of onset, 17 (37%) had been present since birth and 36 (90%) had appeared by 18 months of age (FIGURE 1).

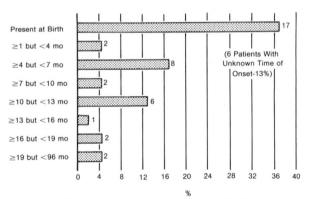

Fig 1.—Age at onset of premature thelarche in 46 girls.

J.L. Mills, et al. [7]

Information on what happens to the breast enlargement is limited because of the variable length of follow-up in existing studies. Available data suggest that breast enlargement may persist for seven years or more [7, 8]. The majority of cases either regress or do not continue to enlarge [2, 7, 9, 12]. Even when complete resolution occurs, however, it may require years. The mean duration of cases which resolved in one series was 23 months (FIGURE 2).

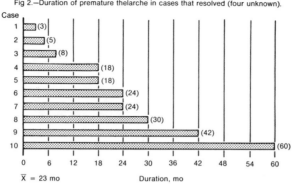

Fig 2.—Duration of premature thelarche in cases that resolved (four unknown).

J.L. Mills, et al. [7]

Finally, little information is available on long term problems associated with premature thelarche. Mills and colleagues [7] did not find significantly higher rates of sexual or medical problems in girls who had premature thelarche, but the period of follow-up was limited.

HORMONE ACTIVITY AND THE REPRODUCTIVE SYSTEM IN EARLY LIFE

It is useful to review interactions of the hormones controlling the reproductive system as background to discussing the alterations reported in girls with premature thelarche. Human female ovarian functions, ovulation and sex hormone production, are normally under the control of the pituitary gonadotropic hormones, luteinizing hormone (LH) and follicle stimulating hormone (FSH). LH and FSH are regulated by hypothalamic secretion of luteinizing hormone releasing hormone (LHRH). Before puberty, hormone regulation occurs by a negative feedback system. When ovarian production of estradiol is below the level considered "appropriate" by the hypothalamus and pituitary, LHRH is released stimulating LH and FSH release which, in turn, stimulates the ovary to produce estradiol. Estradiol concentration in the blood rises, turning off the hypothalamus and pituitary. While this explanation is oversimplified, the most important points are that: 1) gonadotropic hormones can initiate sex hormone production and 2) a small amount of estrogen will turn off gonadotropin production in a young child.

While it was once believed that the whole system of hormonal regulation was quiescent until puberty, it is now appreciated that activity begins far earlier, in fact, even before birth. FSH and LH have been found in the fetal pituitary gland at 10 to 13 weeks of gestation [13]. The gland is capable of releasing these hormones in response to LHRH in the prenatal period as well. Between 12 and 24 weeks gestation, serum gonadotropic hormones may reach levels higher than those seen in normal adult women [13]. Post-natally, LH and FSH rise again as the inhibiting effect of placental steroids wanes. LH usually remains elevated for several months while FSH levels may stay above normal childhood values for up to two years [14].

Not surprisingly, this gonadotropin stimulation results in ovarian growth and development. Follicular development eventually ends in atresia, not ovulation. In the first year of life, ovarian cysts may appear early in the process of atresia [13]. Estradiol production increases during gestation and after delivery, reaching a peak in the first postnatal year.

After this burst of activity in the period from 12 weeks of gestation to the end of the first year of life, the entire system becomes dormant. Until the beginning of puberty, gonadotropin production is low and secretion is easily inhibited by small amounts of sex hormones. The reason that the hypothalamus, pituitary and ovaries become quiescent is no clearer than the reason that they are so active earlier. If the reasons were known, they might provide valuable clues to the etiology of premature thelarche, particularly if premature thelarche is the result of over-activation early in life, or inadequate suppression later.

Why are these hormonal changes important to a discussion of premature thelarche? It is because the ovary is the critical organ in breast development. Estrogens are thought to promote growth of the breast ducts; progesterone is thought to promote lobuloalveolar development [15]. While many hormones may play a role in lactation, including prolactin, insulin and corticosteroids [15], estrogen by itself can cause breast growth. This has been well documented in cases of premature thelarche secondary to exogenous estrogen contamination.

ENDOCRINE FUNCTION IN PREMATURE THELARCHE

Studies of endocrine function in premature thelarche may be grouped into four categories: examinations for physical effects of hormones, measurements of hormone levels, provocative tests for hormones, and direct examinations of other sexual organs. All address the same basic question: To what extent is premature thelarche a condition of sexual activation similar to precocious puberty? It will become evident as each type of evaluation is discussed that the answer is not always clear.

Vaginal Smears-Urine Cytology

It is possible to detect the presence of estrogen in the female by the changes it causes in the vaginal mucosa. The vaginal cells will become cornified by estrogenic stimulation. Either direct examination by vaginal smear or indirect examination of exfoliated cells in the urine will reveal the effect. Many investigators have looked for evidence of estrogen in girls with premature thelarche; curiously, their findings have been totally contradictory. Both Silver et al. [8] and Collett-Solberg et al. [16] reported a highly significant increase in the proportion of superficial cells (indicating an estrogen effect) in the urine of girls with premature thelarche compared to control subjects. In contrast, Kenny et al. [17] found "slight or no estrogen effect."

Vaginal smears indicated estrogenic stimulation in all nine of Pasquino and co-workers' [2] subjects and in 20 of 24 of Dumic and associates' [18, 19] subjects. Yet Landier et al. [9] saw estrogen effects in only two of 22 cases and Dresch et al. [10] saw no effect at all in 17 tested subjects. There are many possible reasons for these contradictory results; two in particular deserve mention. If estrogen is present at some point and then disappears, breast tissue is likely to be palpable after the estrogen effect on the vagina is no longer detectable. Thus, a "fresh" case would have a positive smear or cytology; an "old" case would not. A second possibility is that there are major differences in laboratory technique in different centers.

Estrogen

Rather than look for estrogen effects in vaginal cytology, several investigators have elected to measure plasma estrogen levels directly. Two small series [20, 21] found modest elevations in estradiol in some, but not all girls with premature thelarche. Another [22] reported no significant elevation of estradiol or estrone, but an increase in unbound (active) estradiol. The largest series reported to date initially found modest increases in estrone and estradiol [23]. As their sample size increased, they were able to identify a subset of girls (13 of 61) with clearly elevated estradiol levels (over 40 pg/ml) [19]. All were under two and a half years of age.

It seems reasonable to conclude from these studies that plasma estradiol is elevated in some proportion of girls with premature thelarche. In the early part of normal puberty, estradiol levels are quite variable, rising above pre-pubertal levels primarily after intermittent "spikes" of gonadotropins and then falling back. The finding of high estradiol levels in some, but not all premature thelarche cases is compatible with the findings in the early stages of puberty. The possibility that premature thelarche is an arrested form of precocious puberty will be discussed later.

There are several other plausible explanations for the finding of elevated estradiol levels in some, but not all cases. There may be multiple etiologies; an initially elevated estradiol level may have returned to normal by the time some cases were studied; or perhaps, the free estradiol is critical and those with normal total estradiol have more of the active form.

Luteinizing Hormone and Follicle Stimulating Hormone

It is appropriate to move from a discussion of estrogens to a discussion of the hormones which control ovarian function and estrogen secretion. Basal (unstimulated) blood LH and FSH levels have been measured
by a number of investigators. When girls with premature thelarche have been
compared to pre-pubertal girls, there has been no increase [24, 25,26], or
only a statistically insignificant increase [17], or, in one study, 13
normal and two slightly elevated values [27].

Studies using different techniques have shown similar results. Job et
al. [23] used a urinary gonadotropin bioassay. He reported 20 cases with
less than 3 mouse units per 24 hours, two cases with 3-10 mouse units, and
one with more than ten mouse units. These results indicate that most
subjects had little LH or FSH present. Vanelli and colleagues [12] reported
a pre-pubertal LH/FSH ratio. Lucky et al. [28] found normal bioassayable LH
and immunoassayable LH levels in girls with premature thelarche. Interestingly, bioassayable levels in her cases of precocious puberty were 16 times
higher, suggesting that the LH bioassay might be useful in differentiating
between the two conditions. In summary, it appears that basal LH and FSH
are not increased in most girls with premature thelarche.

To put these findings in perspective, recall that early in normal
puberty gonadotropin levels are usually in the pre-pubertal range. Unless
one happens to be measuring at the time of one of the "spikes," pre-pubertal
levels will be found. Thus, the reports of all low, or a few elevated LH or
FSH values do not exclude the possibility that there is some activation of
the pituitary gonadotropins. A better measure than basal hormone levels is
required. Since in early puberty many "spikes" occur during sleep, one
study measured LH and FSH overnight [29]. The number of subjects was very
small, but the authors found that hormone levels increased during the night.

Luteinizing Hormone Releasing Hormone Studies

Fortunately, there is a more precise way to assess pituitary activity,
the LHRH stimulation test. It is assumed that the pituitary that has been

"activated" by hypothalamic stimulation in the recent past will respond to
an injection of LHRH by secreting more LH and FSH than a pituitary that has
not been stimulated before. When the LHRH stimulation test has been used to
test the state of pituitary activation in premature thelarche the results
have been mixed. Since the small number of girls studied may have
contributed to the confusing findings, the number in each report will be
noted.

Caufriez et al. [24] found that the patterns of LH and FSH response to
LHRH were the same in girls with premature thelarche (N=15) as in control
subjects. Vanelli et al. [12] found peak LH values in three girls with
premature thelarche to be no different than those in control subjects who
were less than one year of age.

In contrast, Reiter and co-workers [30] found a pre-pubertal LH
response but a significantly increased peak FSH response in their premature
thelarche cases (N=3). Pasquino et al. [2] found the same pre-pubertal LH
response, significantly increased peak FSH, and significantly increased FSH
increment. The age distribution of their cases (N=9) was considerably older
than would be expected, suggesting that some selection factors were present.
Beck and Stubbe [29] report a 10 to 15 fold gonadotropin increase with a
marked predominance of FSH in their three subjects, but no control
information is included.

Perhaps the most helpful data come from the investigators at Hopital
Saint-Vincent de Paul, Paris. In their first report [31], they found an
increased FSH and LH response in the two premature thelarche cases studied.
Two years later [23], 12 cases were reviewed; only a moderate increase was
found suggesting "prolongation and/or increase of the physiologic gonadotropic activity." Most recently [9], they published their findings on 29
cases. They concluded that the LH and FSH responses to LHRH were completely
superimposable on the responses of age-matched control subjects.

The results of LHRH testing in premature thelarche in these various
studies are contradictory. As indicated, the small number of subjects in

many studies may contribute to the confusion. Knowing how subjects were selected for study might be enlightening. If premature thelarche is a condition with multiple etiologies, inconsistent test results might be expected. Until the situation is clarified, it seems prudent to accept the largest study's finding that FSH and LH responses to LHRH are not higher than normal in premature thelarche.

Basal and Stimulated Prolactin Levels

It is logical that prolactin, because of its importance in lactation, should be studied in premature thelarche. Like the gonadotropins, it has been measured in both the basal and stimulated states. Basal prolactin levels in seven girls with premature thelarche were not significantly higher than in normal control girls in Caufriez and associates' [24] study. When thyrotropin-releasing hormone has been used to stimulate prolactin, peak values in premature thelarche have not exceeded control standards in any of three reported studies [24, 29, 32]. These investigations demonstrate that prolactin does not play an important role in premature thelarche.

Adrenal Hormones

A review of the literature has identified only one study of adrenal hormones and premature thelarche [18]. Dumic et al. reported high dehydroepiandrosterone (DHEA) levels in 24 girls with premature thelarche. The elevation was statistically significant (p = .04) compared to control subjects. These findings require confirmation. Seven hormones were studied, making it not unlikely that a p value of .04 could occur by chance. Until the reported association between elevated DHEA and premature thelarche is confirmed, it cannot be concluded that the adrenal gland plays a role in this condition.

The Ovaries and Uterus in Premature Thelarche

Ultrasonography and direct surgical examination have produced very interesting information about the appearance of the ovaries and uterus in girls with premature thelarche. Some background information on normal findings in young girls will help in the interpretation of these studies.

Ovarian follicles grow at all times in childhood [33]. Based on findings in anencephalic infants, it appears that gonadotropins are necessary for development of follicles from the pre-antral to the antral stage. In the normal infant all stages of ovarian follicular development short of ovulation occur [34]. Shortly after birth ovarian activity increases; estradiol production is augmented and follicular cysts appear. The number of cysts is highest around four months of age. Regression occurs in later infancy [34]. In summary, the ovary is active and cysts are common in infancy.

The largest series of pelvic ultrasound findings in premature thelarche has been published by Saenz and her co-workers [35]. From a population of 322 cases, 75 were selected for study, of whom 60 had pelvic ultrasound examinations. Forty-one girls had ovarian cysts. In all, 31 cystectomies were performed: all but one had a pathologic diagnosis of follicular cyst. The other case was an ovarian fibroma. No cysts were found in an age and sex matched control group from an unspecified source.

There are several important points to note about this study. First, these may not have been typical cases of premature thelarche. The investigators believe that an exogenous agent was responsible for breast enlargement in this group, whereas, in most cases no exogenous exposure can be identified. Second, this was a selected population. Only those who had pigmentation of the areola and labia minora, and mucus vaginal discharge underwent ultrasound examination. Some had advanced bone age, a finding which would exclude them from our definition of premature thelarche. These factors make it very difficult to relate this study's findings to a general discussion of premature thelarche.

Nonetheless, this study raises very interesting questions. Since estrogen is supposed to turn off the hypothalamic-pituitary-gonadal activating system, why would girls exposed to exogenous estrogen have evidence of ovarian activation, i.e., follicular cysts? How does one explain the high rate of ovarian cysts? Data from the other studies noted

above indicate that cysts are common in young girls. This study's control
data suggest they are not. Does the older age distribution of this
population explain the difference? If so, there seems to be a strong
relationship between ovarian cysts and premature thelarche, at least in
older girls.

Unfortunately, there is little additional information available to
clarify this relationship. Shawker et al. [36] published their ultrasound
findings on precocious puberty and related conditions, however, only three
of their patients had premature thelarche. Unlike the precocious puberty
cases, these girls had ovarian volumes in the pre-pubertal range. No cysts
were reported. Both uterine length and thickness were also pre-pubertal.

What conclusions can be drawn from these studies? Ultrasound may be
useful for distinguishing premature thelarche from precocious puberty if the
reported differences in ovarian and uterine size can be confirmed. The
relationship between premature thelarche and ovarian cysts needs to be
explored in an unselected population where exogenous estrogen is not a major
concern.

POSSIBLE MECHANISMS

The famous fictional detective Sherlock Holmes cautioned, "It is a
capital mistake to theorize before one has data. Insensibly one begins to
twist facts to suit theories, instead of theories to suit facts [37]." Now
that the data have been reviewed, it is proper to speculate on how premature
thelarche happens. Bear in mind that no one really knows the answer and
that there may be many answers since premature thelarche may be several
disorders with the common end point of premature breast development. These
speculations will begin with the breast itself, moving from there to the
organ that most directly influences the breast, the ovary. Next, organs
controlling the ovary will be considered. Finally, "exotic" factors will be
examined.

Perhaps the simplest and in some ways most attractive explanation for premature thelarche is that some girls' breasts are more sensitive to growth promoting agents than others. Muldoon [38] remarks, "A prominent feature of the estrogen receptors of mammary tissue is their ability to exist as different molecular species, each of which may have different degrees of receptor-like activity." Some breasts might be induced to grow by agents which would have no effect on others. Differences in receptor number or structure may explain response or non-response to normal pre-pubertal levels of circulating hormones. Thus, there is reason to believe that premature thelarche could be the result of the high sensitivity of some girls' breasts to stimulants present in all girls.

Others believe that the impetus to breast growth comes from outside the breast itself. As the major source of estrogens, the ovary is the most likely source. Cases of autonomous ovarian function resulting in breast growth and other sexual development have been reported [39]. Ovarian cysts could be a manifestation of either independent or gonadotropin mediated activity.

Premature thelarche could also result from hypothalamic or pituitary overactivity stimulating overproduction of estrogen which, in turn, stimulates the breast. Persistence of hypothalamic-pituitary-gonadal activity beyond the first post-natal months in some girls could explain the peak of premature thelarche in the first 12 to 18 months of life. Similarly, temporary reactivation of the axis, a theoretical process dubbed "arrested precocious puberty" by some, could explain breast development without other signs of puberty. Just as some breasts might be more sensitive to estrogenic stimulation, some ovaries might be more sensitive to gonadotropic stimulation.

Finally, more unusual mechanisms for stimulating breast development ought to be considered. The pituitary might be stimulated to produce gonadotropins by breast milk. This curious possibility has been raised by the finding that LHRH is present in human milk [40]. Breast development following contamination by exogenous estrogen has been well described

elsewhere in this text and will not be reviewed here. Another unusual

abnormality which results in excess estrogen is massive aromatization of

androstenedione to estrone. To the author's knowledge this problem has been

described only in boys [41]. Finally, there are conditions and chemicals

known to produce breast growth that do not appear to be estrogen-mediated.

Refeeding gynecomastia in adult males and gynecomastia in adults using

certain classes of drugs, e.g., phenothiazines, are well known entities.

The possibility that these same mechanisms could produce premature thelarche

has not been explored.

CONCLUSIONS

Despite the efforts of numerous investigators, premature thelarche

remains in many ways a mystery. Its true incidence is unknown. While it

appears to be benign, long-term follow-up data are limited.

Endocrinologic investigations into the etiology of premature thelarche

have not always been enlightening. Attempts to find evidence of estrogen by

vaginal smear and urine cytology have produced contradictory results.

Direct measurements of blood estrogens suggest that levels may be high in

some girls with premature thelarche. Gonadotropin levels in the basal and

stimulated states have been studied. Basal levels have not been elevated.

The more sensitive provocative tests have been inconsistent. By far the

largest study suggests that the hypothalamus and pituitary are not activated

in premature thelarche. There is no definitive evidence that prolactin or

adrenal hormones are etiologically important in premature thelarche.

Direct observation of the ovaries and uterus by ultrasound has just

recently been employed in premature thelarche. Selected cases from one

center have had ovarian cysts while a very small number from another center

have had normal pre-pubertal sized ovaries and uteri.

Because current information on the etiology of premature thelarche is

so limited, speculations abound. It has been suggested that some girls'

426

breasts are more sensitive to the stimulatory effect of normal levels of

circulating hormones. Excessive production of estrogen by autonomously

functioning ovaries could also cause premature thelarche. The hypothalamus

and pituitary could be responsible either by overactivity in early life or

by failure to suppress hormone production at the normal time after infancy.

Finally, the possibility must be entertained that there is another

totally unsuspected etiology or that premature thelarche has multiple

etiologies. The last possibility would account for the inconsistent labo-

ratory findings.

ACKNOWLEDGEMENTS: I am grateful to Drs. Heinz Berendes, Mark Klebanoff,
George Rhoads and Anne Willoughby for their insightful suggestions, and to
Ms. Beverly Trainor and Ms. Diane Wetherill for preparing this manuscript.

REFERENCES

1. W.A. Marshall in: Human Growth volume 2: Postnatal Growth, F. Falkner
   and J.M. Tanner, eds. (Plenum Press, New York and London 1978).
2. A.M. Pasquino, F. Piccolo, A. Scalamandre, M. Malvaso, R. Ortolani, and
   B. Boscherini, Arch. Dis. Child. 55, 941-944 (1980).
3. S. Prushka, G.L. Warne, Unpublished Data.
4. K.G. Nelson, J. Pediatr. 103, 756-758 (1983).
5. J.F. McKiernan and D. Hull, Arch. Dis. Child. 56, 525-529 (1981).
6. J. McKiernan, J. Pediatr. 105, 171 (1984).
7. J.L. Mills, P.D. Stolley, J. Davies, and T. Moshang, Jr., Am. J. Dis.
   Child. 135, 743-745 (1981).
8. H.K. Silver, and D. Sami, Pediatr. 34, 107-111 (1964).
9. F. Landier, J.L. Chaussain, and J.C. Job, Arch. Franc. Ped. 40,
   549-552 (1983).
10. C. Dresch, M. Arnal, and A. Prader, Helvetica Paediatr. Acta 6,
    585-593 (1960).
11. V.J. Capraro, N.P. Bayonet-Rivera, T. Aceto, Jr., and M. MacGillivray,
    Obstet. and Gynecol. Survey 26, 2-7 (1971).
12. M. Vanelli, S. Bernasconi, N. Caronna, P. Balestrazzi, G. Cavagni, M.
    Ziveri, M. Rocca, S. Rossi, and A. Turni, Acta Bio-Medica de l'Ateneo
    Parmense, 52, 153-158 (1981).
13. S.R. Ojeda, W.W. Andrews, J.P. Advis, and S. Smith White, Endocrine
    Reviews, 1, 228-257 (1980).
14. M.M. Grumbach, Hosp. Pract. 15, 51-60 (1980).
15. J.C. Porter, J. Invest. Dermatol. 63, 85-92 (1974).
16. P.R. Collett-Solberg and M.M. Grumbach, J. Pediatr. 66, 883-890 (1965).
17. F.M. Kenny, A.R. Midgley, Jr., R.B. Jaffe, L.Y. Garces, A. Vazquez, and
    F.H. Taylor, J.C.E.M. 29, 1272-1275 (1969).
18. M. Dumic, M. Tajic, D. Mardesic, and Z. Kalafatic, Arch. Dis. Child.
    57, 200-203 (1982).
19. M. Dumic, Arch. Dis. Child. 57, 642 (1982).
20. M.R. Jenner, R.P. Kelch, S.L. Kaplan, and M.M. Grumbach, J.C.E.M. 34,
    521-530 (1972).

21. M.E. Escobar, M.A. Rivarola, and C. Bergada, Acta Endocrinologica 81, 351-361 (1976).
22. N. Radfar, K. Ansusingha, and F.M. Kenny, J. Pediatr. 89, 719-723 (1976).
23. J.C. Job, B. Guilhaume, J.L. Chaussain, P.E. Garnier, Arch. Franc. Ped. 32, 39-48 (1975).
24. A. Caufriez, R. Wolter, M. Govaerts, M. L'Hermite, and C. Robyn, J. Pediatr. 91, 751-753 (1977).
25. R. Penny, H.J. Guyda, A. Baghdassarian, A.J. Johanson, and R.M. Blizzard, J. Clin. Invest. 49, 1847-1852 (1970).
26. H.J. Guyda, A.J. Johanson, C.J. Migeon, and R.M. Blizzard, Pediatr. Res. 3, 538-544 (1969).
27. A.W. Root, T. Moshang, Jr., A.M. Bongiovanni and W.R. Eberlein, Pediatr. Res. 4, 175-186 (1970).
28. A.W. Lucky, B.H. Rich, R.L. Rosenfield, V.S. Fang, and N. Roche-Bender, J. Pediatr. 97, 214-216 (1980).
29. W. Beck, and P. Stubbe, Eur. J. Pediatr. 141, 168-170 (1984).
30. E.O. Reiter, S.L. Kaplan, F.A. Conte, and M.M. Grumbach, Pediatr. Res., 9, 111-116 (1975).
31. J.C. Job, P.E. Garnier, J.L. Chaussain, and P. Canlorbe, Biomedicine, 19, 77-81 (1973).
32. K. Abe, N. Matsuura, Y. Nohara, H. Fujita, K. Fujieda, T. Kato, and Y. Mikami, Tohoku J. Exp. Med., 142, 283-288 (1984).
33. H. Peters, Eur. J. Ob. Gyn. Rep. Bio., 9, 137-144 (1979).
34. M.G. Frost, Eur. J. Ob. Gyn. Rep. Bio., 9, 145 (1979).
35. C.A. Saenz, M.A. Toro-Sola, L. Conde, N.P. Bayonet-Rivera, Bol. Asoc. Med. P. Rico, 74, 16-19 (1982).
36. T.H. Shawker, F. Comite, K.G. Rieth, A.J. Dwyer, G.B. Cutler, Jr., and I. Loriaux, J. Ultrasound Med. 3, 309-316 (1984).
37. A.C. Doyle, The Adventures of Sherlock Holmes, vol. 1, Section 3, 1-28, The A. Conan Doyle Memorial Edition (Doubleday, Doran, New York 1932).
38. T.G. Muldoon, Endocrine Rev., 1, 339-364 (1980).
39. R.G. Wieland, R. Bendezu, M.C. Hallberg, P. Tang, and K. Webster, Am. J. Obstet. Gynecol., 126, 731-733 (1976).
40. T. Baram, Y. Koch, E. Hazum, and M. Fridkin, Science, 198, 300-302 (1977).
41. D.L. Hemsell, C.D. Edman, J.F. Marks, P.K. Siiteri, and P.C. MacDonald, J. Clin. Invest., 60, 455-464 (1977).

DISCUSSION

MCLACHLAN: Your talk was a thorough analysis of the endocrine correlates of premature thelarche. It would be useful to know what is the threshold amount of estrogen needed to trigger breast development in young girls.

MILLS: I agree, but as far I know this information is not yet available.

O'NEILL: Measurement of LH and FSH should be done during the night (sleep) for that is when they first rise. LRH stimulation tests must be done by giving the dose at 90-minute intervals. Sonograms that show a cystic structure in the ovary mean nothing unless they are followed by serial sonograms. Atresia of 600,000 follicles takes place between birth and menarche.

MILLS: There is one study in which sleep LH and FSH were measured by Beck and Stubbe (Eur. J. Pediatr. 141, 168, 1984). They reported an increase above basal levels in their three subjects with premature thelarche. They defined an increase as 40% above basal levels for FSH and 70% for LH. To my knowledge, no one has published data on LRH stimulation tests using multiple doses of LRH in girls with premature thelarche.

Index

Accidental estrogen exposure,
    epidemic, 349
Acetazolamide, 98
Acetylaminofluorene,
    mutagenicity, 150
Acetylation, nuclear histones, 268
Adenocarcinoma
    rete testis, 310
    vaginal, 304, 305, 312
Adenosis,
    vaginal, 304
Adrenal androgens, 203
Adrenal cortex, 1
Adult bladder epithelium
    histochemistry, 274
    histology, 274
Allen, Dr. Edgar, 2
Alphafetoprotein, 24
α-Zearalanol, 169, 194, 239
Anabolic activities,
    mammals, 238
Androgen binding
    autoradiographic studies, 275
Androgen
    receptors, 275, 286
Androgens, 24, 35, 195, 197, 203, 273
    adiol, 204
    adrenal, 203
    antiestrogenic properties, 204
    aromatization, 212, 213
Androstenedione, 216
Animals, 69, 188
    hyperestrogenism, 239
    infertility, 239
    neoplasia, 4
    reproductive tracts, 86
    Rhesus monkey, 3
Antiandrogen, 201
Antiestrogen,
    binding, 263
Antiestrogens, 85, 204, 215, 221, 252,
    262, 263, 268
Aromatization,
    androgens, 212, 213
Autoradiography, 277

β-androstane, 24
Binding, 19, 24, 33, 34, 45, 49, 63,
    66, 67, 111, 156, 192, 226, 236
    conformation, freedom of rotation, 32
    ligand, 46, 63, 226
    progesterone, 253
    triphenylacrylonitrile derivatives, 31
Binding sites,
    liver, 191, 192, 193
Biochanin A, 170, 173, 174, 182, 229, 230

Biological responses, 267
    nafoxidine, 266
    tamoxifen, 266
Bladder
    histochemistry, 274
    histology, 274
Bone
    epiphyseal closure, 1
Breast, 350, 351, 352, 353,
    354, 356, 410, 424
    cancer, 203, 204, 205, 208
    cyst fluid, 204
    estrogen receptor, 257,
        323
    estrogen synthesis, 212
    growth, 425
    gynecomastic, 6
    precocious development,
        356
Breast development,
    premature, 398
Breast enlargement, 367,
    371, 380, 382, 385, 412
    414
Breast estrogens,
    pregnancy, 211
Breast fluids
    serum estrogens, 210
    steroids, 209
Breast sensitivity, 324

Calcium metabolism, 1
Cancer, 3, 78, 203-220
    breast, 203, 204, 205,
        208, 257
    endometrial, 8, 203, 206
Capillary GC/MS, 116
Carcinogens, 22, 146, 160,
    182, 212, 309
Carcinoma,
    renal, 171
Catechol estrogens, 154,
    161, 163
Catechol metabolites, 177
Catecholestrogen formation,
    35
Cell culture, 280
Cell transformation, 153
Cells
    granulosa, 1
    interstitial, 1
    mitotic activity, 1
    natural killer, 331
Cervix, DES, 302

Chlordecone (Kepone), 86, 87, 88, 89
   birds, 87
   mammals, 87
   milk, 87, 91, 95, 99, 100
   ultrastructure, 88
Cimetidine, 406
Clover, 4, 168
Clover disease, 70
Comutagenicity

   estrogens, 161
Contraceptive
   pill, 8
   steroid, 10
Corpora lutea, 290, 327, 337
Coumestans, 69, 168
Coumesterol, 170, 173, 229, 232
Cryptorchid testes, 312
Cryptorchidism, 310, 312
Cysts
   epididymal, 312
Cytochrome P-450
   liver, 198
Cytosol, 26, 193, 194
   assay, 405, 407
Cytosolic receptors, 110, 141, 192,
   193, 399, 401, 404

DDT, 86, 108, 109, 111, 112, 113
   estrogenic effects, 109
Dehydroepiandrosterone sulfate
   (DHEAS), 203
DES, 5, 6, 16-19, 43-45, 47, 48, 50,
   56-58, 60-62, 66, 69, 77, 78, 116,
   119, 122-124, 126, 128, 130, 131,
   133, 136, 137, 139-143, 150, 152,
   161-163, 175, 187, 192, 194,
   288-291, 294-296, 298, 300-305,
   327, 330-333, 335, 338, 340-343,
   363, 382, 402
   in utero, 289
   prenatal exposure, 289
   screening techniques, 117
Diadzein, 221
Diethylstilbestrol, See DES
Digitalis, 406
DLT micro-LC/MS, 116, 120
DMBA, 188
DNA
   synthesis activity, 54, 55, 56
Doisy, Dr. Edward, 2
Drugs
   contaminants, 6
   isoniazide, 6
Ducts
   mullerian, 268, 289
   wolffian, 268, 289
Dysplasia, 319
Early sexual development (ESD), 380

E , peripheral production,
   216
Effect modification, 390
Enantiomers, 59, 61, 62,
   63, 67
Endometrium,
   cancer, 203
Energy calculations, 16,
   18, 19
Energy minimization, 19
Enterodiol, 71, 72, 74, 109
Enterolactone, 71, 72, 74,
   85, 232, 233
Environmental enzymes,
   349-357
Environmental estrogens, 139
Environmental hormone
   contamination, 404
Environmental pollution, 87
Enzymes, reduced
   activities, 344
EPD, 19
Epididymal cysts, 312
Epithelial hyperplasia, 296
Epithelium
   bladder, 274
   vagina, 274
Equol, 74, 78, 80, 84, 85,
   221, 232, 396
   excretion, 74, 75, 80,
   84, 85
Estradiol, 17, 18, 21, 22,
   24, 25, 27, 29, 35, 36,
   51, 53, 69, 78, 88, 89,
   91, 97, 99, 140, 142,
   143, 150, 154, 160, 162,
   163, 170, 174, 191, 209,
   211, 216, 224, 226, 231,
   232, 258, 259, 263, 265,
   268, 277-279, 327, 329,
   333, 334, 336, 337, 363,
   382, 400, 415, 418
Estradiol-receptor complex,
   258, 268
Estriol, 142, 143, 216
Estrogen
   clearance, 86
   contaminants, 86
   hormone action, 45, 110,
   146
   methoxychlor, 7
   mycotoxins, 168-183
   problem epidemiology, 10
   receptor, 45, 110, 139,
   168, 191, 251, 252,
   254, 261, 265
   receptor binding, 111,
   146, 253

Estrogen
  steroid, 7
  stimulation, 64
  synthesis, 86
Estrogens, 1, 2, 17, 18, 69,
  116-138, 281
  agonists, 15
  alphafetoprotein, 24
  animals, 86
  analysis, 116-138
  antagonists, 15
  anti-estrogenic compounds,
    triphenylethylene series, 24
  β-androstane, 24
  binding, 19, 24, 37, 41, 42,
    43, 192
  cancer, 203-220
  carcinogenic, 288
  catechol, 161
  comutagenicity, 16
  conjugation, 187
  developmental biology, 251-272
  8α-D-homoestradiol, 17
  E-pseudodiethylstilbestrol EPD,
    17, 44
  environmental, 139
  estradiol, 17, 18, 21, 22, 24, 25,
    27, 29, 35, 36, 51, 53
  estrone, 2, 69, 142, 143, 150,
    154, 162, 174, 209, 216, 363
  11-keto-9β-estrone, 17
  exogenous, 216, 349
  food, 398
  free, 400
  genotoxicity, 146
  gestrinone, 24, 25
  2/4 hydroxylase, 157
  indenestrol, A, B, IB, IA, I,
    17, 18, 44, 46, 51
  intoxication, 349
  lipoidal, 145
  metabolism, 216
  mice, 277
  mutagenicity, 150, 151
  neoplastic transformation, 155
  non-steroidal, 69-85, 146
  norgestrienone, 24, 25
  nortestosterone, 24
  oxidation, 187
  potency, 147
  prenortestosterone, 24, 25
  pseudo-DES, 45, 64
  reduction, 187
  steroidal, 139, 146
  stilbene, 43, 44, 64
  stilbestrol, 10, 11
  structure-activity relationship, 221

Estrogens
  substitution at C-11
    position, 31
  synthetic moxestrol, 36
  tamoxifen, 21, 85, 103,
    215, 222, 223
  teratogenic, 288
  toxicity, 98
  trans mirestrol, 17
  Z-pseudodiethylstilbestrol
    ZPD, 17, 18
  trans(Z)tamoxifen, 17, 19
  trans-zearalenone, 17
  uterotrophic activity, 31
Estrogen binding, 214, 271
Estrogen exposure,
  accidental, 349
Estrogen metabolism, 7, 35, 86
Estrogen receptors
  binding, triphenylonitrile
    derivative, 31, 66
  hypothalamus, 267
  xenobiotic, 107
Estrogen receptor levels, 324
Estrogen receptor systems,
  113, 214, 283
Estrogen responsive tumors,
  113
Estrogen sulfate, 220, 262
Estrogen synthesis,
  breast, 212
Estrogenic activity, 6, 8,
  15, 16, 24-42, 139, 213
Estrogenic compounds,
  exogenous, 251
Estrogenic xenobiotics, 107-
  115
  structure-activity
    relationships, 107
Estrone, effect, 3, 69, 142,
  143, 163, 204
Estrone sulfate EIS, 213
Estrophiline, 67
Ethinyl estradiol, 231
Evans, Dr. Herbert, 1
Exogenous estrogens, 216

Fetal hypophysis, 267
Fetal hypothalamus, 267
Fetal uterus
  estrogen effects, 259, 263
  progesterone receptors,
    256, 259
Fetus, 252
Fluoroestrogens, 156, 157, 160
(FSH) Follicle stimulating
  hormone, 415

Food, estrogens, 398
Formononetin, 221, 230, 232
Functional defects, DES, 309
Fusarium, 238, 240, 242

Genistein, 229
Genital tract, development, 273
Genital tract abnormalities,
  female, 290
Genotoxicity, 146
Gestrinone, 24, 25
GLC profiles, 75
Glands
  mesenchyme, 273
  ovary, 290
  steroidogenic, 67
Glucocorticoid, 24
Gonadal hormone receptors, 267
Gonadotropin, 334
Gonads, pituitary gonadotropic
  function, 1
Graffian follicle, 1
Granulosa cells, 1
Gynecomastia, 6, 78, 425

Hamsters, 169, 187
HCLA, 190, 195, 196, 197, 201, 202
Hepatic cytochrome P-450, 198
Hepatic estrogen action
  binding sites, 191
  critical period, 190
  imprinting, 190-202, 196
  pituitary-dependent, 190
Hepatic estrogen receptor,
  ontogeny, 192
Hexestrol, stereochemistry, 60
Histidine reversion, 147, 148, 150
Hormone
  GnRH, 371
  metabolites, 187
  receptor, 273
  responsiveness, 273
Hormones, 1, 205, 323,
  developmental period, 190
  estrogen activity, 45
  historical development, 1
  metabolism, 187
  nuclear binding, 252
  ovarian function control, 419
  pituitary gonadotropic, 415
  primary effect, 1
  steroid, 252
H-testosterone, 340, 341
Human chorionic gonadotropin, 327

Hydrogen bond formation
  steric hindrance, 31
2/4 hydroxylase, 157
4-hydroxytamoxifen, 222, 223
  224, 225
Hyperestrogenism, swine, 239
Hypoestrogenity, 84
Hypoglycemia, 404, 411
Hypothalamo-hypophyseal
  gonadal axis, 268

Indanestrol, 46, 49, 55, 57, 67
Indomethacin, 85
Infertility, animals, 239
Insecticides, 86, 288
  chlordecone, 87
Isoflavones, 69, 168
  daidzein, 74, 76, 77
  daidzin, 76
  genistein, 74, 76, 77
  genistin, 76
  glucosile conjugate, 77
  glycitin, 76
  glycitin-7β-glucoside, 76
  precursors, 76, 85

Kepone, 86, 102, 382
  hepatic bioreduction, 103

LC/MS (LC/MS/MS), 116, 120, 132
(LH) luteinizing hormone, 415
LHRH, 327
Ligand
  binding, 46, 226
  radioactive, 29
Ligand structure, 27
Lignans, 71, 84, 85, 349
  enterodiol, 71, 72, 74
  enterolactone, 71, 72, 74
Lipids, 1
Lipoidal estrogens, 145
Liver
  puberty, 190
  sex differentiation, 190, 198
Liver function tests, 378

Male genital tract
  abnormalities,
  mice-seminal vesicles, 306
  mice-testes, 306
Mammary gland, 273, 319, 322,
  324, 413
Mammary gland development,
  inhibition, 324
Mammary tumorigenesis, 320
Mass spectroscopy, 71, 117, 118

433

Mesonephric duct,
    remnants, 301, 302
Methoxime, 154, 165
Methoxychlor, 7, 109, 188, 382
Mice, 5, 86-103
    choroid plexus, 87, 89, 90, 98
    estrogens, 277
    female subfertility, 305
    kepone action, 86-103
    male genital tract
        abnormalities, 306, 390, 310
    neonatal female, 327
    oviductal lesions, 296, 298, 299
    reduced male fertility, 308
    retained testes, 307
    testicular feminization, 274
Microsomes, 112, 166, 175, 187
Mineralocorticoid, 24
Mirex, 87, 102
    photodegradation, 87
Mitotic activity, 1
Monoclonal antibody, 256
Morphogenesis, 273
Mouse, genital tract
    development, 288
Moxestrol, 36, 161, 201, 277
Müllerian ducts, 268, 289
    paramesonephric, 289
Mycotoxins, 239, 349
    estrogenic, 168-183, 239, 381

Nafoxidine, 49, 50, 264, 266
Natural killer cells, 331
Neonatal castrates, testosterone,
    194, 198
Neonatal estrogen exposure, 320,
    327, 330
Neonatal vagina, epithelium, 276
Neoplasia, 3, 4
Neoplasmic transformation, 149
Neoplastic transformation, 155
Nervous system, behavioral
    patterns, 1
Newborns, 252, 259, 262, 263
Non-steroidal estrogens, 69
Norgestrienone, 24, 25
Nortestosterone, 24
Nuclear binding, hormone, 252
Nuclear estrogen, receptor
    levels, 58, 61, 64
Nuclear histones, acetylation, 268

Oocytes, 290
Ornithine decarboxylase (ODC), 52
Osteoporosis, phytoestrogens, 85
Ovarian follicles, 290

Ovarian cysts, mesonephric
    remants, 291, 381, 422
Ovarian rete, 290
Ovarian steroid synthesis,
    338
Ovaries, DES exposure, 336
Ovary
    corpora lutea, 290, 327, 337
    cysts, 291
    interstitial tissue, 327
    oocytes, 290
    postpubertal, 335
Oviduct
    developmentally arrested,
        293, 295
    malformation, 293, 312
    structural malformation, 312
    teratogenic defect, 291
Oviduct morphogenesis,
    DES, 293

Papanicolaou, Dr. George, 1
Paraovarian cysts,
    mesonephric, 312
Pelvic sonograms, 404, 405
Pesticides, estrogenic, 364
Phenolic steroids, equol,
    75, 76, 78
Phenothiazines, 326, 425
Phytoestrogens, 77, 78, 79,
    80, 84, 168-183, 221, 229,
    349, 396
Pituitary cells, 221
Pituitary gonadotropic
    function, 1
Pituitary gonadotropic
    hormones, 415
Plauts
    edible, 69
    estrogenic substances, 4
    estrogenic substances,
        clover, 4, 5, 69
Postmenopausal women, 204,
    206
Precocious breast develop-
    ment, 356
Precocious puberty, Puerto
    Rico, 361, 361, 380
Pregnancy, breast
    estrogens, 211
Pre-hormones, 262, 268
Premarin, 7
Premature adrenarche,
    Puerto Rico, 361, 407
Premature breast
    development, 398, 412

Premature sexual development, 349
  Puerto Rico, 349, 404, 406
Premature thelarche, 349, 354
  380, 381, 410, 412, 413, 414,
  415, 416, 417, 418, 419, 420,
  421, 423, 424, 426, 427
  endocrinology, 412-427
  Puerto Rico, 358, 359, 360, 362,
  364, 365, 366, 369, 370, 374,
  376, 380, 381, 383, 387, 388,
  392, 394, 396, 397, 407, 409,
  410
Prenortestosterone, 24, 25
Prepubertal gynecomastia, Puerto
  Rico, 361
Proestrogens, 187
Progesterone, 172, 253, 262, 263,
  326, 327, 329, 342
  binding globulin PBG, 253
  receptors, 255, 256, 259, 260,
  264
Prohormones, 251
Prolactin, 221, 329, 378
  synthesis, 221
Prostate, 273
  histochemistry, 274
  histology, 274
  production, 78
Prostaglandin synthase, 35
Protein, soy, 74, 77
Pseudoprecocious puberty
  Puerto Rico, 361, 407
  premature sexual development,
  358-379
Puberty, 380

Radioactive ligand, 29
Radioimmunoassay, 399
Rat uterine cytosol receptors, 141
Receptors
  progesterone, 172
  conformational changes, 15, 16, 24
  cytosolic, 15, 26, 110
  estrogenic, 110
  glucocorticoid, 35
  estrogen, 45, 86
  hormone, 273
  levels, 46, 53
  protein, 15, 24
  stability, 27
  steroid, 15, 24, 34, 60
  steroid screening, 34
  temperature dependent, 15
Reproductive failure, 86
Reproductive tract, dysfunction, 305
Resorcylic acid lactones, 69, 168

Rhesus monkey, 3
RNA, polymerase I and II, 268

Salpingitis, isthmica
  nodosa, 299, 312
Secretory cytodifferentiation
  bladder, 274
  vagina, 274
Selected ion monitoring, See
  SIM
Seminal vesicles,
  abnormalities, 306
Serum estrogens, breast
  fluids, 210, 211
Serum prolactin levels, 378
Sex differentiation, 251, 289
  290
Sex hormone
  action, 282
  binding globulin SHBG, 206,
  207
Sexual activation, 417
Sexual development,
  premature, 80, 349
SHBG, 206, 207
SIM, 116, 124, 125, 126, 128
Sonograms, pelvic, 404, 405,
  407
Soy ingestion, GLC
  profiles, 75
(SRM)LC/MS/MS, 116, 120
Steric hindrance, hydrogen
  bond formation, 31
Steroid hormones, 252, 287
Steroid synthesis, ovarian,
  338
Steroid, urinary, 71
Steroidogenesis, 68
Steroids
  androgen, 24
  breast fluids, 209
  structure affinity, 27
  substitution, 30
Stilbestrol, 10, 11
Subfertility, female mice, 305
Swine, hyperestrogenism, 239

Tamoxifen, 215, 222, 223, 224,
  225, 226, 227, 235, 236,
  237, 252, 264, 265, 266,
  272
Tandem mass spectrometry, 116
Testes
  abnormalities, 306, 312
  cryptorchid, 312
Testicular lesions, 312
Testosterone, 330

Thelarche, premature, 349, 359
Thrombotic disorders, 10
Thymidine labeling, 282
Tissue
    breast, 323
    differentiation, 251
    fetal, 251
    fluid balance, 1
    genital tract, 251
    hamster kidney, 172, 187
    hamster liver, 187
    liver, 7, 190
    liver zeranol, 116
    mitotic activity, 3
    muscular elements, 1
    ovary, 290
    proliferation, 251
    recombinants, 274
    uterus, 7
    vagina, 277
TPE, 38
Triphenylacrylonitrile derivatives,
    31
Triphenylethylene structure, 264
Tumorigenesis, mammary 320
Tumors, estrogen responsive, 113

Urinary steroid, 71, 72
Urogenital sinus epithelium,
    273, 274
Uterine cytosol estrogen
    receptors, 146
Uterine differentiation, 276
Uterine wet weight, 327
Uterotrophic activity, 31
Uterotrophic response, 27
Uterotropic stimulation, 47
Uterus
    DES, 302
    engorgement, 2

Vagina
    chlordecone, 94, 99
    DES, 302
    Estradiol, 94
Vaginal bleeding, 368
Vaginal cells, microridges, 96
Vaginal cytology, 377, 418
Vaginal mucosa, 417
Vitamins, 6
Vagina, cornification, 2
Vaginal, adenocarcinoma, 304,
    305, 312

Vaginal adenosis, 304
Vaginal stroma, 276

Wolffian ducts, 268, 289
    mesonephric, 289
Women, postmenopausal, 204,
    206

Xearalenol, 142
Xenobiotics, 108
X-ray crystallographic data,
    15, 18
X-ray data, 15, 16, 19

Zearalenone, 69, 169, 174,
    175, 238, 239, 240, 241,
    242, 243, 244, 245, 246,
    364, 386
    metabolism, 241
Zearalenol, 69, 116, 140, 239
    240, 363, 382
ZPD, 19
Zeranol, 116, 119, 120, 121,
    126, 131, 133, 137, 138,
    401